Handbook of Drug Delivery and Nanomedicine

Handbook of Drug Delivery and Nanomedicine

Editor: Miranda Cowan

AMERICAN
MEDICAL PUBLISHERS
www.americanmedicalpublishers.com

AMERICAN
MEDICAL PUBLISHERS
www.americanmedicalpublishers.com

Cataloging-in-Publication Data

Handbook of drug delivery and nanomedicine / edited by Miranda Cowan.
p. cm.
Includes bibliographical references and index.
ISBN 979-8-88740-069-3
1. Drug delivery systems. 2. Nanomedicine. 3. Pharmaceutical technology. 4. Nanotechnology--Therapeutic use.
5. Pharmacology. I. Cowan, Miranda.
RS199.5 .H36 2023
615.6--dc23

American Medical Publishers,
41 Flatbush Avenue,
1st Floor, New York,
NY 11217, USA

ISBN 979-8-88740-069-3 (Hardback)

Contents

Preface VII

Chapter 1 **Nanostructured Polymeric, Liposomal and other Materials to Control the Drug Delivery for Cardiovascular Diseases** 1
Dimitrios Skourtis, Dimitra Stavroulaki, Varvara Athanasiou, Panagiota G. Fragouli and Hermis Iatrou

Chapter 2 **Long-Lasting, Antinociceptive Effects of pH-Sensitive Niosomes Loaded with Ibuprofen in Acute and Chronic Models of Pain** 26
Francesca Marzoli, Carlotta Marianecci, Federica Rinaldi, Daniele Passeri, Marco Rossi, Paola Minosi, Maria Carafa and Stefano Pieretti

Chapter 3 **Latest Advances in the Development of Eukaryotic Vaults as Targeted Drug Delivery Systems** 38
Amanda Muñoz-Juan, Aida Carreño, Rosa Mendoza and José L. Corchero

Chapter 4 **Interaction of Poly(L-lysine)/Polysaccharide Complex Nanoparticles with Human Vascular Endothelial Cells** 54
Dominik Weber, Bernhard Torger, Karsten Richter, Michelle Nessling, Frank Momburg, Beatrice Woltmann, Martin Müller and Reinhard Schwartz-Albiez

Chapter 5 **Stable, Monodisperse and Highly Cell-Permeating Nanocochleates from Natural Soy Lecithin Liposomes** 71
Martina Asprea, Francesca Tatini, Vieri Piazzini, Francesca Rossi, Maria Camilla Bergonzi and Anna Rita Bilia

Chapter 6 **Novel Formulations of C-Peptide with Long-Acting Therapeutic Potential for Treatment of Diabetic Complications** 85
Natalia Zashikhina, Vladimir Sharoyko, Mariia Antipchik, Irina Tarasenko, Yurii Anufrikov, Antonina Lavrentieva, Tatiana Tennikova and Evgenia Korzhikova-Vlakh

Chapter 7 **Transferrin Functionalized Liposomes Loading Dopamine HCl: Development and Permeability Studies across an *In Vitro* Model of Human Blood–Brain Barrier** 107
Antonio Lopalco, Annalisa Cutrignelli, Nunzio Denora, Angela Lopedota, Massimo Franco and Valentino Laquintana

Chapter 8 **In Vitro Anticancer Activity of Extracellular Vesicles (EVs) Secreted by Gingival Mesenchymal Stromal Cells Primed with Paclitaxel** 117
Valentina Coccè, Silvia Franzè, Anna Teresa Brini, Aldo Bruno Giannì, Luisa Pascucci, Emilio Ciusani, Giulio Alessandri, Giampietro Farronato, Loredana Cavicchini, Valeria Sordi, Rita Paroni, Michele Dei Cas, Francesco Cilurzo and Augusto Pessina

Chapter 9 **Nanocarrier Lipid Composition Modulates the Impact of Pulmonary Surfactant Protein B (SP-B) on Cellular Delivery of siRNA** 130
Roberta Guagliardo, Pieterjan Merckx, Agata Zamborlin, Lynn De Backer, Mercedes Echaide, Jesus Pérez-Gil, Stefaan C. De Smedt and Koen Raemdonck

Chapter 10 **Silver Nanoparticles: Synthetic Routes, In Vitro Toxicity and Theranostic Applications for Cancer Disease** 146
Valeria De Matteis, Mariafrancesca Cascione, Chiara Cristina Toma and Stefano Leporatti

Chapter 11 **The Use of Artificial Gel Forming Bolalipids as Novel Formulations in Antimicrobial and Antifungal Therapy** 169
Nathalie Goergen, Matthias Wojcik, Simon Drescher, Shashank Reddy Pinnapireddy, Jana Brüßler, Udo Bakowsky and Jarmila Jedelská

Chapter 12 **Easy Synthesis and Characterization of Holmium-Doped SPIONs** 185
Magdalena Osial, Paulina Rybicka, Marek Pękała, Grzegorz Cichowicz, Michał K. Cyrański and Paweł Krysiński

Chapter 13 **Syringeable Self-Organizing Gels that Trigger Gold Nanoparticle Formation for Localized Thermal Ablation** 200
Sonia Cabana-Montenegro, Silvia Barbosa, Pablo Taboada, Angel Concheiro and Carmen Alvarez-Lorenzo

Chapter 14 **Gadolinium-Doped Gallic Acid-Zinc/Aluminium-Layered Double Hydroxide/Gold Theranostic Nanoparticles for a Bimodal Magnetic Resonance Imaging and Drug Delivery System** 214
Muhammad Sani Usman, Mohd Zobir Hussein, Sharida Fakurazi, Mas Jaffri Masarudin and Fathinul Fikri Ahmad Saad

Permissions

List of Contributors

Index

Preface

This book aims to highlight the current researches and provides a platform to further the scope of innovations in this area. This book is a product of the combined efforts of many researchers and scientists, after going through thorough studies and analysis from different parts of the world. The objective of this book is to provide the readers with the latest information of the field.

Nanomedicine is the medical application of nanotechnology for achieving innovation in healthcare. The introduction of nanomedicine in drug delivery has the potential to enable early detection and prevention of various diseases. In recent years, nanomedicine has been extensively used to improve diagnosis, treatment and follow-up of diseases, including cancer, as well as cardiovascular, neurodegenerative, musculoskeletal and inflammatory diseases. Nanomedicine has several benefits, since it combines therapeutic and diagnostic modalities into one agent. It provides the possibility of site-specific targeting that reduces the side-effects produced by crude drug by minimizing undesired exposure to the healthy cells. The application of nanotechnology in drug delivery allows for the transportation of drugs across epithelial and endothelial barriers. It can act as a key instrument in regenerative, targeted and personalized medicine by delivering novel drugs and treatments. This book aims to shed light on the role of nanomedicine in drug delivery. A number of latest researches have been included to keep the readers up-to-date in this area of study. This book aims to serve as a resource guide for students and experts alike and contribute to the growth of the discipline.

I would like to express my sincere thanks to the authors for their dedicated efforts in the completion of this book. I acknowledge the efforts of the publisher for providing constant support. Lastly, I would like to thank my family for their support in all academic endeavors.

Editor

1

Nanostructured Polymeric, Liposomal and Other Materials to Control the Drug Delivery for Cardiovascular Diseases

Dimitrios Skourtis [1], Dimitra Stavroulaki [1], Varvara Athanasiou [1], Panagiota G. Fragouli [2] and Hermis Iatrou [1,*]

1 Industrial Chemistry Laboratory, Department of Chemistry, National and Kapodistrian University of Athens, Panepistimiopolis, Zografou, GR–15771 Athens, Greece; skourtisd@chem.uoa.gr (D.S.); dimistavrou@chem.uoa.gr (D.S.); bathanas@chem.uoa.gr (V.A.)

2 Dyeing, Finishing, Dyestuffs and Advanced Polymers Laboratory, University of West Attica, DIDPE, 250 Thevon Street, GR–12241 Athens, Greece; pgfragouli@uniwa.gr

* Correspondence: iatrou@chem.uoa.gr;

Abstract: Cardiovascular diseases (CVDs) are the leading cause of death globally, taking an estimated 17.9 million lives each year, representing one third of global mortality. As existing therapies still have limited success, due to the inability to control the biodistribution of the currently approved drugs, the quality of life of these patients is modest. The advent of nanomedicine has brought new insights in innovative treatment strategies. For this reason, several novel nanotechnologies have been developed for both targeted and prolonged delivery of therapeutics to the cardiovascular system to minimize side effects. In this regard, nanoparticles made of natural and/or synthetic nanomaterials, like liposomes, polymers or inorganic materials, are emerging alternatives for the encapsulation of already approved drugs to control their delivery in a targeted way. Therefore, nanomedicine has attracted the attention of the scientific community as a potential platform to deliver therapeutics to the injured heart. In this review, we discuss the current types of biomaterials that have been investigated as potential therapeutic interventions for CVDs as they open up a host of possibilities for more targeted and effective therapies, as well as minimally invasive treatments.

Keywords: cardiovascular; drug delivery systems; liposomes; polymeric nanoparticles; myocardial infarction

---

1. Introduction

Cardiovascular diseases (CVDs) encompass all pathologies of the heart or circulatory system, including coronary artery disease (CAD), myocardial infarction (MI), heart failure and peripheral vascular disease. These diseases are the primary mortality cause worldwide and significantly impact patients' quality of life. More than 17.9 million people died from CVDs in 2016, representing above of one third of global deaths. Of these deaths, 85% are due to heart attack and stroke [1]. In Europe, 45% of all deaths are due to CVDs, accounting for 3.9 million deaths per year [2]. In the economic sector, the direct healthcare expenditure related to CVD treatment is estimated to cost the EU economy over 100 billion euros every year. Unfortunately, these figures are expected to increase over the next years due to an increase in CVD risk factors, such as obesity and diabetes, as well as an expansion of the elderly population [3]. To date, available therapies such as heart transplantation, pharmacological interventions, coronary artery bypass graft surgery, and ventricular assistant devices have significantly prolonged patients' longevity. However, cost effective and less invasive treatments with higher efficacy are vital for the future.

In recent decades, the continuous progress of nanotechnology has led to a dramatic expansion of potential biomedical applications of nanomaterials. Nanoparticles have been widely employed in the diagnosis, imaging and treatment of many diseases, such as cancer. Nanomedicine for curing cancer is the main field of research for decades and several nanomedical products (e.g., Doxil, Abraxane) have been approved by the US FDA and the EMA for their clinical use in humans and many others are in advanced stages of clinical trials [4]. On the contrary, the field of cardiovascular nanomedicine has recently started growing and is still in its infancy. Nonetheless, an increase in research publications with promising lab-scale results has been reported, especially in recent years.

In this context, we report the efforts made for development of nanostructured biocompatible nanomaterials, both natural and synthetic, which exhibit great potential in cardiac or vascular repair and regeneration, either as a carrier for drug delivery or as an extracellular matrix substitute scaffold.

2. Cardiac Targeting Strategies and Nanomedicine

The major priority for a fully functional heart is a sufficient blood flow to the left ventricular. The blood which passes through the left side of the heart contains vital oxygen. When plaque builds up and hardens the arteries (atherosclerosis) that give the heart oxygen and nutrients, narrowed or clogged arteries are formed. As a consequence, the blood volume which reaches the heart is significantly reduced or blocked and this perfusion imbalance between supply and demand leads to MI [5]. After MI, the cardiac muscle is damaged and cardiomyocyte loss happens. Unfortunately, adult cardiomyocytes have poor proliferation ability and scar formation takes place, leading to myocardial hypertrophy, ventricular dilation, perivascular fibrosis and infract wall thinning [6]. For this reason, preventing the loss of cardiomyocyte in the early stages of an acute MI is necessary to achieve long-term efficacy in the treatment of coronary heart disease. If no action is taken, the heart will no longer pump adequately and heart failure will occur.

Current conventional CVDs treatment require the use of drugs in high concentration which results in toxicity to other organs. Therefore, a targeted delivery system should be used to accumulate CVD drugs selectively in the heart. Novel effective treatments have been presented by using nanomedicine. Drug delivery systems (DDSs) provide a new drug delivery avenue for the treatment of CVDs with the development of nanotechnology, demonstrating great advantages over conventional treatments. DDSs are a class of nanoconstructs, usually consisting of biocompatible polymers, lipids or inorganic compounds, that encapsulate hydrophobic or hydrophilic drugs and have the potential to increase their stability and water solubility, minimize their excretion of the body, control their biodistribution, and reduce inactivation or degradation, thereby improving their safety and effectiveness [7]. Apart from drugs, DDSs can also transfer to the site of interest cells, genes or other therapeutic molecules, administered in various ways, offering a plethora of options for the development of sufficient medication.

Contrary to DDS systems that have been developed for cancer treatment, where the drugs lead to tumor cell death, in CVDs the drugs lead to tissue regeneration and control of the proliferation of cardiomyocytes. In cancer treatment, the nanoparticles should escape the endothelium in the blood compartment to reach cancer tissue; therefore, prolonged circulation is required for the synthetic nanocarriers. In the case of CVDs, the nanoparticles delivered through the systemic circulation will eventually reach the myocardium within 20–25 min, since the human heart can pump 250 mL of blood per minute [8]. Nanoparticles must present high stability in order to withstand to the dynamic environment of the bloodstream and the pressure within the heart compartment, while they must not activate the immune system response, a significant extracellular barrier.

Extracellular biological barriers are common for all DDS systems including opsonization and subsequent sequestration by the mononuclear phagocyte system or nonspecific distribution of therapeutics to healthy organs as well as inadequate accumulation to target tissue. Additional extracellular obstacles are the hemorheological-blood vessel flow and pressure gradients, which are more pronounced in the heart compartment. Common intracellular obstacles involve cellular internalization, the escape from endosomal and lysosomal compartments and the presence of multidrug resistance proteins/pumps, which are all factors that inhibit the proper therapeutic outcome of nanomedicine [9].

Targeting is of primary importance for site specific drug delivery, because it implies selective accumulation of the cargo in the diseased tissue, with minimal effect on the healthy tissues. Currently, two strategies are employed, passive and active targeting [10]. In passive targeting, nanoparticles with certain characteristics, like predetermined size and surface charge, tend to accumulate nonspecifically in the diseased tissue, much more than they do in healthy tissue [11]. Especially in tumor tissues, polymeric drug delivery systems increase by 10 to 100-fold the concentration of the drug compared to results following administration of an aqueous solution of the pure drug. This observation can be interpreted by an increase in permeability of the tumor vessels, whose endothelial cells are poorly aligned with wide fenestrations and lack a smooth muscle lining. This phenomenon is usually referred as the enhanced permeability and retention (EPR) effect and was first explored in solid tumors [12]. The EPR effect has been observed not only in tumor growth, but also in chronic inflammation and infection cases, as well as in ischemic tissues and injured myocardial cells [13–15]. MI could cause many pathophysiological changes, including the enhanced permeability of endothelial cell membranes. Several angiogenic factors and vasoactive substances are upregulated after MI in ischemic tissue. This could activate and mobilize endothelial cells to form new leaky vessels, resulting in EPR-attributed nanoparticle localization. For example, vascular endothelial growth factor (VEGF), which is produced to promote angiogenesis and restore oxygen supply to the damaged tissue, is known to increase vascular permeability after MI [16]. However, this is a field of great controversy and there are many contradicting results for this targeting approach [17,18]. In contrast to the EPR effect in tumors, the post-MI EPR effect does not last long and begins to diminish after 24–48 h with partial functional recovery observed after two weeks [15]. A long period of treatment is generally required to treat and heal the heart after an ischemic episode to prevent negative left ventricular remodeling. This time window may be too short for the delivery of the necessary therapeutics through passive targeting strategies [19].

The most promising method, with interesting preliminary results, is active targeting drug delivery. In most cases, a typical nanoparticle carrier consists of a polymer or lipid matrix loaded with a certain medicine. In order to prevent rapid clearance of nanoparticles by the reticulo-endothelial system (RES), the surface of the nanoparticle is often coated with polyethylene glycol (PEG), a biocompatible, FDA-approved material, which increases circulatory half-life of the DDS. A vital step in nanocarrier fabrication is the functionalization of its surface with targeting moieties binding to the outer surface of the particle. Targeting ligands are usually peptides, antibodies, aptamers, inhibitors or small molecules that ensure specific interaction of the nanoparticle with specific molecules on the surface membrane of the targeting cells [20,21]. This is a common strategy for heart targeting, because during and after MI many receptors are overexpressed and appear on the surface of cardiac cells in response to stress, so they can be targeted by their complementary molecules. For instance, atrial natriuretic peptide (ANP) has been used as a targeting moiety for natriuretic peptide type-A receptors that are expressed on the surface of cardiomyocytes in case of ischemia [22,23]. The nanocarriers can also be labeled with radioactive isotopes or fluorescent dyes, which allows visualization of their accumulation in the diseased tissue. Therefore, innovative formulations through nanomedicine, like polymeric hydrogels, liposomic vesicles, gold or multifunctional silica nanoparticles that can go through a plethora of modifications have significant prospects to overcome physiological barriers and improve therapeutic outcomes in patients, and they will be discussed below [24].

Apart from the targeting, the endocytosis of therapeutic nanoparticles remains a major issue. The plasma membrane is a highly selective and effective barrier that protects all living cells from the surrounding environment and strongly limits the entry and exit of large macromolecules. Therefore, drug delivery systems need to overcome this barrier to intrude living cells. It is well known that nanoparticulate systems are able to enter cells, often through several endocytic pathways, like receptor-mediated endocytosis, macropinocytosis, clathrin-mediated endocytosis, caveolae-mediated endocytosis and phagocytosis. However, passive penetration of the plasma membrane may also occur as an alternative route. Particularly, during the receptor-mediated endocytosis of engineered NPs, receptors in the cell membrane freely diffuse to encounter and bind ligands decorated on NPs surface. The formation of ligand–receptor bonds provides a driving force for the membrane to wrap around NPs. Therefore, both receptor diffusion kinetics and thermodynamic driving force are of great importance to determine endocytosis efficiency. Afterwards, pinching-off of the membrane-bound NP carrier leads to the formation of an early stage endosome in cytoplasm and finally endosomal release of the NP during the late stage of endosome occurs. In this way, the cargo is released in cytosol. The properties of NPs, such as size, shape, rigidity and surface charge, could greatly affect their interactions with the surrounding environment and determine their fate during the drug delivery process. The effects of these factors in the endocytosis pathway are extensively investigated in the computational works of Ying Li et al. [25–27].

3. Types of Nanoconstructs for CVDs

Recently, the interest in developing DDS for targeting the cardiovascular system has increased exponentially. Many types of nano-based structures have been developed and can be utilized for the transport of drugs for this purpose. Liposomes, polymer–drug conjugates, polymeric micelles, nanoshells, and magnetic or hybrid carriers are some of these and all can be used for drug delivery [28]. In this section, we report the emerging research progress and results on heart-targeted nanoscale DDS (Scheme 1).

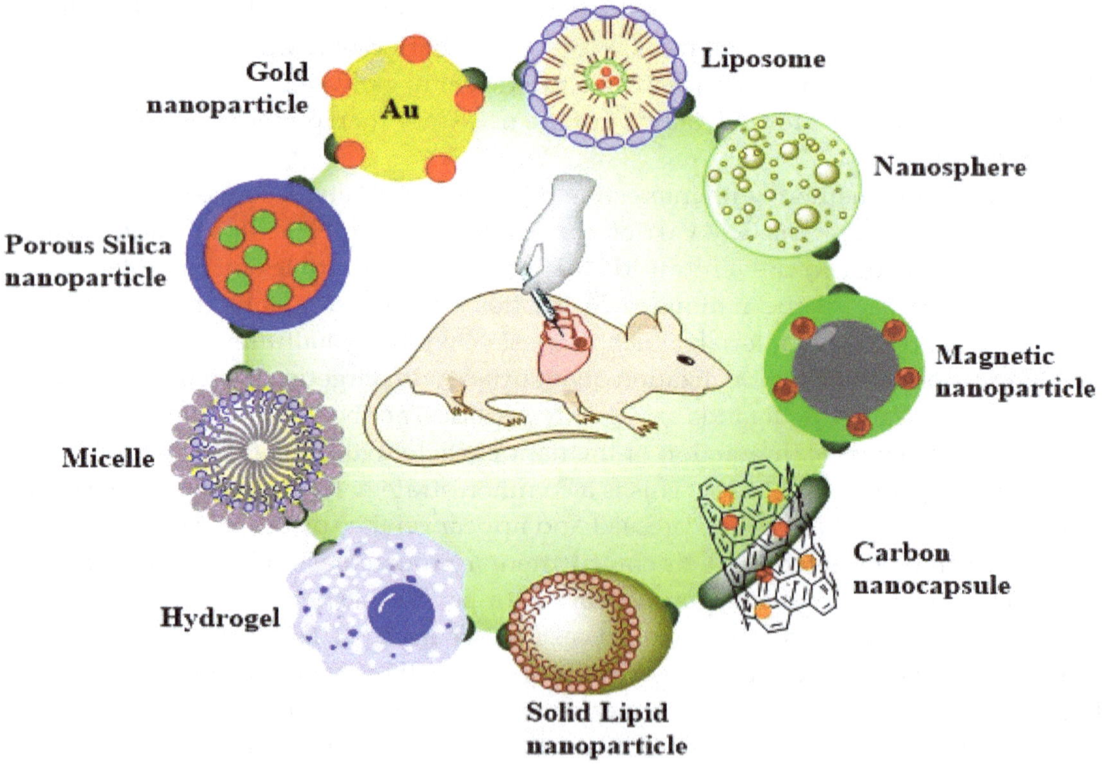

Scheme 1. Overview of the DDS types to treat heart diseases.

3.1. Liposomes

Among them, lipid-based nanoparticles are currently the most commonly used nanoconstructs for drug delivery. Many products based on liposomes have been available on the market for the past decade and some others are currently in clinical development. Liposomes are spherical structures that, most of the time, form vesicles. They are composed of a phospholipid bilayer membrane inside of which aqueous solutions can be entrapped. Their biocompatible and biodegradable composition, as well as their unique ability to encapsulate both hydrophilic and hydrophobic pharmaceutical agents, make liposomes excellent nanocarriers. Liposomes are often coated with biocompatible polymers, such as PEG, to prolong their circulation time and increase stability in aqueous environments. The polymer coating can also be modified to carry a functional group, which can be used as a surface marker [29]. Many experimental attempts to treat the infarcted heart include supplying growth factors, cytokines, drugs, and other biomolecules to the damaged cells in the infarcted tissue.

Dvir and coworkers designed a nanoparticulate system that could specifically target cardiac cells. These particles are angiotensin II type 1 (AT1) nano-liposomes that contain a targeting amino acid sequence (Gly-Gly-Gly-Gly-Asp-Arg-Val-Tyr-Ile-His-Pro-Phe) for AT1 receptor binding. This peptide was conjugated to carboxylic groups on the PEG-HSPC liposomes. AT1 receptors found to be overexpressed in heart after MI or heart failure. The AT1 particles with 142 nm size exhibited great targeting capability in vitro and in vivo. The authors first found in vitro that there was a 3-fold increase in the expression of the AT1 receptor in cardiac cells subjected to hypoxia (ventricular myocytes) compared with cells growing under normal conditions, and 83% of total amount of NPs accumulated in these cells. Furthermore, in in vivo experiments, fluorescent liposomes were injected in mice 1, 4 and 7 days after MI and it was found that NPs amassed predominantly in the left ventricle of the infarcted heart. This finding shows the ability of these particles to specifically target the injured myocardium and may be exploited to deliver therapeutic agents to it [30].

Yu et al., reported the fabrication of oleate adenosine prodrug lipid nanocarriers functionalized with atrial natriuretic peptide (ANP) for the treatment of MI. Adenosine is an endogenous nucleoside that regulates the proper function of the heart and brain, but its short plasma half-life hindered its clinical use. In this study, this nucleoside was conjugated to oleate acid in order to achieve better stability and sustained release. In addition, ANP, which has cardioprotective properties and its receptors are overexpressed in the endocardium of the ischemic heart [31], was conjugated to polyethylene glycol-distearoylphosphatidylethanolamine (PEG-DSPE) to get ANP-PEG-DSPE. Afterwards, lipid nanocarriers were formed via the solvent evaporation method incorporating adenosine oleate prodrug inside of their core. In vitro drug release and cell uptake studies showed that 80% of the drug was released within 48 h and high cellular uptake efficiency was observed without cytotoxic effects. In vivo experiments indicated that the infarct size was significantly inhibited and nanoparticles accumulated predominantly in the infarcted myocardium. Therefore, ANP-modified oleate adenosine lipid nanocarriers are candidates for novel drug delivery to the heart in a receptor-dependent manner due to their therapeutic efficiency and targeting ability [23].

Takahama and colleagues also presented a study in which they investigated whether liposomal adenosine has fewer side effects and offers better cardioprotection than free adenosine. For this purpose, they synthesized liposomes consisting of DSPE-PEG, cholesterol, hydrogenated soy phosphatidyl choline (HSPC) and adenosine via the hydration method. The PEGylated liposomes with a diameter of 134 nm accumulated specifically in ischemic myocardium of rats at 3 h after MI, taking advantage of the enhanced permeability effect of the affected tissue. Intravenous infusion of free adenosine led to a decrease in blood pressure and heart rate in a dose dependent manner, while liposomal adenosine did not. Radioisotope-labeled adenosine encapsulated in liposomes exhibited prolonged circulation time in comparison with the free form. Moreover, liposomal adenosine significantly reduced MI size showing increasing cardioprotective effects [32].

Dong et al. reported the synthesis of a novel solid lipid nanoparticle (SLN) system, as a transferring agent of Puerarin (7,4′-dihydroxyisoflavone-8b-glucopyranoside, PUE) for MI treatment. This SLN system consisted of two different parts and was fabricated following the solvent evaporation method. The solid core was consisted of Compritol®888 ATO and soya lecithin and the PEG-DSPE compartment modified with cyclic arginyl-glycyl-aspartic acid (RGD) peptide was exploited for stabilization and targeting purposes. The RGD peptide was used as targeting moiety for $\alpha v\beta 3$ integrin, which is overexpressed on endothelial cells. The size of these nanoparticles (RGD/PEG-PUE-SLN) loaded with

PUE was about 110 nm, and the zeta potential was negative (−26 mV), ensuring the inhibition of platelet activation and the major protection of the heart. The encapsulation efficiency was about 85.7% for RGD/PEG-PUE-SLN and the loading capacity was 16.5%. In vitro tests showed no cytotoxicity of the SLNs and rapid drug release was observed at the first 12 h, followed by a sustained release in 48 h. In vivo studies revealed that the RGD/PEG-PUE-SLN accumulated mainly in the infarcted heart and PUE concentration was 23-fold higher than free PUE. RGD/PEG-PUE-SLN also minimized the infarct size to 6.2%, indicating the potential of this system for MI treatment [33].

Another target-specific lipid nanoparticle was reported by Dasa for the delivery of small molecule drugs after MI. This team synthesized liposomes with different targeting 7-mer peptides (obtained by phage display biopanning) with affinity for cell types present in heart after MI. The most effective system was a I-1 peptide functionalized liposome consisting of dioleoylphosphatidylcholine (DOPC) cholesterol and DSPE-PEG, 100–120 nm in size, that showed specific interaction with cardiomyocytes, but not exclusively. These liposomes were used to deliver in mice AZ7379, a PARP-1 (Poly(ADP-ribose) polymerase 1) inhibitor. PARP-1 is a nuclear enzyme that is activated in response to oxidative stress and catalyzes the formation of poly (ADP-ribose). The cardiomyocyte-targeted delivery of AZ7379 promotes cardiomyocyte-specific inhibition of PARP-1, with 9-fold higher efficiency 24 h post injection than negative control liposomes. Free AZ7379 showed very limited inhibition [34].

Wang and his group recently investigated the development of a dual modified liposome carrier with improved heart delivery capability. The targeting ligands on the surface of the NPs were two peptides, PCM (WLSEAGPVVTVRALRGTGSW) and TAT (YGRKKRRQRRR). PCM is a 20-mer peptide with the ability to bind primary cardiomyocytes with high affinity and TAT is an 11-mer peptide that can promote the intracellular penetration through nonspecific endocytosis. The liposomes composed of soybean phospholipids, cholesterol and DSPE-PEG had a size slightly over 100 nm, negative zeta potential (−10 mV) and were stable for at least 30 days in vitro. These particles showed no cytotoxic effects at a concentration bellow 0.8 mM and in vitro and in vivo experiments with fluorescent coumarin-6 exhibited high cellular internalization. Thus, this novel dual-modified delivery system provides better cardiomyocytes targeting ability and it would be able to deliver therapeutic agents to the heart effectively [35].

A similar approach was followed by Ko for gene delivery to the ischemic heart by double-targeted lipoplexes. In this case, TAT peptide and anti-myosin monoclonal antibody (mAb 2G4) were employed as targeting moieties. Anti-myosin mAb 2G4 is a highly specific antibody that has the ability to recognize and bind ischemic cells with damaged plasma membranes when intracellular myosin becomes exposed to the extracellular surface and thus allows for the antibody binding. TAT- and TAT-mAb 2G4 lipoplexes were fabricated with the addition of a cationic lipid (DOTAP) in a very small ratio to the other components, in order to complex with a negative charged plasmid DNA. Both lipoplexes exhibited in vitro transfection to rat hypoxic cardiomyocytes, with double modified NPs showing enhanced transfection and four-fold higher green fluorescence protein (GFP) expression. However, no synergistic effect was observed for the two ligands. In vivo, fluorescent polyplexes administered in an MI rat model showed preferential accumulation in the ischemic area of the heart and expression of the GFP gene, making this system a candidate for the potential delivery of therapeutic genes to the ischemic myocardium [36].

The targeting efficiency of mAb 2G4 for the cardiac myosin was exploited by Liang and coworkers for the synthesis of ATP-containing immunoliposomes. In the ischemic heart, myocardial adenosine triphosphate (ATP) utilization is reduced due to inadequate contractile function, while the need for ATP remains high. This imbalance between supply and demand for ATP deteriorates left ventricular cardiac function. Free ATP cannot be administered because of its short circulation half-life and, because of its strong negatively charged nature, cannot enter into cells through their membrane. So, in this study, ATP was encapsulated in liposomes containing phosphatidylcholine, cholesterol, PEG-DSPE and 2G4-PEG-PE. Liposomes were produced via the freeze-thawing method and after ATP entrapment only minor ATP leakage was observed after 24 h at 37 °C. The specific binding of

2G4-immunoliposomes to myosin was evaluated using ELISA. The results showed strong binding to the myosin monolayer [37]. In vivo experiments using these NPs with or without the targeting antibody were conducted by Verma et al. in rabbits after an acute myocardial infarction. Infusion of ATP-NPs followed by 30 min of coronary artery occlusion and 3 h of reperfusion, resulted in a significant decrease (over 50%) in the size of irreversibly damaged myocardium within the total area at risk. These NPs accumulated in the heart due to the EPR effect and seem to have a cardioprotective effect by supplying the myocardium with the required energy [38]. Some myosin specific liposomes demonstrated even better cardioprotection by significantly restoring the systolic and diastolic function of the heart. At the end of reperfusion, the left ventricular pressure recovered to more than 80%, while the left ventricular end diastolic pressure reduced considerably [39]. In addition, the delivery of Coenzyme Q10 (CoQ10) with similar liposomes was investigated by the same team. Intracoronary infusion of CoQ10 loaded liposomes in rabbits with MI resulted in a 50% reduction in infarct size, which could in turn be sufficient for potential recovery from an infarction in a clinical situation [40].

Scott and coworkers focused their efforts on developing anti-P-selectin conjugated lipid nanocarriers to treat rat MI. Anti-P-selectin was used as targeting ligand because it has been reported that P-selectin is upregulated in endothelial cells after ischemic or inflammatory events in several tissues. In particular, P-selectin is expressed in the region between the healthy and necrotic tissue (border zone) in infarcted heart as observed by immunohistochemical analysis. Liposomes were fabricated using HSPC, cholesterol and DSPE-PEG and anti-P-selectin was conjugated to the surface of the nanocarriers by thiol group modifications. Anti-P-selectin coated NPs were administered instantly or 4 h after MI. The immediately infused liposomes showed a significant increase in accumulation (83%) to the infarct region as compared to the non-infarcted area after 24 h circulation, while the 4 h post-MI infused liposomes showed a 92% increase in adhesion. Exploiting this property, vascular endothelial growth factor (VEGF), a proangiogenic compound, was encapsulated to the liposomes in an attempt to revascularize the infarcted myocardium. Administration of a single dose of 0.12 $\mu g\ kg^{-1}$ targeted VEGF immunoliposomes resulted in significant improvements in cardiac function and vascular structure up to 4 weeks after MI. VEGF enhanced systolic function and fractional shortening of the infarcted tissue, while a raise in number of anatomical and perfused vessels in myocardium border zone was noticed. At this point, is very important to note that in many VEGF therapies initiated many days after MI, no therapeutic effects were detected. Therefore, the immediate exposure of the heart tissue to VEGF, which could delay the myocardial apoptosis and cardiac remodeling is of primary importance [41,42].

In addition, an interesting study was reported by Liu for the therapy of arrhythmia to the ischemic heart. They synthesized antibody modified liposomes for the targeted delivery of anti-miR-1 antisense oligonucleotides AMO-1 to the ischemic myocardium. It is well established that microRNA-1 (miR-1) can be found in cardiac and skeletal muscle tissues and is overexpressed in the ischemic heart. The suppression of miR-1 by AMO-1, an anti-miR-1 antisense oligonucleotide, can lead to the therapy of cardiac arrhythmia. Furthermore, cardiac troponin I (cTn-I) is a specific marker which is expressed only in damaged heart tissues. Based on this, anti-cTn-I antibody was harnessed as a targeting moiety. The liposomes, containing egg phosphatidylcholine, cholesterol and DSPE-PEG, were fabricated via the thin film hydration method, and the antibody was conjugated using DSPE-PEG-MAL. The NPs had a slightly negative surface charge, a size close to 100 nm, high AMO-1 entrapment efficiency (>60%) and 23% in vitro release rate in 24 h. Time lapse live cell imaging and in vivo imaging utilized to monitor anti-cTn-I NPs and both demonstrated high accumulation in the heart and specifically in the cytoplasm of myocardial cells. After administration of AMO-I loaded NPs in rats, electrocardiograph recordings exhibited repression of arrhythmogenesis. To conclude, anti-cTnI liposomes not only delivered AMO-1 to infarcted myocardium in rats, but also relieved cardiac arrhythmia via the silencing of miR-1 in the ischemic heart [43]. All efforts presented above are summarized in Table 1.

Table 1. Summary of liposomic nanoparticles and their therapeutic effects.

Liposome	Targeting Method	Drug/Cargo	Therapeutic Effect	Reference
PEG-HSPC	Active targeting of AT1 receptor	-	Targeting of injured myocardium	[30]
PEG-DSPE	Active targeting of ANP receptor	Adenosine	Infarct size inhibition	[23]
PEG-DSPE, HSPC	Passive targeting of myocardium	Adenosine	Ischemic myocardium accumulation and cardioprotection	[32]
PEG-DSPE, 888ATO, soya lecithin	Active targeting of $\alpha v\beta 3$ integrin	Puerarin	Infarct size reduction	[33]
PEG-DSPE, DOPC, cholesterol	Active targeting of Poly(ADP-ribose) polymerase 1	AZ7379 (Poly(ADP-ribose) polymerase 1 inhibitor)	Cardiomyocyte inhibition of PARP-1	[34]
PEG-DSPE, cholesterol	Active cardiomyocyte targeting	-	High cardiomyocyte internalization	[35]
PEG-PE, POPC, DOTAP	Active ischemic cell targeting	Plasmid DNA	Ischemic heart accumulation	[36]
PEG-DSPE, PEG-PE, cholesterol, PC	Active targeting of myosin	ATP or Q10 coenzyme	Reduction in ischemic area	[37–39]
PEG-DSPE, HSPC, cholesterol	Active targeting of P-Selectin	VEGF	Cardiac function and vascular structure improvement	[41,42]
PEG-DSPE, PC, cholesterol	Active targeting of cardiac troponin-I	AMO-1	Therapy of cardiac arrhythmia	[43]

3.2. *Polymeric Nanoparticles*

Biodegradable polymeric nanoconstructs have been extensively investigated as drug carriers. This type of nanocarrier includes copolymers consisting of two or more blocks with different hydrophobicity. In aqueous environments, these copolymers usually form micellar structures composed of a hydrophilic shell and a hydrophobic core. Inside the hydrophobic core, water-insoluble drugs can be hosted, while the hydrophilic corona can be additionally modified for the attachment of water-soluble drugs or targeting moieties. [44]. However, this is not always the case. To date, many other polymeric nanoconstructs have been synthesized with very different structures. For instance, polymers can form hydrogels [45–47], network-like scaffolds [48], microparticles [49], nanospheres or nanoshells that are suitable not only for the release of hydrophobic but also hydrophilic drugs, proteins, genes, nucleic acids or genes. [50]. The release of encapsulated drugs occurs at a controlled rate in a time or environment dependent manner. The kinetics of the release of nanoparticle-bound drugs depend on the duration of nanoparticles residence in the organism and characteristics of their microenvironment. In general, biodegradable polymer formulations maintain the desired therapeutic drug concentration in the tissue of interest for a longer period of time than other nanocarriers. This feature makes them suitable platforms for the transport of highly toxic, poorly soluble, and unstable drugs.

Poly(D,L-lactic acid), poly(D,L-glycolic acid) (PLGA) is a copolymer that has been widely used for medical applications due to its low toxicity, high biocompatibility and biodegradability and because it is an FDA approved material. In this route, many research groups have focused their attempts on developing PLGA based nanomedicine materials. For example, Chang and coworkers presented the synthesis of insulin-like growth factor-1 (IGF-1) complexed PLGA NPs for early cardioprotection after acute MI. IGF-1 is crucial in regulating heart function and it has been found to promote cardiomyocyte proliferation. In humans, IGF-1 treatment enhances cardiac function after infarction. In order to maintain its biological function, anionic IGF-1 formed complexes with PLGA via electrostatic interactions. Because PLGA is also negatively charged, polyethylenimine conjugation was utilized to render PLGA's surface cationic and to achieve PLGA-IGF-1 complexation. Various-sized NPs were synthesized (1 μm, 200 nm, 70 nm), with the smallest ones (70 nm) found to have the best binding capability and activated the most Akt phosphorylation in cultured cardiomyocytes. After a single intramyocardial injection in mice, IGF-1-PLGA NPs prolonged IGF-1 retention time to at least

24 h, inhibited cardiomyocyte apoptosis, reduced infarct size and prevented ventricular dilation and wall thinning 21 days after MI. These results highlight the potential of nanomedicine in treating cardiovascular diseases and encourage its translation into clinical applications [51].

Administration of statins at the time of reperfusion exhibited no therapeutic effects in animals and in patients with acute MI. Nevertheless, Nagaoka and his team found that nanoparticle delivered Pitavastatin presented cardioprotective effects. They synthesized Pitavastatin-PLGA NPs that accumulated in the infarcted region of the myocardium of a rat MI model due to its enhanced vascular permeability. After single intravenous injection at reperfusion, Pitavastatin NPs reduced the size of infarct after 24 h and improved left ventricular function. They also induced phosphorylation of Akt and GSK3β and inhibited inflammation and cardiomyocyte necrosis in the infarcted heart, while the free Pitavastatin drug failed to show any cardioprotection. Moreover, Pitavastatin NPs have successfully completed phase I clinical trials at a university hospital, suggesting that this nanoparticle-based technology can serve as novel therapeutic treatment for ischemic injury [52].

In coronary artery disease (CAD) and peripheral artery disease (PAD), therapeutic angiogenesis has appeared as a potential clinical approach for the recovery of ischemic tissues, including the direct administration of pro-angiogenic growth factors to promote the synthesis of growth factors by target tissues. In this context, adrenomedullin-2 (ADM-2) has been recently identified as a new angiogenic factor able to regulate blood flow and cardiovascular function. Due to its short biological half-life and low plasma stability, ADM-2 has, up to now, limited applications. For this reason, Quadros and coworkers tried to encapsulate this peptide into PLGA nanoformulations that could serve as delivery system for heart repair. PLGA-ADM-2 NPs, prepared by a double emulsion method, had a size of 300–350 nm, negative surface charge, good colloidal stability and did not present toxicity in cardiomyocyte cells. The entrapment efficiency of ADM-2 reached circa 70%, as identified by ELISA, and in vitro peptide release showed a 60% release in the first 3 days followed by a slower release rate in the next 3 weeks. In vitro experiments in EA.hy926 endothelial cells also exhibited enhanced cell proliferation (1.4 fold higher), rendering AMD-2-PLGA NPs a novel approach for therapeutic angiogenesis in CVDs [53].

In a pioneering work, Nguyen et al. presented a system for potential treatment of heart failure following a MI based on intravenous administration of enzyme responsive nanoparticles. These nanomaterials have the ability to respond to the enzymatic conditions present in the heart after an acute MI by changing their structure from discrete micellar nanostructures to network-like scaffolds. It is worth noting that these nanosystems (Figure 1), consisting of brush peptide–polymer amphiphiles based on a polynorbornene backbone with peptide targeting sequences specific for recognition by matrix metalloproteinases MMP-2 and MMP-9, have the ability to remain stable during blood circulation conditions until they reach the infarct region through the vascular leakage after MI. At this site, their structure is altered, and it has been found that they remain on the injured tissue for up to 28 days after injection. In previous work, super resolution fluorescence microscopy measurements showed that the responsive nanoparticles are MMP-9 activated and they are kept assembled into scaffolds at the injection site for 7 days, while the non-responsive particles were inactive in the presence of MMP-9 and were cleared within 1 h. Furthermore, the efficacy of the system was also studied in rats with MI and it was indicated that the responding particles were activated in the presence of MMPs and remained aggregated in network-like scaffolds for 6 days, in contrast with the reduced aggregation observed in non-responsive particles. Finally, after injecting responsive and non-responsive particles into the tail vein of healthy rats as well as in 24 h post-MI rats, a targeted and prolonged accumulation of responsive particles in the diseased heart tissue was demonstrated for 28 days. In conclusion, MMP-responsive nanoparticles exploit the EPR effect for initial passive targeting and present a very promising approach to deliver therapeutics to the heart after MI in an effective and controlled manner [48].

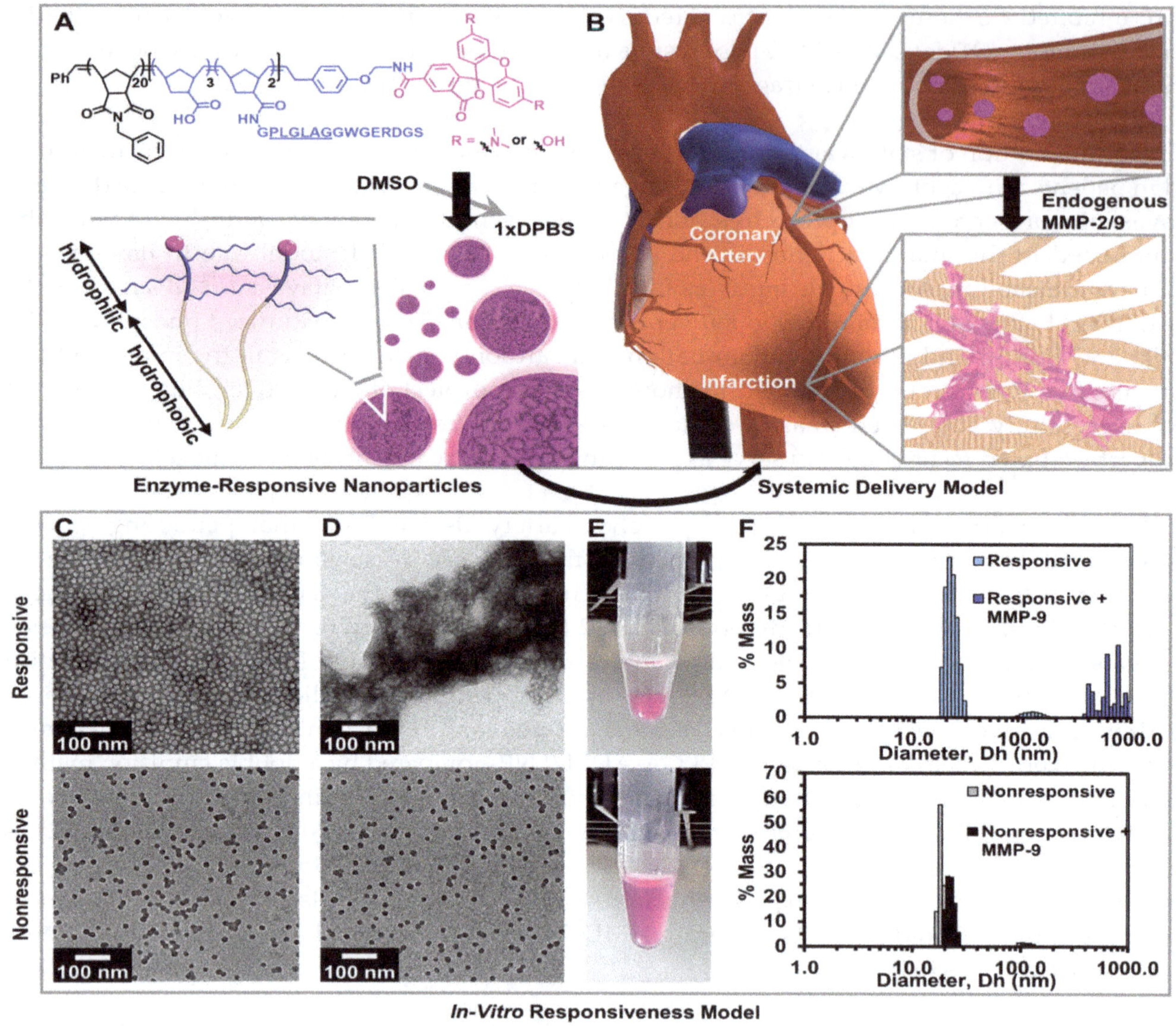

Figure 1. Responsive nanoparticles target, accumulate, and are retained within an acute MI due to enzyme-induced aggregation. (**A**) Diagram of a dye-labeled brush peptide–polymer amphiphile (PPA) containing an MMP-2 and MMP-9 specific recognition sequence, shown underlined. PPAs self-assemble into nanoparticles through hydrophobic–hydrophilic interactions when dialyzed into aqueous buffer. (**B**) Schematic of nanoparticles freely circulating in the bloodstream (not to scale) upon systemic delivery. Nanoparticles enter the infarct tissue through the leaky acute MI vasculature, and up-regulated MMPs within the infarct induce the formation of an aggregate-like scaffold. (**C**) In vitro, responsive (top) and non-responsive (bottom) nanoparticles are monodisperse micelles with diameters of 15–20 nm, and (**D**) upon activation, only responsive nanoparticles form an aggregate-like scaffold. (**E**) Corresponding images of nanoparticle solutions following activation. (**F**) Dynamic light scattering of nanoparticles before and after MMP activation. Reproduced with permission from [48], Wiley-VCH, 2015.

Furthermore, for the promotion of angiogenesis in the infarcted tissue, Garbern and her team designed a pH- and temperature responsive nanocarrier for the delivery of basic fibroblast growth factor (bFGF). They used the random copolymer poly(*N*-isopropylacrylamide-*co*-propylacrylic acid-*co*-butyl acrylate) (p[*N*IPAAm-*co*-PAA-*co*-BA]), synthesized by reversible addition fragmentation chain transfer (RAFT) polymerization, because of its ability to undergo a sol–gel phase transition. This polymer is liquid at pH = 7.4 and becomes a gel at pH = 6.8, exploiting the lower pH of the ischemic region. In vivo experiments in rat hearts showed that the injectable hydrogel enhanced local accumulation of bFGF in the apex of the heart, with minor diffusion to other regions of the tissue.

In addition, the retention of bFGF 7 days post injection was 10-fold higher with hydrogel than with saline delivery, and, after 28 days of treatment, the relative blood flow was significantly increased (2-fold increase) as compared to day 0. In addition, capillary and arteriolar densities were increased by over 30%, while fractional shortening, determined by echocardiography, was remarkably increased following treatment with this polymeric hydrogel [46].

A different approach was followed by Sy for the inhibition of cardiac dysfunction after MI. They presented the synthesis of poly(cyclohexane-1,4-diylacetone dimethylene ketal) (PCADK) microparticles and the encapsulation of SB239063, a p-38 inhibitor, into these particles. The p38 mitogen-activated protein kinase pathway plays a key role in activating macrophages and in inducing cardiomyocyte apoptosis. For this reason, PCADK-p38 particles of 10–20 μm size formed via a single emulsion/evaporation method and the encapsulation efficiency of the inhibitor reached nearly 50% with a concentration in microparticles of 3–5 μg of inhibitor per mg of polymer. In vitro experiments in cultured macrophages showed that PCADK-p38 microparticles prevented p-38 phosphorylation by TNF-a stimulation, reduced superoxide production (an inflammatory effector) and at the same time an accelerated release of the inhibitor was observed, possibly due to intracellular release after phagocytosis. In addition, PCADK-p38 microparticles did not induce any inflammatory response in vitro and in vivo. After a single intramyocardial injection in mice, the microparticles remained in the heart for days and seriously inhibited p-38 phosphorylation within the infarct zone, whereas free SB239063 had no effect. At 21 days postinfarction, an obvious improvement in fractional shortening and a reduction in fibrosis were observed [49]. A similar study was presented by Gray for the development of smaller (<500 nm) *N*-acetylglucosamine functionalized PCADK nanoparticles. These NPs carried the same inhibitor, but *N*-acetylglucosamine on their surface promoted cell internalization. In vitro and in vivo experiments also showed promising results, as administration of PCADK NPs reduced apoptotic events and infarct size and improved acute cardiac function [54].

Somasuntharam and coworkers developed a nanocarrier for the delivery of Nox2-siRNA to the infarcted heart environment through particles based on acid-sensitive polyketals, in order to silence the Nox2 gene in cardiac macrophages. Nox2 is a catalytic subunit for nicotinamide adenine dinucleotide phosphate (NADPH) oxidase, responsible for reactive oxygen species production, and Nox2-NADPH upregulation mainly occurred in the infarcted myocardium. Silencing of this gene has been found to have cardioprotective properties. So, polyketal PK3 copolymer was used for the incorporation of Nox2-siRNA in the nanoparticles. The encapsulation efficiency of siRNA within the PK3 particles was found to be 40%, while their average size was 500 nm. The internalization of siNox2 loaded particles by macrophages was found to be over 80%, as determined by flow cytometry. Further experiments in the mouse macrophage cell line RAW 264.7 also confirmed that PK-siNox2 particles suspended Nox2 mRNA expression by over 40%. In vivo experiments in mice also showed lower levels of Nox2 mRNA expression and echocardiography data evidenced that cardiac function improved significantly after NPs intramyocardial administration. This promising Nox2-siRNA delivery system is stable during blood circulation, leading to a reduction in oxidative stress and protection of the heart from failure [55].

Huang et al., reported the synthesis of cysteine–arginine–glutamic acid–lysine–alanine (CREKA)-modified NPs for the delivery of thymosin beta 4 (Tβ4) to the infarcted myocardium. Tβ4 is a 43 amino acid, expressed in the embryonic heart, responsible for epicardial and coronary artery growth and overexpressed in the infarcted heart. Recent research has uncovered that Tβ4 enhances heart function by protecting cardiomyocytes from apoptosis and by activating epicardial progenitor cells. However, free Tβ4 administration is unfeasible due to short circulation half-life. Fibrin is predominantly expressed in the early stages of MI in the injured area of the heart and constitutes a potential target for DDS. CREKA, a fibrin targeted peptide and Tβ4 were both conjugated to the outer area of poly(ethylene glycol)–poly(lactic acid) (PEG-PLA) NPs via EDC/NHS and maleimide–thiol reactions, respectively. The NPs produced by an emulsion/solvent evaporation protocol had a size of 100 nm and negative zeta potential (−10 mV). Ex vivo heart imaging experiments revealed that CREKA-NPs accumulated in the infarcted area, and this mostly occurred 24 h after administration.

Interestingly, bare NPs (without CREKA) also accumulated in the same area because of the EPR effect. Tail vein injection of CREKA-NPs in mice showed multiple therapeutic effects, such as reduction in end diastolic and systolic diameter, 30% reduction in infarct size, increased wall thickness, increased vessel and arteriole density and cell proliferation in the peri-infarct area. All these results indicate that this delivery system is very promising for further clinical applications [56].

Diabetic cardiomyopathy (DCM) is a CVD caused by diabetes and it has many adverse effects in heart function, like systolic/diastolic cardiac changes and atherosclerotic heart disease that later leads to heart failure or ischemia. To tackle DCM, Tong and coworkers developed curcumin polymeric carriers consisting of a triblock copolymer poly(γ-benzyl L-glutamate)-poly(ethylene glycol)-poly(γ-benzyl L-glutamate) (PBLG-PEG-PBLG) (P). The copolymer was synthesized by the ring opening polymerization of the BLG-N-carboxy anhydride with H_2N-PEG-NH_2 as the macroinitiator. The curcumin incorporated particles had a diameter of 30 nm and the loading capacity of curcumin was over 30%. These particles showed very limited cell toxicity in vitro in high concentrations and curcumin release was achieved within 3 days. In previous studies, curcumin was found to have therapeutic effects on diabetes and to alleviate DCM. Indeed, it was found that curcumin loaded NPs reduced pathological morphological damage of cardiac tissue and increased H_2S levels that play a vital role in the inhibition of apoptosis in cardiomyocytes [57].

Hardy et al. designed a double loaded drug delivery system against L-type Ca^{2+} channel. The L-type Ca^{2+} is the main source for calcium in cardiomyocytes. When ischemia reperfusion injury occurs, increasing levels of intracellular calcium and reactive oxygen species are the two main factors contributing to cardiac hypertrophy, inflammation and cell apoptosis. To deal with this, they designed poly(glycidyl methacrylate) (PGMA) nanoparticles loaded either with curcumin or resveratrol and a peptide derived against the alpha-interacting domain of the L-type Ca^{2+} channel (AID), with amino acid sequence QQLEEDLKGYLDWITQAE, that has been found to reduce heart injury post reperfusion. The NPs constructed through oil in water emulsion process and AID peptide were electrostatically attached to the surface of NPs after modification of PGMA with positively charged polyethylenimine. The loading efficiency of resveratrol was quite low (1% *w*/*w*) with fast release rate compared to curcumin and AID loading that reached 12% *w*/*w* with a sustained release profile within 60 min of reperfusion. The curcumin-AID NPs were found to be more effective in minimizing oxidative stress and superoxide production ex vivo in rat hearts, while resveratrol NPs were found to have only an initial therapeutic effect, preventing their further application as potential DDS. Importantly, AID in combination with curcumin proved to ameliorate ischemia reperfusion injury via different mechanisms, rendering them as vital components of an effective DDS [58].

In 2010, Nam et al., reported the synthesis of a primary cardiomyocyte specific peptide-functionalized poly (cystamine bisacrylamide-diaminohexane, CBA-DAH) (PCD) polymer in order to deliver Fas siRNA selectively and efficiently in cardiomyocytes. The delivery of Fas siRNA leads to the silence of Fas gene expression and inhibits cardiomyocyte apoptosis. This cardiomyocyte-targeted Fas siRNA delivery system presented not only high transfection efficiency, but also low cytotoxicity. PCM peptide indicated high selectivity for cardiomyocytes and z potential measurements showed that the binding of PCM to the polymer, via amino groups, led to a reduction in cationic charges, impairing their ability to incorporate negatively charged genes. Therefore, it was necessary to introduce unmodified PCD, in a ratio of 1:1 *w*/*w* with the PCM-PCD, in order to increase the positive charge and obtain stable nanoparticles with a diameter of less than 200 nm. These polymers can form complexes with polyanionic genes efficiently, like Fas siRNA. Transfection experiments and cellular uptake studies confirmed that the biodegradable PCM-modified polymer could bind specifically to H9C2 cells, revealing the cardiomyocyte-targeting ability of PCM-PCD nanoparticles. Flow cytometry measurements in H9C2 cells indicated the efficiency of Fas gene silencing by PCM-polymer/Fas siRNA complexes to inhibit apoptosis under hypoxic conditions. Quantitative real-time PCR analysis showed a 77% reduction in Fas gene expression in H9C2 cells treated with Fas siRNA, delivered using the PCM-PCD/PCD carrier. The PCM-modified polymer/Fas siRNA polyplexes facilitate Fas gene silencing and increase cardiomyocyte viability under hypoxic conditions. To conclude, PCM modification is a promising method for cardiomyocyte targeting, and siRNA delivery with PCM-PCD polymers inhibits cardiomyocyte apoptosis [59].

Another interesting aspect for treating MI is the restoration of mechanical and electrical function of the heart by exploiting the conductive properties of some nanoformulations. As an example, a soft conductive hydrogel was presented by Bao and his group as an electrical signal transmitter for the infarcted myocardium (Figure 2). They synthesized an injectable hydrogel consisting of a multi-armed PEGDA700-Melamine (PEG-MEL) crosslinker, stabilized through π–π interactions between the triazine rings of melamine, that was used to conjugate a thiol modified hyaluronic acid (HA). Moreover, the addition of graphene oxide (GO) has provided soft ($G' = 25$ Pa) and conductive ($G = 2.84 \times 10^{-4}$ S cm^{-1}) properties and enhanced mechanical stress stability. To improve the healing ability of the hydrogel, adipose tissue-derived stromal cells (ADSCs) were incorporated. After an injection in the MI area in a rat model, an overall enhancement of cardiac function was observed. In particular, the ejection fraction (EF) and fractional shortening (FS) greatly improved in a one month period (EF = 78% and FS = 53%), the size of infarction and fibrosis reduced and the vascular density increased. Eventually, the overexpression of Connexin 43 and α-Smooth Muscle Actin confirmed the efficient transmission of electrical and mechanical signals to the heart [45].

The insufficient propagation of electrical signals to the heart after MI can also cause cardiac arrhythmia. For this reason, Zhang and coworkers designed an injectable conductive hydrogel that ameliorates arrhythmia and preserves cardiac function (Figure 3). This group synthesized a conductive poly-3-amino-4-methoxybenzoic acid-gelatin (PAMB-G) copolymer through an oxidative polymerization method. The PAMB is the conductive ingredient, while gelatin improves the biocompatibility of the whole system. The copolymer formed a hydrogel after crosslinking of the polymer chains by using EDC/NHS chemistry. An injection to the scar zone of the heart in a rat model one week after MI, showed that the hydrogel enhanced electrical impulse transmission and activated isolated contracting regions. In addition, four weeks after treatment, regional electrical field potential amplitude around the infarcted area was greatly increased and electrocardiograph recordings indicated that fewer premature ventricular contractions occurred. Except for that, PAMB-G treated hearts presented higher fractional shortening and ejection fraction, lower left ventricular internal systolic and diastolic dimensions and a smaller fibrotic area, all resulting in cardiac function enhancement [47]. In Table 2 a synopsis of the polymeric nanostructures discussed in this section is presented.

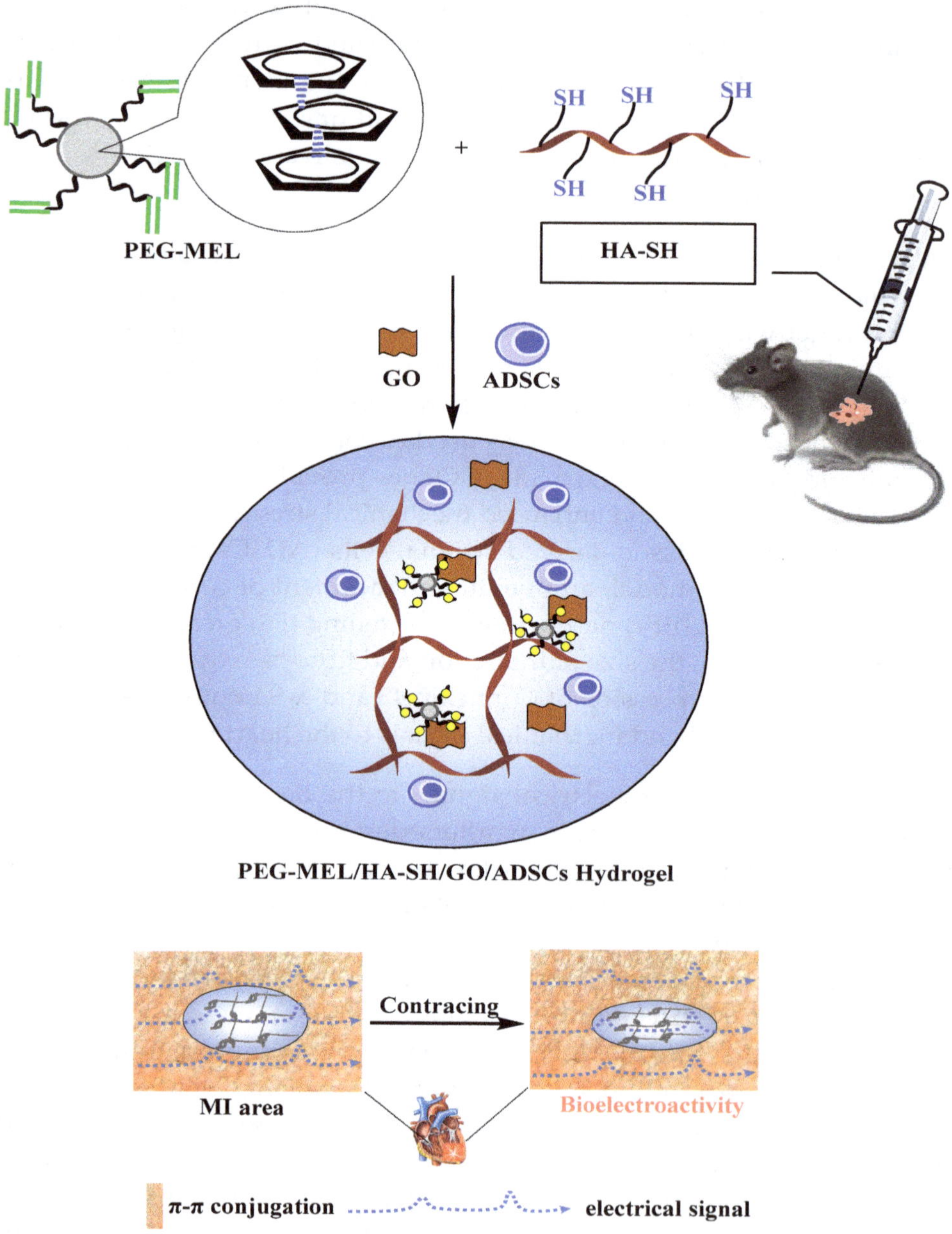

Figure 2. Schematic sketch illustrating the application of this soft and conductive PEG-MEL/HA-SH/GO hydrogel system encapsulating ADSCs for cardiac repair by injection into the MI area of Sprague-Dawley (SD) rats, with the objective of enhancing the transmission of mechanical and electrical signals to rebuild cardiac function. Adapted from [45], Elsevier 2017.

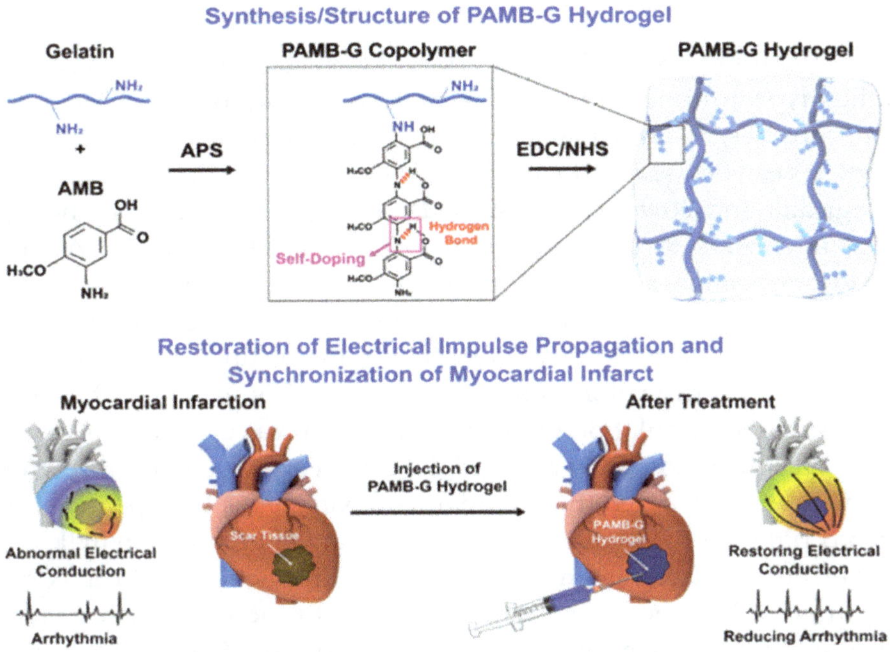

Figure 3. Synthesis and structure of PAMB hydrogel and mechanism of its restoring electrical impulse propagation and synchronizing myocardial contraction following a myocardial infarction. Reproduced with permission from [47], Elsevier, 2019.

Table 2. Summary of polymeric nanoparticles and their therapeutic effects.

Polymer	Targeting Method	Drug/Cargo	Therapeutic Effect	Reference
PLGA	Passive	Insulin-like growth factor-1	Inhibition of cardiomyocyte apoptosis	[51]
PLGA	Passive	Pitavastatin	Infarct size reduction and cardioprotection	[52]
PLGA	Passive	Adrenomedullin-2	Therapeutic angiogenesis	[53]
Poly(norbornene)	Active targeting of metalloproteinases MMP-2, MMP-9	-	Efficient targeting of ischemic zones	[48]
p[NIPAAm-*co*-PAA-*co*-BA]	Passive	Basic Fibroblast Growth Factor	Promotion of angiogenesis and blood flow restoration	[46]
PCADK	Passive	SB239063 (p38 inhibitor)	Inhibition of cardiac dysfunction	[49]
Polyketal derivatives	Passive	Nox2-siRNA	Oxidative species reduction and cardioprotection	[55]
PEG-PLA	Active targeting of fibrin	Thymosin beta 4	Overall improvement in cardiac structure	[56]
PBLG-PEG-PBLG	Passive	Curcumin	Cardiac damage reduction and inhibition of cardiomyocyte apoptosis	[57]
PGMA	Active targeting of L-type Ca^{2+} channels	Curcumin or Resveratrol	Oxidative stress reduction	[58]
Poly(cystamine bisacrylamide -diaminohexane)	Active targeting of cardiomyocytes	Fas siRNA	Inhibition of cardiomyocyte apoptosis	[59]
PEG-MEL, GO, HA	Injection to the site	Adipose tissue-derived stromal cells	Improvement of mechanical and electrical heart function	[45]
Poly(3-amino-4 -methoxybenzoic acid-gelatin)	Injection to the site	-	Enhancement of electrical impulse propagation	[47]

3.3. Other Types

Apart from polymeric and lipid NPs, other types of nanoconstructs have also been developed for drug delivery to the myocardium. Some of them may contain inorganic components such as silica, gold or carbon nanocapsules, and others may contain biomaterials, such as alginate salts or chitosan.

Silica nanoparticles can be used for heart-targeted drug delivery in both passive and active ways. In particular, Galagudza and coworkers designed adenosine loaded silica nanoparticles for the passive delivery of adenosine to the ischemic-reperfused cardiac tissue. As mentioned before, adenosine is a cardioprotective agent and its incorporation to the NPs was achieved through adsorption on their surface. The NPs mean diameter was 6–13 nm, presenting no toxic effects in vitro and in vivo. However, their long-term toxicity remains unclear due to their capture by the liver. After intravenous administration of adenosine-silica NPs in rats with ischemic-reperfusion injured hearts, augmented accumulation in the infarcted area was observed. Adenosine bounded to NPs restored blood pressure and notably reduced the infarct size in comparison with free adenosine administration. It must be emphasized that in order to maximize the therapeutic effects of the DDS, it must be administered right after ischemia or at the beginning of reperfusion [60].

In contrast, Ferreira and her team developed multifunctional silica NPs loaded with a cardioprotective compound for active targeting delivery to the endocardial layer of the injured heart (Figure 4). The synthesized bare silica NPs with initial size of 165 nm were further functionalized with PEG and ANP peptide to reach a final size of 200 nm. The zeta potential of the NPs after ANP modification turned from negative (−30 mV) to positive (>25 mV) due to positively charged amines in the peptide sequence, thus reducing the stealth properties of the system that contribute to the possible formation of protein corona. However, ANP functionalized NPs presented enhanced long-term colloidal stability, no hemotoxicity and retained cardiac cell viability. In vitro experiments confirmed that these NPs interacted preferentially with cardiomyocytes and non-myocytes through the binding of ANP to the natriuretic peptide receptors that are overexpressed in the infarcted region. Furthermore, ^{111}In-labeled NPs were used for in vivo imaging experiments that again showed significant accumulation of the nanocarrier in the ischemic area and particularly in the endocardial layer of the left ventricle, underlining the targeting potential of ANP. At the final stage, the NPs were loaded with a hydrophobic small molecule (trisubsituted-3,4,5-isoxazole, C1) with cardioprotective properties. After intravenous administration of C1-NPs in a MI model in mice and in rats, a significant increase in the left ventricular ejection fraction and fractional shortening was observed. In addition, C1 decreased ERK1/2 phosphorylation, which is a key pathway leading to cardiac hypertrophy. In this way, the development of this nanocarrier provides a targeted therapeutic option against cardiac remodeling and further research should be conducted to study the effects of the delivery of other therapeutic molecules with this promising system [22].

The same group also developed a dual drug loaded dextran-based system for cellular reprogramming of cardiac fibroblasts into cardiac myocytes, for cardiac regeneration purposes after MI. The spermine acetalated dextran-based nanomaterial (AcDXSp) was prepared with an oil-in-water single emulsion method and was further functionalized with PEG and ANP to increase its stability and its specificity for cardiac cells, respectively. Two small hydrophobic molecules (CHIR99021 and SB431542) were incorporated to these NPs in a ratio of 1:2 in order to induce cardiomyocytes' proliferation. SB431542 is a TGF-β inhibitor and CHIR99021 is a Wnt activator, both capable of increasing the efficiency of direct reprogramming of fibroblasts into cardiomyocytes. The final size of these NPs was below 400 nm, with a positive surface charge and minimal toxicity to cardiomyocytes. In addition, the pH responsive nature of this nanomaterial can provide a triggered release of the drugs in the cytoplasm of cardiac cells upon internalization into the acidic subcellular compartments. It was found that at pH = 5, the release was much faster than at pH = 7.4. Finally, in vitro administration of dual-loaded dextran NPs to rat cardiac cells indicated that CHIR99021, on the one hand, stabilized β-catenin, and SB431542, on the other hand, prevented the translocation of Smad3 to the nucleus of fibroblasts, both modulating different pathways for fibroblast reprogramming and increasing heart regeneration potential [61]. Recently, Torrieri and coworkers presented an advanced approach for this system, aiming for better targeting efficiency. Instead of using only ANP peptide for accumulation in cardiac cells, they also exploited linTTP1 peptide (AKRGARSTA) for targeting macrophages, associated with atherosclerotic plaques. This system was found to be safe for macrophages cell lines and primary macrophages, presenting no toxicity. In vitro experiments with macrophages indicated that the NPs could associate well with them and especially with M2-like macrophages, making them a possible target for efficient delivery. Interestingly, it was found that this system showed higher association versus uptake ratio towards M2-like macrophages and enhanced delivery of the drugs by dual targeting procedure [62].

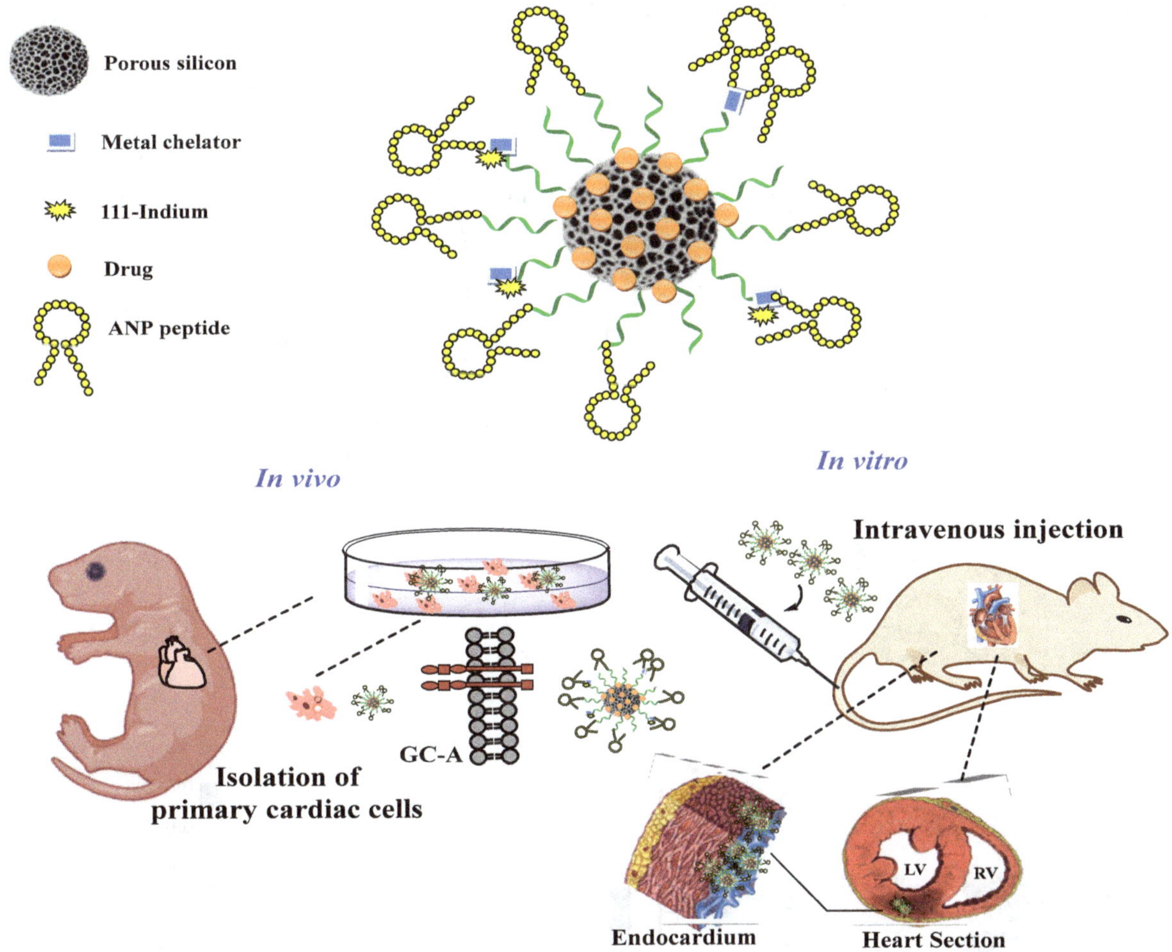

Figure 4. This schematic representation of the engineered multifunctional nanoparticle and its components, as well as an overview of the conducted in vitro and in vivo studies and the main findings of this study. Adapted from [22], Wiley-VCH, 2019.

Gold NPs are already known for their various applications in many fields of material science, as they have unique optical and physical properties. They are also an emerging type of DDS that can be easily functionalized and serve as vehicles for various therapeutic agents, as well as for imaging and diagnosis of diseases. Due to their potential biomedical applications, such as in photothermal therapy [63], many researchers are trying to develop gold-based nanosystems for curing different diseases. Recently, Somasuntharam and coworkers presented a very promising system for the treatment of inflammatory response caused during acute MI (Figure 5). They synthesized 80 nm sized (as determined by dynamic light scattering) gold NPs functionalized on their surface with deoxyribozyme (Dz) (Dz-AuNPs). DNAzymes are DNA oligonucleotides that are capable of inhibiting the activation of tumor necrosis factor α (TNF-α), a key factor implicated in many pathological processes, such as cellular inflammation, causing damage to the infarcted myocardium. Dz-AuNPs possess enhanced stability, cytocompatibility and in vitro studies showed that they are able to internalize in cardiomyocytes and in macrophages. Ex vivo fluorescent imaging revealed predominant accumulation in heart and secondary accumulation in liver and kidney. In vivo experiments in a rat model of acute MI exhibited a 50% reduction in TNF-α, followed by several beneficial effects, such as reduction in pro-inflammatory cytokines that regulate cell survival or apoptosis and trigger oxidative stress. Furthermore, echocardiography and pressure–volume catheter analysis followed by hemodynamic measurements showed a 40% improvement in cardiac function, while many cardiac indices, such as ejection fraction, end-diastolic/systolic pressure, end systolic volume, all improved. All these features indicate that Dz-AuNPs seem to be a potent vehicle for MI treatment by reducing local inflammatory responses and improving cardiac cell survival [64].

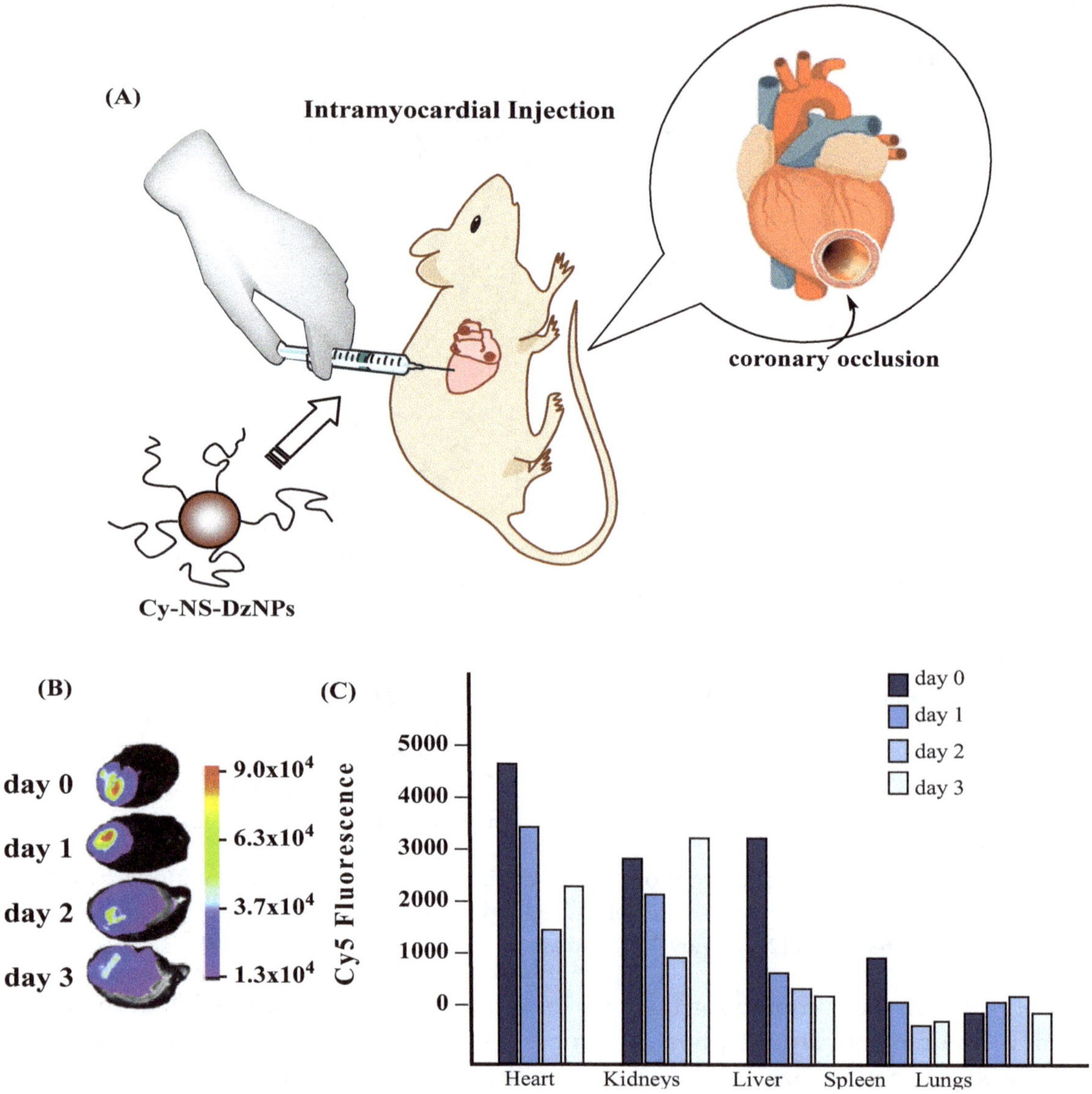

Figure 5. Ex-vivo fluorescence imaging of organs from animals injected with Cyanine 5-Non-Specific (Cy5-NS)-deoxyribozyme Nanoparticles (DzNP). (**A**) Schematic of ligation of the coronary artery to cause permanent ligation MI in rats followed by particle injection. (**B**) Fluorescence images of hearts from each day following injection. The heat map indicates the Cy5 emission intensity in arbitrary units. (**C**) Fluorescence intensity of all organs imaged from days 0, 1, 2 and 3. The Cy5 fluorescence intensity is expressed in arbitrary units. A total of four rats were used where each time point consists of fluorescence from an individual rat. Adapted from [65], NRC, 2018.

In a different study, Tian et al., reported the effect of bare 10 nm sized PEG-coated gold nanoparticles in MI in mice. The results showed that AuNPs accumulated in the heart, specifically after infarction, decreased infarct size, inhibited heart fibrosis by reducing gene expression of collagen I and collagen III, limited inflammation by TNF-α reduction and improved contractile function. However, administration of AuNPs had no effect on cardiac cell apoptosis and could not ameliorate cardiac hypertrophy post-MI [65].

An interesting work was referred by Ruvinov for the development of an injectable system consisting of an alginate biomaterial which could bind, with great affinity, to both insulin-like growth factor-1 (IGF-1) and hepatocyte growth factor (HGF). These factors have cytoprotective, anti-fibrotic and pro-angiogenic properties and have been utilized for infarct repair. With the use of this biomaterial, the two factors could be co-delivered to the injured area of the heart, leading to an efficient system for MI treatment. IGF-1 and HGF were reversibly bounded to alginate sulfate and both retained their bioactivity after bioconjugation, while at the same time they were protected from proteolysis in the MI environment. Release studies showed that the release of IGF-1 was quicker than the release of HGF, leading to sequential delivery. In vitro experiments revealed that after treatment with this double-loaded biomaterial, cardiomyocyte apoptosis was inhibited. The therapeutic potential of this dual IGF-1/HGF alginate biomaterial was proved in a rat model of acute MI after an intramyocardial injection. Specifically, four weeks after administration, scar thickness was increased, infarct expansion was prevented, scar fibrosis was decreased, vessel density increased and finally tissue restoration was achieved [66].

Hao's group reported the synthesis of an alginate hydrogel to study the effect of delivery and sequential release of vascular endothelial growth factor-A_{165} (VEGF-A_{165}) and platelet-derived growth factor-BB (PDGF-BB) to the heart after MI. These two factors both play a key role in angiogenesis. The hydrogel was prepared by combining alginate with two different molecular weights (5000 Da and 250,000 Da) and in vitro studies were conducted to monitor the release kinetics. It was found that VEGF-A_{165} released first, followed by a slower release of PDGF-BB. Both factors exhibited a sustained release for a 30-day period. Four weeks after intramyocardial administration, increased capillary densities were observed in periinfarct tissue sections and higher α-actin smooth muscle cell vessel density was noticed. In addition, the dual factor delivery increased the systolic velocity–time integral, a marker for proper cardiac function. In summary, single injection of this double loaded hydrogel induced angiogenesis and improved cardiac function in a rat model of MI and it was found to have enhanced therapeutic effects compared to single factor administration [67].

Recently, Tang and his team proposed for the first time the use of carbon nanocapsules (CNCs) as drug delivery systems for thromboembolism treatment in mice. Carbon nanocapsules were found to be biocompatible systems when injected intravenously, in contrast with carbon nanotubes that are toxic. Specifically, they developed heparin-conjugated CNCs (CNC-H), which exhibited high antithrombotic activity. Heparin is commonly used as an anticoagulant and has thrombolytic properties. It was conjugated to the surface of CNCs via EDC after acid modification of their surface. The diameter of CNC-H did not exceed 50 nm and drug loading was found to be circa 40%, as determined by TGA. Release experiments showed a burst release at the beginning, followed by a slower release rate. In vivo administration of CNC-H retarded thrombus formation, retained blood flow to acceptable levels and prolonged blood flow decrease [68].

Cell transplantation is an alternative method for the treatment of cardiac injury. However, the low cell survival and retention induced by this approach hampers its further application. Lu and coworkers have reported for the first time the preparation of a temperature-responsive chitosan hydrogel that protects and delivers embryonic stem cells (ESCs) to the damaged myocardium. Chitosan is a biocompatible and biodegradable material that is liquid at 4 °C and becomes solid at 37 °C within 15 min. This in situ gelation process makes chitosan a potent scaffold for the delivery of therapeutics to the area of interest. ESCs survived well when incorporated into the hydrogel in vitro. Four weeks after injection of the hydrogel into the infarct wall, graft size and cell retention increased.

Echocardiography experiments exhibited a significant improvement in end-systolic/diastolic diameter, ejection fraction, and fractional shortening of the heart. Moreover, the infarct size was reduced by over 50%, the ventricular wall thickness was increased by over 50%, as compared with control groups, and the microvessel density was higher. Overall, this chitosan-based vehicle efficiently delivered stem cells to the affected area and considerably enhanced the heart function, making it a potential candidate for injured myocardium treatment [69].

A different method for cell replacement was followed by Ottersbach et al. They used embryonic cardiomyocytes (eCMs) and embryonic stem cell-derived cardiomyocytes (ES-CM) loaded with silica-coated magnetic NPs (SOMag5 MNPs) to increase their engraftment to the damaged myocardium. SOMag5 MNPs exhibited good loading and magnetization properties, while cytotoxic effects were absent (200 pg Fe/cell). With the application of magnetic field by a custom made 1.3 T magnet, at 5 mm distance and for 10 min, they achieved a 7-fold and 3.4-fold increase in engraftment of eCMs and ES-CM 2 weeks and 8 weeks after transplantation in rats. The MNPs were localized, mainly intra- and peri-cellularly, and accumulated in the heart, specifically to the left ventricle, even two months post-operation. The viability and the proliferation rate of the engrafted cells increased significantly, while better differentiation and an augmentation of cell to cell contacts was noticed. Furthermore, the left ventricle function strongly improved, as the left ventricular ejection fraction increased and end diastolic pressure and volume reduced. Overall, this novel nanosystem gives insight into a new cell transplantation approach for cardiomyoplasty [70]. A similar study was also presented by Zhang who labeled endothelial progenitor cells with silica-coated MNPs to restore cardiac function [71].

A short time ago, Miragoli and his team presented an unconventional approach for the delivery of a therapeutic peptide to the heart via inhalation. Treatment with inhalation delivery of drugs is common for respiratory diseases, although no such therapies have been found to treat cardiovascular diseases, until now. This team designed negatively charged calcium phosphate NPs (CaPs) that are bioresorbable, biocompatible and smaller than 50 nm. These particles, loaded with a cell-penetrating mimetic peptide (R7W-MP, DQRPDREAPRS), can be translocated from the pulmonary tree to the bloodstream and then to the heart. CaPs-R7W NPs can be internalized in cardiomyocytes by passing through their cell membrane, as in vitro experiments showed, and release their cargo. In vivo biodistribution studies revealed that NPs were rapidly deposited to the myocardium, as confirmed by fluorescence molecular tomography imaging and transmission electron microscopy. Notably, echocardiography showed that after administration of CaPs-R7W NPs in rats suffering from diabetic cardiomyopathy, complete restoration of heart contractility and function was achieved. These data underscore the importance of this DDS, as its non-invasive method and its efficacy open avenues for the treatment of CVDs [72].

4. Conclusions

The aim of this review is not only to provide an account of acquired knowledge on nanostructured materials developed for targeted drug delivery, but also to show that this concept can be easily applied to cardiovascular diseases. In the future, new revolutionized nanomaterials may play a key role in the establishment of innovative treatment for the challenge of current CVDs. All in all, it is clear that the application of nanotechnology to medicine is at the forefront of innovation for modern health care and represents a promising approach for efficient delivery of therapeutics.

Author Contributions: Conceptualization, H.I.; methodology, D.S. (Dimitrios Skourtis); formal analysis, P.G.F.; writing—original draft preparation, D.S. (Dimitrios Skourtis); writing—review and editing, P.G.F., D.S. (Dimitra Stavroulaki) and V.A.; supervision, H.I.; project administration, H.I.; funding acquisition, H.I. All authors have read and agreed to the published version of the manuscript.

Acknowledgments: The authors acknowledge the Stavros Niarchos Foundation grant for funding.

Abbreviations

ADM-2	Adrenomedullin-2
ADSCs	Adipose Tissue-Derived Stromal Cells
ANP	Atrial Natriuretic Peptide
AT1	Angiotensin II receptor Type 1
bFGF	basic Fibroblast Growth Factor
CAD	Coronary Artery Disease
CNCs	Carbon Nanocapsules
cTn1	Cardiac Troponin I
CVDs	Cardiovascular Diseases
Cy5	Cyanine 5
DCM	Diabetic Cardiomyopathy
DDSs	Drug Delivery Systems
DOPC	Dioleoylphosphatidylcholine
DSPE	Distearoylphosphatidylethanolamine
Dz	Deoxyribozyme
eCMs	Embryonic Cardiomyocytes
EDC	1-Ethyl-3-(3-dimethylaminopropyl)carbodiimide
EF	Ejection Fraction
ELISA	Enzyme-Linked Immunosorbent Assay
EMA	European Medicines Agency
EPR	Enhanced Permeability and Retention
ESCs	Embryonic Stem Cells
FDA	Food and Drug Administration
FS	Fractional Shortening
GFP	Green Fluorescent Protein
GFP	Green Fluorescent Protein
GO	Graphene Oxide
HA	Hyaluronic Acid
HGF	Hepatocyte Growth Factor
HSPC	Hydrogenated Soy Phosphatidylcholine
IGF-1	Insulin-Like Growth Factor-
mAb	Monoclonal Antibody
MAL	Maleimide
MEL	Melamine
MI	Myocardial Infarction
MMP	Matrix Metalloproteinases
MNPs	Magnetic Nanoparticles
NADPH	Nicotinamide Adenine Dinucleotide Phosphate
NHS	*N*-Hydroxysuccinimide
NPs	Nanoparticles
NS	Non-Specific
(p[*N*IPAAm-*co*-PAA-*co*-BA])	Poly(*N*-isopropylacrylamide-*co*-propylacrylic acid-*co*-butyl acrylate)
PAD	Peripheral Artery Disease
PAMB-G	Poly-3-amino-4-methoxybenzoic acid-gelatin
PBLG	Poly(gamma-benzyl L-glutamate)
PCADK	Poly(cyclohexane-1,4-diylacetone dimethylene ketal)
PCM	Primary Cardiomyocyte
PGMA	Poly(glycidyl methacrylate)
PLA	Poly(lactic acid)
PLGA	Poly(D,L-glycolic acid)
PUE	Puerarin
RAFT	Reversible Addition Fragmentation Chain Transfer

RES	Reticulo-Endothelial System
RGD	Arginyl-Glycyl-Aspartic Acid
SD	Sprague-Dawley
SLN	Solid Lipid Nanoparticle
TGA	Thermogravimetric Analysis
TNF-α	Tumor Necrosis Factor α
Tβ4	Thymosin beta 4
VEGF	Vascular Endothelial Growth Factor

References

1. World Health Organization. Cardiovascular Diseases (CVDs) Fact Sheet. 2017. Available online: https://www.who.int/news-room/fact-sheets/detail/cardiovascular-diseases-(cvds) (accessed on 25 May 2019).
2. Timmis, A.; Townsend, N.; Gale, C.; Grobbee, R.; Maniadakis, N.; Flather, M.; Wilkins, E.; Wright, L.; Vos, R.; Bax, J.; et al. European Society of Cardiology: Cardiovascular Disease Statistics 2017. *Eur. Heart J.* **2018**, *39*, 508–579. [CrossRef] [PubMed]
3. Heidenreich, P. Heart Failure Prevention and Team-based Interventions. *Heart Fail. Clin.* **2015**, *11*, 349–358. [CrossRef] [PubMed]
4. Bobo, D.; Robinson, K.J.; Islam, J.; Thurecht, K.J.; Corrie, S.R. Nanoparticle-Based Medicines: A Review of FDA-Approved Materials and Clinical Trials to Date. *Pharm. Res.* **2016**, *33*, 2373–2387. [CrossRef] [PubMed]
5. Thygesen, K.; Alpert, J.S.; White, H.D. Universal definition of myocardial infarction. *J. Am. Coll. Cardiol.* **2007**, *50*, 2173–2195. [CrossRef] [PubMed]
6. Sun, Y.; Weber, K.T. Infarct scar: A dynamic tissue. *Cardiovasc. Res.* **2000**, *46*, 250–256. [CrossRef]
7. Gupta, P.; Garcia, E.; Sarkar, A.; Kapoor, S.; Rafiq, K.; Chand, H.S.; Jayant, R.D. Nanoparticle based treatment for cardiovascular diseases. *Cardiovasc. Haematol. Disord. Drug Targets* **2019**, *19*, 33–44. [CrossRef]
8. Ramanathan, T.; Skinner, H. Coronary blood flow. *Contin. Educ. Anaesth. Critic. Care Pain* **2005**, *5*, 61–64. [CrossRef]
9. Blanco, E.; Shen, H.; Ferrari, M. Principles of nanoparticle design for overcoming biological barriers to drug delivery. *Nat. Biotechnol.* **2015**, *33*, 941–951. [CrossRef]
10. Attia, M.F.; Anton, N.; Wallyn, J.; Omran, Z.; Vandamme, T.F. An overview of active and passive targeting strategies to improve the nanocarriers efficiency to tumour sites. *J. Pharm. Pharmacol.* **2019**, *71*, 1185–1198. [CrossRef]
11. Lundy, D.J.; Chen, K.H.; Toh, E.K.; Hsieh, P.C. Distribution of Systemically Administered Nanoparticles Reveals a Size-Dependent Effect Immediately following Cardiac Ischaemia-Reperfusion Injury. *Sci. Rep.* **2016**, *6*, 25613. [CrossRef]
12. Matsumura, Y.; Maeda, H. A new concept for macromolecular therapeutics in cancer chemotherapy: Mechanism of tumoritropic accumulation of proteins and the antitumor agent smancs. *Cancer Res.* **1986**, *46*, 6387–6392. [PubMed]
13. England, C.G.; Im, H.J.; Feng, L.; Chen, F.; Graves, S.A.; Hernandez, R.; Orbay, H.; Xu, C.; Cho, S.Y.; Nickles, R.J.; et al. Re-assessing the enhanced permeability and retention effect in peripheral arterial disease using radiolabeled long circulating nanoparticles. *Biomaterials* **2016**, *100*, 101–109. [CrossRef] [PubMed]
14. Sun, G.; Lin, X.; Hong, Y.; Feng, Y.; Ruan, K.; Xu, D. PEGylation for drug delivery to ischemic myocardium: Pharmacokinetics and cardiac distribution of poly(ethylene glycol)s in mice with normal and ischemic myocardium. *Eur. J. Pharm. Sci.* **2012**, *46*, 545–552. [CrossRef] [PubMed]
15. Horwitz, L.D.; Kaufman, D.; Keller, M.W.; Kong, Y. Time course of coronary endothelial healing after injury due to ischemia and reperfusion. *Circulation* **1994**, *90*, 2439–2447. [CrossRef]
16. Lukyanov, A.N.; Hartner, W.C.; Torchilin, V.P. Increased accumulation of PEG-PE micelles in the area of experimental myocardial infarction in rabbits. *J. Control. Release* **2004**, *94*, 187–193. [CrossRef]
17. Nichols, J.W.; Bae, Y.H. EPR: Evidence and fallacy. *J. Control. Release* **2014**, *190*, 451–464. [CrossRef]
18. Danhier, F. To exploit the tumor microenvironment: Since the EPR effect fails in the clinic, what is the future of nanomedicine? *J. Control. Release* **2016**, *244*, 108–121. [CrossRef]
19. Sindhwani, S.; Syed, A.M.; Ngai, J.; Kingston, B.R.; Maiorino, L.; Rothschild, J.; MacMillan, P.; Zhang, Y.; Rajesh, N.U.; Hoang, T.; et al. The entry of nanoparticles into solid tumours. *Nature Mater.* **2020**, *19*, 566–575. [CrossRef]

20. Ho, Y.T.; Poinard, B.; Kah, J.C. Nanoparticle drug delivery systems and their use in cardiac tissue therapy. *Nanomedicine* **2016**, *11*, 693–714. [CrossRef]
21. Pala, R.; Anju, V.T.; Dyavaiah, M.; Busi, S.; Nauli, S.M. Nanoparticle-Mediated Drug Delivery for the Treatment of Cardiovascular Diseases. *Int. J. Nanomed.* **2020**, *15*, 3741–3769. [CrossRef]
22. Ferreira, M.P.A.; Ranjan, S.; Kinnunen, S.; Correia, A.; Talman, V.; Makila, E.; Barrios-Lopez, B.; Kemell, M.; Balasubramanian, V.; Salonen, J.; et al. Drug-Loaded Multifunctional Nanoparticles Targeted to the Endocardial Layer of the Injured Heart Modulate Hypertrophic Signaling. *Small* **2017**, *13*. [CrossRef]
23. Yu, J.; Li, W.; Yu, D. Atrial natriuretic peptide modified oleate adenosine prodrug lipid nanocarriers for the treatment of myocardial infarction: In vitro and in vivo evaluation. *Drug Des. Dev. Ther.* **2018**, *12*, 1697–1706. [CrossRef] [PubMed]
24. Kumar, A.; Chen, F.; Mozhi, A.; Zhang, X.; Zhao, Y.; Xue, X.; Hao, Y.; Zhang, X.; Wang, P.C.; Liang, X.J. Innovative pharmaceutical development based on unique properties of nanoscale delivery formulation. *Nanoscale* **2013**, *5*, 8307–8325. [CrossRef] [PubMed]
25. Li, Y.; Kroger, M.; Liu, W.K. Endocytosis of PEGylated nanoparticles accompanied by structural and free energy changes of the grafted polyethylene glycol. *Biomaterials* **2014**, *35*, 8467–8478. [CrossRef] [PubMed]
26. Shen, Z.; Ye, H.; Kroger, M.; Li, Y. Aggregation of polyethylene glycol polymers suppresses receptor-mediated endocytosis of PEGylated liposomes. *Nanoscale* **2018**, *10*, 4545–4560. [CrossRef]
27. Shen, Z.; Ye, H.; Yi, X.; Li, Y. Membrane Wrapping Efficiency of Elastic Nanoparticles during Endocytosis: Size and Shape Matter. *ACS Nano* **2019**, *13*, 215–228. [CrossRef] [PubMed]
28. Wang, A.Z.; Gu, F.; Zhang, L.; Chan, J.M.; Radovic-Moreno, A.; Shaikh, M.R.; Farokhzad, O.C. Biofunctionalized targeted nanoparticles for therapeutic applications. *Expert Opin. Biol. Ther.* **2008**, *8*, 1063–1070. [CrossRef] [PubMed]
29. Nekkanti, V.; Kalepu, S. Recent advances in liposomal drug delivery: A review. *Pharm. Nanotech.* **2015**, *3*, 35–55. [CrossRef]
30. Dvir, T.; Bauer, M.; Schroeder, A.; Tsui, J.H.; Anderson, D.G.; Langer, R.; Liao, R.; Kohane, D.S. Nanoparticles targeting the infarcted heart. *Nano Lett.* **2011**, *11*, 4411–4414. [CrossRef] [PubMed]
31. Cannone, V.; Cabassi, A.; Volpi, R.; Burnett, J.C., Jr. Atrial Natriuretic Peptide: A Molecular Target of Novel Therapeutic Approaches to Cardio-Metabolic Disease. *Int. J. Mol. Sci.* **2019**, *20*, 3265. [CrossRef] [PubMed]
32. Takahama, H.; Minamino, T.; Asanuma, H.; Fujita, M.; Asai, T.; Wakeno, M.; Sasaki, H.; Kikuchi, H.; Hashimoto, K.; Oku, N.; et al. Prolonged targeting of ischemic/reperfused myocardium by liposomal adenosine augments cardioprotection in rats. *J. Am. Coll. Cardiol.* **2009**, *53*, 709–717. [CrossRef] [PubMed]
33. Dong, Z.; Guo, J.; Xing, X.; Zhang, X.; Du, Y.; Lu, Q. RGD modified and PEGylated lipid nanoparticles loaded with puerarin: Formulation, characterization and protective effects on acute myocardial ischemia model. *Biomed. Pharmacother.* **2017**, *89*, 297–304. [CrossRef] [PubMed]
34. Dasa, S.S.K.; Suzuki, R.; Gutknecht, M.; Brinton, L.T.; Tian, Y.; Michaelsson, E.; Lindfors, L.; Klibanov, A.L.; French, B.A.; Kelly, K.A. Development of target-specific liposomes for delivering small molecule drugs after reperfused myocardial infarction. *J. Control. Release* **2015**, *220*, 556–567. [CrossRef] [PubMed]
35. Wang, X.; Huang, H.; Zhang, L.; Bai, Y.; Chen, H. PCM and TAT co-modified liposome with improved myocardium delivery: In vitro and in vivo evaluations. *Drug Deliv.* **2017**, *24*, 339–345. [CrossRef]
36. Ko, Y.T.; Hartner, W.C.; Kale, A.; Torchilin, V.P. Gene delivery into ischemic myocardium by double-targeted lipoplexes with anti-myosin antibody and TAT peptide. *Gene Ther.* **2009**, *16*, 52–59. [CrossRef]
37. Liang, W.; Levchenko, T.; Khaw, B.A.; Torchilin, V. ATP-containing immunoliposomes specific for cardiac myosin. *Curr. Drug Deliv.* **2004**, *1*, 1–7. [CrossRef]
38. Verma, D.D.; Hartner, W.C.; Levchenko, T.S.; Bernstein, E.A.; Torchilin, V.P. ATP-loaded liposomes effectively protect the myocardium in rabbits with an acute experimental myocardial infarction. *Pharm. Res.* **2005**, *22*, 2115–2120. [CrossRef]
39. Verma, D.D.; Levchenko, T.S.; Bernstein, E.A.; Mongayt, D.; Torchilin, V.P. ATP-loaded immunoliposomes specific for cardiac myosin provide improved protection of the mechanical functions of myocardium from global ischemia in an isolated rat heart model. *J. Drug Target.* **2006**, *14*, 273–280. [CrossRef]
40. Verma, D.D.; Hartner, W.C.; Thakkar, V.; Levchenko, T.S.; Torchilin, V.P. Protective effect of coenzyme Q10-loaded liposomes on the myocardium in rabbits with an acute experimental myocardial infarction. *Pharm. Res.* **2007**, *24*, 2131–2137. [CrossRef]

41. Scott, R.C.; Wang, B.; Nallamothu, R.; Pattillo, C.B.; Perez-Liz, G.; Issekutz, A.; Del Valle, L.; Wood, G.C.; Kiani, M.F. Targeted delivery of antibody conjugated liposomal drug carriers to rat myocardial infarction. *Biotechnol. Bioeng.* **2007**, *96*, 795–802. [CrossRef]
42. Scott, R.C.; Rosano, J.M.; Ivanov, Z.; Wang, B.; Chong, P.L.; Issekutz, A.C.; Crabbe, D.L.; Kiani, M.F. Targeting VEGF-encapsulated immunoliposomes to MI heart improves vascularity and cardiac function. *FASEB J.* **2009**, *23*, 3361–3367. [CrossRef] [PubMed]
43. Liu, M.; Li, M.; Sun, S.; Li, B.; Du, D.; Sun, J.; Cao, F.; Li, H.; Jia, F.; Wang, T.; et al. The use of antibody modified liposomes loaded with AMO-1 to deliver oligonucleotides to ischemic myocardium for arrhythmia therapy. *Biomaterials* **2014**, *35*, 3697–3707. [CrossRef] [PubMed]
44. Torchilin, V.P. Micellar nanocarriers: Pharmaceutical perspectives. *Pharm. Res.* **2007**, *24*, 1–16. [CrossRef] [PubMed]
45. Bao, R.; Tan, B.; Liang, S.; Zhang, N.; Wang, W.; Liu, W. A pi-pi conjugation-containing soft and conductive injectable polymer hydrogel highly efficiently rebuilds cardiac function after myocardial infarction. *Biomaterials* **2017**, *122*, 63–71. [CrossRef] [PubMed]
46. Garbern, J.C.; Minami, E.; Stayton, P.S.; Murry, C.E. Delivery of basic fibroblast growth factor with a pH-responsive, injectable hydrogel to improve angiogenesis in infarcted myocardium. *Biomaterials* **2011**, *32*, 2407–2416. [CrossRef] [PubMed]
47. Zhang, C.; Hsieh, M.H.; Wu, S.Y.; Li, S.H.; Wu, J.; Liu, S.M.; Wei, H.J.; Weisel, R.D.; Sung, H.W.; Li, R.K. A self-doping conductive polymer hydrogel that can restore electrical impulse propagation at myocardial infarct to prevent cardiac arrhythmia and preserve ventricular function. *Biomaterials* **2020**, *231*, 119672. [CrossRef]
48. Nguyen, M.M.; Carlini, A.S.; Chien, M.P.; Sonnenberg, S.; Luo, C.; Braden, R.L.; Osborn, K.G.; Li, Y.; Gianneschi, N.C.; Christman, K.L. Enzyme-Responsive Nanoparticles for Targeted Accumulation and Prolonged Retention in Heart Tissue after Myocardial Infarction. *Adv. Mater.* **2015**, *27*, 5547–5552. [CrossRef]
49. Sy, J.C.; Seshadri, G.; Yang, S.C.; Brown, M.; Oh, T.; Dikalov, S.; Murthy, N.; Davis, M.E. Sustained release of a p38 inhibitor from non-inflammatory microspheres inhibits cardiac dysfunction. *Nat. Mater.* **2008**, *7*, 863–868. [CrossRef]
50. Perez, C.; Sanchez, A.; Putnam, D.; Ting, D.; Langer, R.; Alonso, M.J. Poly(lactic acid)-poly(ethylene glycol) nanoparticles as new carriers for the delivery of plasmid DNA. *J. Control. Release* **2001**, *75*, 211–224. [CrossRef]
51. Chang, M.Y.; Yang, Y.J.; Chang, C.H.; Tang, A.C.; Liao, W.Y.; Cheng, F.Y.; Yeh, C.S.; Lai, J.J.; Stayton, P.S.; Hsieh, P.C. Functionalized nanoparticles provide early cardioprotection after acute myocardial infarction. *J. Control. Release* **2013**, *170*, 287–294. [CrossRef]
52. Nagaoka, K.; Matoba, T.; Mao, Y.; Nakano, Y.; Ikeda, G.; Egusa, S.; Tokutome, M.; Nagahama, R.; Nakano, K.; Sunagawa, K.; et al. A New Therapeutic Modality for Acute Myocardial Infarction: Nanoparticle-Mediated Delivery of Pitavastatin Induces Cardioprotection from Ischemia-Reperfusion Injury via Activation of PI3K/Akt Pathway and Anti-Inflammation in a Rat Model. *PLoS ONE* **2015**, *10*, e0132451. [CrossRef]
53. Quadros, H.C.; Santos, L.M.F.; Meira, C.S.; Khouri, M.I.; Mattei, B.; Soares, M.B.P.; de Castro-Borges, W.; Farias, L.P.; Formiga, F.R. Development and in vitro characterization of polymeric nanoparticles containing recombinant adrenomedullin-2 intended for therapeutic angiogenesis. *Int J. Pharm* **2020**, *576*, 118997. [CrossRef]
54. Gray, W.D.; Che, P.; Brown, M.; Ning, X.; Murthy, N.; Davis, M.E. N-acetylglucosamine conjugated to nanoparticles enhances myocyte uptake and improves delivery of a small molecule p38 inhibitor for post-infarct healing. *J. Cardiovasc. Transl. Res.* **2011**, *4*, 631–643. [CrossRef] [PubMed]
55. Somasuntharam, I.; Boopathy, A.V.; Khan, R.S.; Martinez, M.D.; Brown, M.E.; Murthy, N.; Davis, M.E. Delivery of Nox2-NADPH oxidase siRNA with polyketal nanoparticles for improving cardiac function following myocardial infarction. *Biomaterials* **2013**, *34*, 7790–7798. [CrossRef] [PubMed]
56. Huang, Z.; Song, Y.; Pang, Z.; Zhang, B.; Yang, H.; Shi, H.; Chen, J.; Gong, H.; Qian, J.; Ge, J. Targeted delivery of thymosin beta 4 to the injured myocardium using CREKA-conjugated nanoparticles. *Int. J. Nanomed.* **2017**, *12*, 3023–3036. [CrossRef] [PubMed]
57. Tong, F.; Chai, R.; Jiang, H.; Dong, B. In vitro/vivo drug release and anti-diabetic cardiomyopathy properties of curcumin/PBLG-PEG-PBLG nanoparticles. *Int. J. Nanomed.* **2018**, *13*, 1945–1962. [CrossRef] [PubMed]
58. Hardy, N.; Viola, H.M.; Johnstone, V.P.; Clemons, T.D.; Cserne Szappanos, H.; Singh, R.; Smith, N.M.; Iyer, K.S.; Hool, L.C. Nanoparticle-mediated dual delivery of an antioxidant and a peptide against the L-Type

Ca2+ channel enables simultaneous reduction of cardiac ischemia-reperfusion injury. *ACS Nano* **2015**, *9*, 279–289. [CrossRef]

59. Nam, H.Y.; McGinn, A.; Kim, P.H.; Kim, S.W.; Bull, D.A. Primary cardiomyocyte-targeted bioreducible polymer for efficient gene delivery to the myocardium. *Biomaterials* **2010**, *31*, 8081–8087. [CrossRef]
60. Galagudza, M.; Korolev, D.; Postnov, V.; Naumisheva, E.; Grigorova, Y.; Uskov, I.; Shlyakhto, E. Passive targeting of ischemic-reperfused myocardium with adenosine-loaded silica nanoparticles. *Int. J. Nanomed.* **2012**, *7*, 1671–1678. [CrossRef]
61. Ferreira, M.P.; Talman, V.; Torrieri, G.; Liu, D.; Marques, G.; Moslova, K.; Liu, Z.; Pinto, J.F.; Hirvonen, J.; Ruskoaho, H. Dual-drug delivery using dextran-functionalized nanoparticles targeting cardiac fibroblasts for cellular reprogramming. *Adv. Funct. Mater.* **2018**, *28*, 1705134. [CrossRef]
62. Torrieri, G.; Fontana, F.; Figueiredo, P.; Liu, Z.; Ferreira, M.P.A.; Talman, V.; Martins, J.P.; Fusciello, M.; Moslova, K.; Teesalu, T.; et al. Dual-peptide functionalized acetalated dextran-based nanoparticles for sequential targeting of macrophages during myocardial infarction. *Nanoscale* **2020**, *12*, 2350–2358. [CrossRef] [PubMed]
63. Huang, X.; El-Sayed, M.A. Gold nanoparticles: Optical properties and implementations in cancer diagnosis and photothermal therapy. *J. Adv. Res.* **2010**, *1*, 13–28. [CrossRef]
64. Somasuntharam, I.; Yehl, K.; Carroll, S.L.; Maxwell, J.T.; Martinez, M.D.; Che, P.L.; Brown, M.E.; Salaita, K.; Davis, M.E. Knockdown of TNF-alpha by DNAzyme gold nanoparticles as an anti-inflammatory therapy for myocardial infarction. *Biomaterials* **2016**, *83*, 12–22. [CrossRef] [PubMed]
65. Tian, A.; Yang, C.; Zhu, B.; Wang, W.; Liu, K.; Jiang, Y.; Qiao, Y.; Fu, H.; Li, Z. Polyethylene-glycol-coated gold nanoparticles improve cardiac function after myocardial infarction in mice. *Can. J. Physiol. Pharmacol.* **2018**, *96*, 1318–1327. [CrossRef] [PubMed]
66. Ruvinov, E.; Leor, J.; Cohen, S. The promotion of myocardial repair by the sequential delivery of IGF-1 and HGF from an injectable alginate biomaterial in a model of acute myocardial infarction. *Biomaterials* **2011**, *32*, 565–578. [CrossRef]
67. Hao, X.; Silva, E.A.; Mansson-Broberg, A.; Grinnemo, K.H.; Siddiqui, A.J.; Dellgren, G.; Wardell, E.; Brodin, L.A.; Mooney, D.J.; Sylven, C. Angiogenic effects of sequential release of VEGF-A165 and PDGF-BB with alginate hydrogels after myocardial infarction. *Cardiovasc. Res.* **2007**, *75*, 178–185. [CrossRef] [PubMed]
68. Tang, A.C.; Chang, M.Y.; Tang, Z.C.; Li, H.J.; Hwang, G.L.; Hsieh, P.C. Treatment of acute thromboembolism in mice using heparin-conjugated carbon nanocapsules. *ACS Nano* **2012**, *6*, 6099–6107. [CrossRef] [PubMed]
69. Lu, W.N.; Lu, S.H.; Wang, H.B.; Li, D.X.; Duan, C.M.; Liu, Z.Q.; Hao, T.; He, W.J.; Xu, B.; Fu, Q.; et al. Functional improvement of infarcted heart by co-injection of embryonic stem cells with temperature-responsive chitosan hydrogel. *Tissue Eng. Part A* **2009**, *15*, 1437–1447. [CrossRef] [PubMed]
70. Ottersbach, A.; Mykhaylyk, O.; Heidsieck, A.; Eberbeck, D.; Rieck, S.; Zimmermann, K.; Breitbach, M.; Engelbrecht, B.; Brugmann, T.; Hesse, M.; et al. Improved heart repair upon myocardial infarction: Combination of magnetic nanoparticles and tailored magnets strongly increases engraftment of myocytes. *Biomaterials* **2018**, *155*, 176–190. [CrossRef]
71. Zhang, B.F.; Jiang, H.; Chen, J.; Hu, Q.; Yang, S.; Liu, X.P. Silica-coated magnetic nanoparticles labeled endothelial progenitor cells alleviate ischemic myocardial injury and improve long-term cardiac function with magnetic field guidance in rats with myocardial infarction. *J. Cell Physiol.* **2019**, *234*, 18544–18559. [CrossRef]
72. Miragoli, M.; Ceriotti, P.; Iafisco, M.; Vacchiano, M.; Salvarani, N.; Alogna, A.; Carullo, P.; Ramirez-Rodriguez, G.B.; Patricio, T.; Esposti, L.D.; et al. Inhalation of peptide-loaded nanoparticles improves heart failure. *Sci. Transl. Med.* **2018**, *10*. [CrossRef] [PubMed]

2

Long-Lasting, Antinociceptive Effects of pH-Sensitive Niosomes Loaded with Ibuprofen in Acute and Chronic Models of Pain

Francesca Marzoli [1], Carlotta Marianecci [2], Federica Rinaldi [3], Daniele Passeri [4], Marco Rossi [4,5], Paola Minosi [1], Maria Carafa [2] and Stefano Pieretti [1,*]

[1] Istituto Superiore di Sanità, National Center for Drug Research and Evaluation, 00161 Rome, Italy; francesca.marzoli@iss.it (F.M.); paola.minosi@iss.it (P.M.)
[2] Department of Drug Chemistry and Technology, Sapienza University of Rome, 00185 Rome, Italy; carlotta.marianecci@uniroma1.it (C.M.); maria.carafa@uniroma1.it (M.C.)
[3] Center for Life Nano Science@Sapienza, Istituto Italiano di Tecnologia (ITT), 00161 Rome, Italy; federica.rinaldi@uniroma1.it
[4] Department of Basic and Applied Sciences for Engineering, Sapienza University of Rome, 00161 Rome, Italy; daniele.passeri@uniroma1.it (D.P.); marco.rossi@uniroma1.it (M.R.)
[5] Research Center for Nanotechnology Applied to Engineering, Sapienza University of Rome (CNIS), 00185 Rome, Italy
* Correspondence: stefano.pieretti@iss.it;

Abstract: Ibuprofen is one of the non-steroidal anti-inflammatory drugs (NSAIDs) widely used to treat pain conditions. NSAIDs encounter several obstacles to passing across biological membranes. To overcome these constraints, we decided to study the effects of a new pH-sensitive formulation of niosomes containing Polysorbate 20 derivatized by Glycine and loaded with ibuprofen (NioIbu) in several animal models of pain in mice. We performed two tests commonly used to study acute antinociceptive activity, namely the writhing test and the capsaicin test. Our results demonstrated that NioIbu, administered 2 h before testing, reduced nociception, whereas the free form of ibuprofen was ineffective. In a model of inflammatory pain, hyperalgesia induced by zymosan, NioIbu induced a long-lasting reduction in hyperalgesia in treated mice. In a model of neuropathic pain induced by sciatic nerve chronic constriction, NioIbu reduced both neuropathy-induced allodynia and hyperalgesia. The results obtained in our experiments suggest that pH-sensitive niosomes containing Polysorbate 20 derivatized by Glycine is an effective model for NSAIDs delivery, providing durable antinociceptive effects and reducing the incidence of side effects.

Keywords: Ibuprofen; pH-sensitive niosomes; Pain; Analgesia; NSAIDs

---

1. Introduction

The non-steroidal anti-inflammatory drug (NSAID) Ibuprofen (α-methyl-4-(2-methylpropyl) benzeneacetic acid, IBU) is commonly used in the treatment of pain, fever, and inflammatory diseases. Ibuprofen was discovered in 1960 for the treatment of some pain conditions and inflammatory autoimmune diseases, such as rheumatoid arthritis [1]. In 1961, Ibuprofen became available in tablet form, and in 1983 was launched as a topical formulation. Ibuprofen is an analgesic drug that inhibits the production of cyclooxygenase (Cox-2) pathway-derived prostaglandins, which increase in inflamed tissues and control inflammatory disorder [2,3]. As is well-known, prostanoids mediate the sensation of peripheral and central pain, increasing membrane excitability and reducing the threshold of nociceptor stimulation [4].

While ibuprofen is completely absorbed after oral administration [5], the plasma level is still low several hours after topical application [6]. Various studies have reported different techniques to increase the permeability of cell membranes and the transdermal transport of ibuprofen and other drugs: preparing colloidal microstructures with lysinate and lecithin [7,8], nanoscaled emulsion with palm olein esters [9], iontophoresis [10], and using surfactants and various vehicles, such as the niosomes [11,12]. Niosomes are unilamellar or multilamellar non-ionic surfactant vesicles similar to liposomes that can be used as therapeutic nanocarriers. The main characteristic of these vesicles is their capability to encapsulate both hydrophilic and lipophilic drugs. Hydrophilic drugs are encapsulated in the inner core where the aqueous compartment is located, while lipophilic drugs are encapsulated into the lipophilic domain of the bilayer [13–15].

The basic components of niosomes are non-ionic surfactants in addition to cholesterol (Chol). The surfactants are mainly composed of two distinct regions and are classified as anionic, cationic, amphoteric, and non-ionic according to the feature of the hydrophilic head, which contains sulfonate or ammonium salts of fatty and zwitterionic acids. Non-ionic surfactants have no charge groups in their hydrophilic heads and are able to form niosomal vesicles that represent an innovative system with better performance compared to conventional drug delivery systems. Indeed, niosomes are more stable than liposomes. They show greater bioavailability compared with conventional dosage forms because they are able to increase the permeation of drugs through the skin [16]. Furthermore, they can be employed for oral and parenteral administration, protecting drugs from biological enzymes and the environment. Moreover, the surfactants employed in the preparation of niosomes are less expensive and more versatile than the phospholipids used for liposomal formulations [17]. To obtain a site-specific drug release, pH-sensitive molecules can be added to the formulation or used to derivatize the surfactants employed. It is well known that some pathological states are associated with pH profiles different from that of normal tissues. Examples include ischemia, infection, inflammation, and cancer, which are often associated with acidosis. Extracellular pH values ranging from 5.5 to 7.0 have been detected in inflamed tissues associated with bacterial infections [18], atherosclerotic plaque, [19], and cancers [20]. This pH gradient is of particular importance since several drugs and drug carriers are taken up by endocytosis and found and/or trapped within endosomes and lysosomes. In this context, niosomes with increased affinity for an acidic pH microenvironment can take advantage of pathological conditions of inflammation for selective targeting. Recently, Rinaldi et al. [21,22] have described the formulation of pH-sensitive niosomes containing Polysorbate 20/Chems (Tween 20, Tw20) or Polysorbate 20 derivatized by Glycine (Tw20-Gly) as an effective strategy for the delivery of anaesthetics and anti-inflammatory drugs. In particular, the preparation steps (panel A) and mechanism of bilayer destabilization (panel B) are shown in Figure 1.

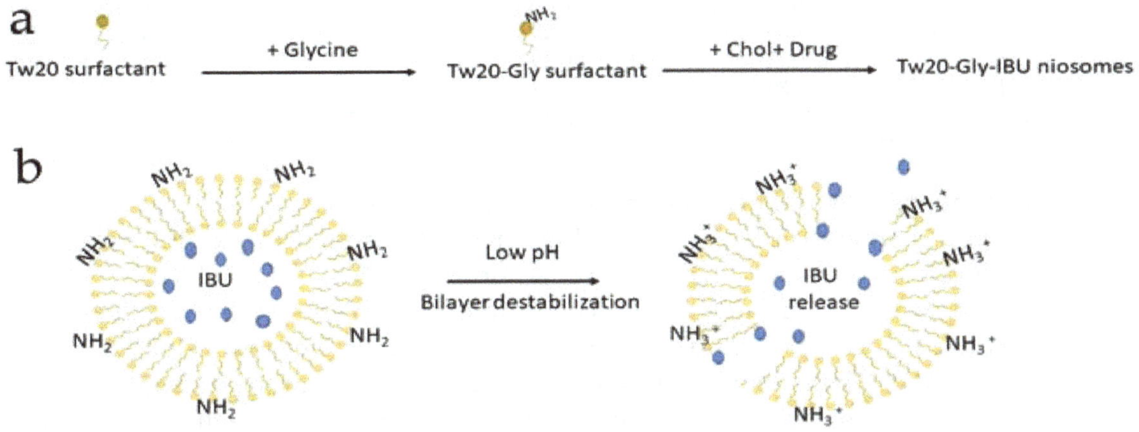

Figure 1. Cartoon describing: (**a**) niosomal preparation by a derivatized surfactant; and (**b**) bilayer destabilization at an acidic pH and consequent drug release. IBU is for Ibuprofen.

In this paper, the well-characterized and selected samples of the previous research study [16,17] were newly prepared to compare the analgesic activity of pH-Tw20Gly niosomes loaded with ibuprofen (NioIbu) to that of free ibuprofen in animal models of acute and chronic pain. We showed that NioIbu strongly increases Ibuprofen's analgesic activity, promoting a longer duration of action of this drug. We suggest that NioIbu is a new and more effective strategy to treat pain arising from chronic inflammatory conditions.

2. Materials and Methods

2.1. Materials

Tween 20 (Tw20), Cholesterol >99% (Chol), *N*-(2-Hydroxyethyl)piperazine-*N*′-(2-ethanesulfonic acid) (HEPES) >99.5%, Sephadex G75, Glycine (Gly), and all other chemicals and solvents of the highest purity and of spectroscopic grade were purchased from Sigma-Aldrich (Sigma-Aldrich S.r.l., Milan, Italy). Water was purified through a Millipore Milli-Q system (Merck S.p.a., Milan, Italy).

2.2. Nanovesicle Formulation and Characterization

Niosomes based on a polysorbate-20 glycine derivative (Tw20Gly) were prepared by the thin film evaporation method at different Ibuprofen loading concentrations (Table 1) and purified by glass chromatography, as previously described [21,22]. A Nano ZS90 Dynamic light scattering LS (Malvern Instruments Ltd., Malvern, UK) at a scattering angle of 90.0° and a LS50B spectrofluorometer (PerkinElmer, MA, USA), were both employed for the physico-chemical characterization of vesicles (hydrodimanic diameter, size distribution, zeta potential, bilayer properties, stability, and in vitro release studies) [21]. Drug entrapment within non-ionic surfactant vesicles was determined using high-performance liquid chromatography (HPLC). HPLC analyses were carried out with a Perkin-Elmer 250 liquid chromatography apparatus (PerkinElmer, MA, USA), equipped with a Perkin-Elmer 235 photo-diode array detector, a 20-µl-loop Rheodyne injector and a computer hardware, as previously described, on purified niosomes after disruption with isopropanol (vesicle dispersion/isopropanol 1:1 *v*/*v* final ratio) [23].

Table 1. Sample composition (NioIbu 5% has been the analyzed formulation). Nio, pH-Tw20Gly niosomes; NioIbu, pH-Tw20Gly niosomes loaded with different percentages of Ibuprofen Hepes solutions. Tw 20, is for Tween 20; Chol, is for Cholesterol; IBU, is for Ibuprofen.

Sample	Tw20 (mM)	Tw20-Gly (mM)	Chol (mM)	IBU (% *p*/*v*)
Nio	3.75	11.25	7.5	=
NioIbu 1%	3.75	11.25	7.5	1
NioIbu 3%	3.75	11.25	7.5	3
NioIbu 5%	3.75	11.25	7.5	5
NioIbu 7%	3.75	11.25	7.5	7

Atomic force microscopy (AFM) topographical characterization has been carried out using a standard AFM setup (Dimension Icon, Bruker Inc. in 'soft tapping' mode, Billerica, MA, USA) equipped with standard silicon cantilevers (OTESPA, Bruker Inc., Billerica, MA, USA). Analysis of niosomal dimensions was carried out by means of atomic force microscopy (AFM) by imaging the samples in tapping mode after deposition on a Si substrate. A diameter and height of nine isolated niosomes were measured. These allowed us to determine the surface of the niosomes deposited on the substrate (which obviously lost their original spherical shape) given by the sum of areas of the surface of the spherical cap and of the base circle. Assuming that the flattening of niosomes resulted in the modification of shape and volume without significantly affecting the surface area, the diameter of niosomes in solution was evaluated as that of a sphere having the same surface area.

2.3. Animals and Treatments

We used male CD-1 mice (Harlan, Italy) weighing 25 g in all of the experiments. Mice were housed in colony cages under standard conditions of light, temperature, and relative humidity for at least 1 week before the start of experimental sessions. All experiments were performed according to Legislative Decree 26/14, which implements the European Directive 2010/63/UE on laboratory animal protection in Italy, and were approved by the local ethics committee. Animal studies are reported in accordance with the ARRIVE (Animal Research: Reporting of In Vivo Experiments) guidelines [24].

In all experiments, NioIbu 5%, diluted to obtain the same drug concentration, was compared to: (i) Hepes buffer (HB), (ii) an "unstructured" surfactant formulation (TG), composed of surfactant and cholesterol, and (iii) an "unstructured" surfactant formulation (TG-Ibu), composed of surfactant, cholesterol, and ibuprofen at the same concentrations as the ones present in NioIbu, but not organized in vesicular systems.

2.4. Writhing Test

The procedure was similar to the one previously described [25]. After 1 h of adaptation to transparent cages, mice received a subcutaneous (s.c.) injection of 1500 L of HB, TG, TG-Ibu, and NioIbu into the loose skin over the interscapular area. One hundred and twenty minutes after sample injection, mice received an intraperitoneal (i.p.) injection (10 mL/kg) of 0.6% acetic acid solution. A writhe is characterized by a wave of abdominal muscle contractions accompanied by body elongation and the extension of one or both hind limbs. The number of writhes in a 20-min period was counted, starting 5 min after acetic acid injection.

2.5. Capsaicin-Induced Paw Licking

The method used was similar to the one previously described [26]. Mice were allowed to adapt to transparent cages individually for 1 h before testing. Then, s.c. injections of samples (HB, TG, TG-Ibu, and NioIbu, 40 μL) were performed in the dorsal surface of mice hind paw for 120 min before 1.6 μg of capsaicin (20 μL). A micro syringe with a 26-gauge needle was used to inject capsaicin and samples. The time (in seconds) the animals spent licking the injected paw, for a total period of 5 min, was registered and considered as indicative of pain. Capsaicin was dissolved in DMSO as a stock solution and stored at −20 °C. On the test day, this solution was diluted in order to obtain the final concentration of 1.6 μg/20 μl in DMSO:saline (1:3 *v:v*).

2.6. Zymosan-Induced Hyperalgesia

In these experiments, 20 μL of zymosan A (2.5% *w/v* in saline) were administered s.c. into the dorsal surface of one hind paw. Then, thermal thresholds were determined, as previously reported [27]. Briefly, mice were placed in clear plastic boxes with a glass floor and allowed to acclimatize to their surroundings for at least 1 h in a temperature-controlled (21 °C) experimental room for three consecutive days prior to testing. On the test day, the animals were acclimatized to the experimental room 1 h before paw withdrawal latency (PWL) was measured. Attention was taken to start the test when the animal was not walking, with its hind paw in contact with the glass floor of the apparatus. A radiant heat source was directed at the mouse footpad until an aversive action was observed, such as paw withdrawal, foot drumming, or licking. A timer automatically measured in seconds the paw withdrawal latency. The heat source was set to an intensity of 30 and a cutoff time of 15 s was used to prevent tissue damage. Animals were first tested to determine their baseline PWL; after zymosan injection, the PWL (s) of each animal in response to the plantar test was determined again at 1, 2, 3, 4, 5, 24, and 48 h. In these experiments, HB, TG, TG-Ibu, and NioIbu were injected s.c. in a volume of 40 L in the dorsal surface of mice hind paw, 15 min before zymosan injection.

2.7. Neuropathy-Induced Allodynia and Hyperalgesia

The chronic constriction injury (CCI) model was carried out as previously described [28], with slight modifications [23]. Briefly, mice were anesthetized with chloralium hydrate-xylazine (400 + 10 mg/kg, i.p.). The right sciatic nerve was exposed at the mid-thigh level and, in the vicinity of the sciatic nerve trifurcation, was loosely tied with two ligatures of nylon black monofilament (9–0 non-absorbable, S&T, Neuhausen, Switzerland). Ligatures spaced 1.5–2 mm apart. Then, the muscles and the skin were closed with sutures. These animals were used in two nociceptive tests in the following order: mechanical allodynia followed by thermal hyperalgesia. The threshold for mechanical allodynia was assessed with the dynamic plantar aesthesiometer (Ugo Basile, Italy). Animals were trained on the apparatus, consisting of clear cages with a wire mesh floor, for 3 days before experimental sessions to allow for acclimatization. When the animal was at rest, a straight metal filament exerting an increasing upward force at a constant rate (5 g/s) with a maximum cutoff force of 50 g was placed under the plantar surface of the hind paw. Measurement was stopped when the paw was withdrawn and the results were expressed in grams. The measurement was repeated three times for each paw and averaged.

The development of thermal hyperalgesia was measured by subjecting the injured animals to the plantar test, as described in the "Zymosan-induced hyperalgesia" section.

Behavioural assessments of CCI-induced allodynia and thermal hyperalgesia were carried out 10 days after nerve injury, and behavioural responses compared with the ones measured before surgery. In these experiments, s.c. injection volumes of 40 L of HB, TG, TG-Ibu, and NioIbu were performed in the dorsal surface of mice hind paw.

2.8. Data Analysis and Statistics

Experimental data are presented as mean ± standard error of the mean (s.e.m.). Statistically significant differences between groups were calculated with an analysis of variance (ANOVA) followed by Tukey's post-hoc comparisons. Data were analyzed using the GraphPad Prism 6.03 software. The criterion for significance was set at $P < 0.05$. The data and statistical analysis conformed to the recommendations on experimental design and analysis in pharmacology [29].

3. Results

3.1. Nanovesicle Formulation and Characterization

All in vivo tests were performed by administration of well-characterized (Table 2) and stable (at least 3 months when stored at 4 °C) pH-sensitive vesicles (Nio, NioIbu). AFM characterization indicates that niosomes have a spherical shape (Figure 2). In agreement with DLS, AFM images indicate that NioIbu nanovesicles are smaller and have a less-uniform size than the Nio ones. Sizes deduced from AFM images seem underestimated with respect to the DLS results. In particular, for both the samples, the diameter evaluated by AFM is 70% of that evaluated by DLS, probably due to the approximations assumed in the model. In particular, Ibuprofen-loaded vesicles show the appropriate dimensions and zeta potential to be tested in animal studies. Drug entrapment efficiency is useful to perform in vivo studies, and the bilayer fluidity is quite high to ensure drug release, as reported in Rinaldi et al. [21]. This selection was carried out based on the best in-vitro performance of the sample, in particular in terms of the percentage of released drug [21]; in this previous study, sample characterization in the presence of different pH conditions was carried out, and the pH sensitivity of the selected formulation was confirmed.

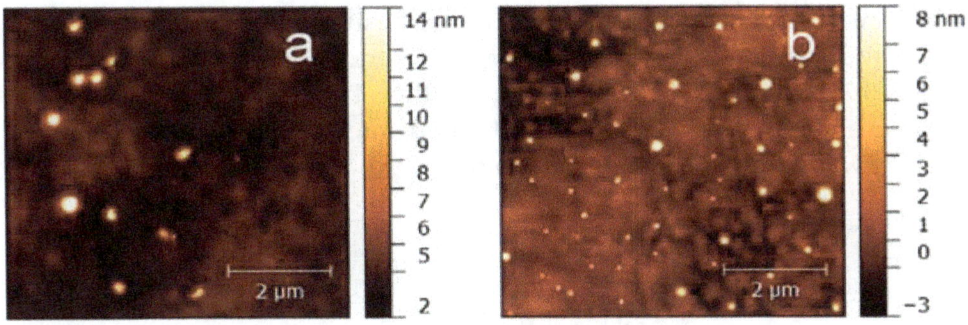

Figure 2. AFM images of Nio (**a**) and NioIbu (**b**) samples.

Table 2. Vesicle characterization. Nio, pH-Tw20Gly niosomes; NioIbu, pH-Tw20Gly niosomes loaded with a 5% Ibuprofen Hepes solution.

Niosomes	Diameter (nm)	AFM Diameter (nm)	ζ Potential (mV)	Polydispersity Index	Fluorescence Anisotropy (AU)	Loaded Drug Conc. (mg/mL)
Nio	215.0 ± 3.0	152 ± 18	−41.0 ± 1.2	0.160 ± 0.08	0.17 ± 0.01	–
NioIbu 5%	122.1 ± 19.6	89 ± 24	−40.2 ± 0.1	0.404 ± 0.05	0.20 ± 0.04	0.37 ± 0.05

3.2. *Writhing Test*

The in vivo antinociceptive activity of NioIbu was first assessed through a writhing test (Figure 2). As detailed in the experimental procedure section, acetic acid was used to induce peripheral pain. Analgesic activity was determined by recording the decrease in the number of writhes after acetic acid injection. The acetic-acid-induced writhing test in mice is the most commonly used method for measuring preliminary antinociceptive activity, since, in this test, both central and peripheral analgesics are detected. In these experiments, tested mice were injected with acetic acid 120 min after drug treatment. Statistical analysis revealed significant differences between treatments [$F_{(3, 28)} = 5.545$, $P = 0.0041$]. In this test, the administration of TG or TG-Ibu did not change the response to acetic acid in mice (Figure 3). Strong inhibition of the number of writhes was instead observed when NioIbu was administered 120 min before the acetic acid (Figure 3). In comparison with the TG group, NioIbu significantly reduced the number of writhes ($P < 0.05$), and the inhibition ratio was 52.5.

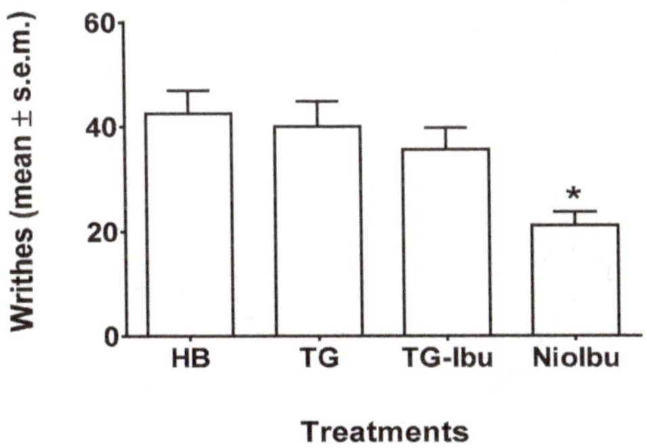

Figure 3. Effects of Hepes buffer (HB), the unstructured surfactant formulation (TG), the unstructured surfactant formulation with the same Ibuprofen (IBU) concentration (TG-Ibu), and TW20-Gly loaded with IBU (NioIbu) on the number of writhes induced by acetic acid. Samples were subcutaneously injected 120 min before acid acetic injection. * is for $P < 0.05$ versus TG. $N = 8$.

3.3. *Capsaicin Test*

In order to better evaluate the antinociceptive activity of ibuprofen-loaded vesicles, we also performed the capsaicin test (Figure 4). This test reflects acute pain responses related to neurogenic inflammation. In sensory neurons, capsaicin is an activator of the TRPV1 channels present in C-fibers and, to a lesser extent, Aδ. After injection, capsaicin shows a biphasic effect, i.e., it stimulates TRPV1 located in sensory neurons, producing a rapid phase of burning sensation, and local vascular and extravascular responses, followed by a persistent desensitization with concomitant long-lasting analgesia. Statistical analysis revealed significant differences between treatments, as revealed by ANOVA ($F_{(3, 36)} = 10.22$, $P < 0.0001$). In this test, neither TG nor TG-Ibu reduced the duration of the licking response as compared with the HB-treated mice (Figure 4). A statistically significant antinociceptive effect was shown for NioIbu (inhibition ratio, 55.4%, $P < 0.001$) versus TG-treated mice.

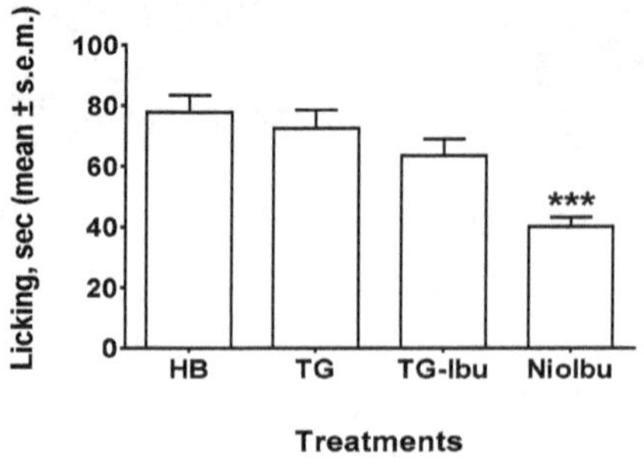

Figure 4. Effects of Hepes buffer (HB), the unstructured surfactant formulation (TG), the unstructured surfactant formulation with the same Ibuprofen (IBU) concentration (TG-Ibu), and TW20-Gly loaded with IBU (NioIbu) on the time spent licking the capsaicin-injected paw. Samples were injected subcutaneously in the dorsal surface of the hind paw 120 min before capsaicin injection. *** is for $P < 0.001$ versus TG. $N = 10$.

3.4. *Zymosan-Induced Hyperalgesia*

A s.c. injection of zymosan into mice footpad induces persistent dose- and time-dependent thermal and mechanical hyperalgesia associated with inflammation up to 24 h after treatment (Figure 5). Primary hyperalgesia in the hind paw inflammation model is thought to result from a release of pro-inflammatory mediators that include bradykinin, cytokines, and prostaglandins [30,31]. The reduction in latency response to a thermal stimulus applied to a paw and induced by zymosan was measured as a percentage. In these experiments, samples were injected into the dorsal surface of the right hind paw 15 min before zymonsan injection. As observed in the writhing and capsaicin test, TG and TG-Ibu did not affect the decrease in nociceptive threshold induced by zymosan. On the contrary, the highest increase in pain threshold was observed in NioIbu-treated mice. (Figure 5). Furthermore, the increase in the nociceptive threshold induced by NioIbu was long-lasting, since two-way ANOVA revealed significant differences from 3 to 24 h after NioIbu treatment ($F_{(10, 135)} = 3.44$, $P = 0.0005$).

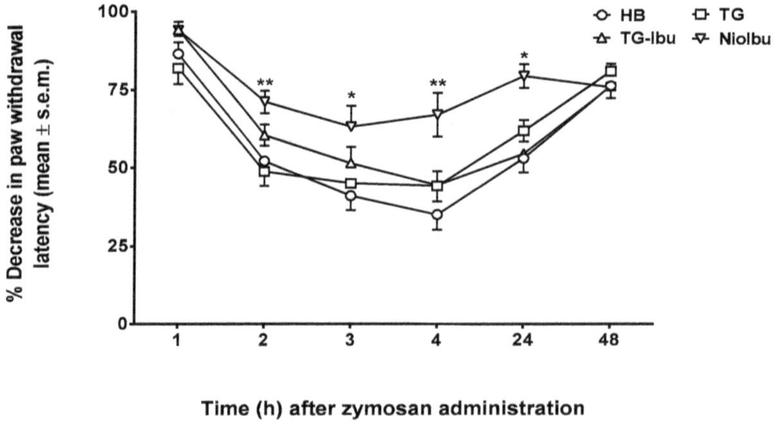

Figure 5. Effects of Hepes buffer (HB), the unstructured surfactant formulation (TG), the unstructured surfactant formulation with the same Ibuprofen (IBU) concentration (TG-Ibu), and TW20-Gly loaded with IBU (NioIbu) on zymosan-induced hyperalgesia. * is for $P < 0.05$ and ** is for $P < 0.01$ versus TG. $N = 10$.

3.5. Neuropathy-Induced Allodynia and Hyperalgesia

Neuropathic pain is a chronic condition caused by injury to the nervous system. This condition is characterized by spontaneous pain, as well as by exaggerated pain responses to painful stimuli (hyperalgesia) and to normally non-painful stimuli (allodynia). In our experiments, allodynia and hyperalgesia were measured 10 days after nerve injury, because this is when the pain threshold reaches the minimum value. The results obtained in these experiments are shown in Figures 6 and 7. When allodynia was measured (Figure 6), two-way ANOVA showed a significant difference between treatments ($F_{(12, 126)} = 4.453$; $P < 0.0001$). A Tukey's multiple comparison test demonstrated that NioIbu significantly increased paw withdrawal latency from 1 to 3 h after treatment, whereas TG-Ibu induced a transient, not significant increase in the nociceptive threshold (Figure 6).

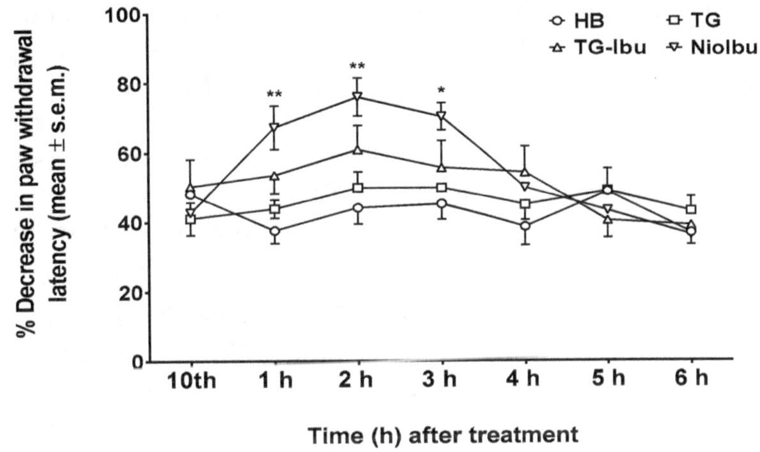

Figure 6. Effects of Hepes buffer (HB), the unstructured surfactant formulation (TG), the unstructured surfactant formulation with the same Ibuprofen (IBU) concentration (TG-Ibu), and TW20-Gly loaded with IBU (NioIbu) on allodynia induced by a chronic constriction injury of the right sciatic nerve. * is for $P < 0.05$ and ** is for $P < 0.01$ versus TG. $N = 8$.

In the same way, two-way ANOVA revealed significant differences in pain threshold when hyperalgesia was measured ($F_{(12, 126)} = 6.811$; $P < 0.0001$) (Figure 7). NioIbu increased the pain threshold from 2 h up to 4 h after treatment, whereas the increase in the pain threshold observed 1 h after TG-Ibu administration was not statistically significant.

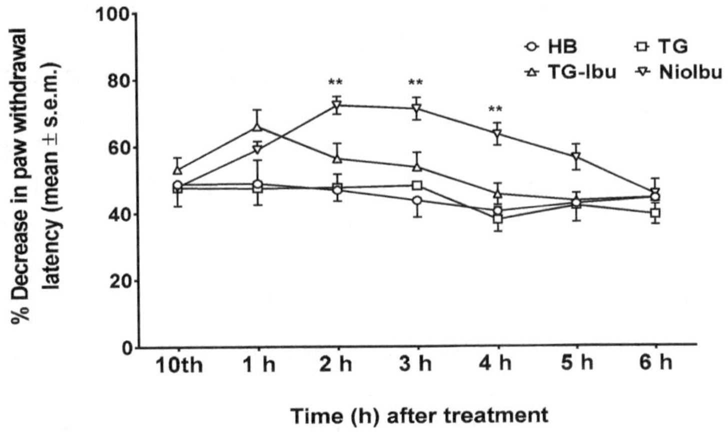

Figure 7. Effects of Hepes buffer (HB), the unstructured surfactant formulation (TG), the unstructured surfactant formulation with the same Ibuprofen (IBU) concentration (TG-Ibu), and TW20-Gly loaded with IBU (NioIbu) on hyperalgesia induced by a chronic constriction injury of the right sciatic nerve. * is for $P < 0.05$ and ** is for $P < 0.01$ versus TG. $N = 8$.

4. Discussion

Several researchers have focused on alternative drug delivery systems to overcome the difficulties associated with the distribution and effectiveness of analgesic drugs. This is mainly due to the low capability of analgesic drugs to pass across biological membranes [32]. One of the strategies adopted to overcome these limitations was loading the drugs into liposomes, which are spherical vesicles composed of phospholipids, such as phosphatidylcholine and phosphatidyl-serine, and possibly other lipids as well [33]. However, liposomes have high production costs due to the phospholipids employed and tend to fuse or aggregate, resulting in an early release of the vesicle payload. Moreover, phospholipids are prone to oxidative degradation. Finally, liposomes have low solubility and stability, and their applicability is limited because they have short half–lives in blood circulation [13,34,35]. To overcome these constraints, we decided to use a new non-toxic drug delivery system, the niosomes. These carriers offer several advantages compared to liposomes: a higher capability to entrap lipophilic, hydrophilic, and amphiphilic drugs; an ability to reach the site of action via oral, parenteral, and topical routes of administration; and a lower cost. [36]. Recently, Di Marzio et al. [13] described specific pH-sensitive, non-ionic surfactant vesicles with polysorbate-20 (Tween-20)/Chems as a good delivery system for analgesic drugs, which increase the stability and affinity in the tissue pH alterations that occur during inflammatory pathologic conditions [37]. These vesicles showed the ability to control and sustain release as well as to protect drugs from catalytic enzymes, thereby increasing drug stability.

Niosomes containing pH-sensitive components, such as TW20Gly, that protonate at lower pH [35] showed bilayer destabilization, leading to localized drug release. This approach could be useful in targeting inflamed tissues. In this study, we evaluated the antinociceptive effects of s.c. injections of Ibuprofen-loaded, pH-sensitive niosomes in comparison with the free form of the drug. To address this issue, we utilized mice under different pain stimuli. This work demonstrates that the use of these nanocarriers enhances the therapeutic efficacy of Ibuprofen, since Ibuprofen-loaded niosomes were effective in reducing pain in laboratory mice. The use of nanovesicles as delivery systems has already been successfully exploited to supply compounds topically and orally. In fact, some studies showed that NSAID-loaded vesicles have better performance in terms of prolonged drug release [38] and improved therapeutic effects [39] compared with the free form of the same compound. Considering that niosomes are a very promising system to administer compounds of different features topically or orally [40–42], we evaluated the capability of niosomes to increase antinociceptive effects of Ibuprofen also in terms of lasting effects after s.c injection. Writhing and capsaicin tests are screening assays commonly used to study peripheral and central antinociceptive activity. Our results showed that, when Ibuprofen-loaded niosomes were administered, there was an increase in the positive response time. In fact, when Ibuprofen was given 120 min earlier, the antinociceptive activity was maintained only in the niosomal form and not in the free form. The capsaicin test confirmed the long-lasting effects of Ibuprofen-loaded niosomes. Similar results were obtained with diclofenac-loaded liposomes administered orally, as reported by Goh et al. [43]. Consistently, in a formalin test, Ibuprofen-loaded niosomes displayed a peripheral antinociceptive activity and were more effective than free Ibuprofen in suppressing inflammatory pain. The niosomal form also had a long-lasting action, while the free form was probably rapidly catabolized [16]. Therefore, the encapsulation of the drug into niosomes significantly enhances drug efficacy and increases the durability of antinociceptive effects. This allows for a reduction in doses and, consequently, might also reduce the drug's side effects.

Some studies reported that nano-formulations reduce hyperalgesic responses to thermal stimuli more efficiently than free drugs [44,45]. Our results on zymosan-induced hyperalgesia are in line with these studies and demonstrate that Ibuprofen-loaded, pH-sensitive niosomes were able to reduce nociception up to 24 h after administration. These results confirm that niosomes release the encapsulated drug efficiently when behavioural experiments were performed. Similarly, Ibuprofen-loaded niosomes decrease neuropathic pain, since the treatment reduced both hyperalgesia and allodynia induced by chronic sciatic nerve constriction.

The increase in drug activity when released by niosomes could be explained by the capability of niosomes to transport lipophilic drugs, in this case Ibuprofen, across tissue membranes. This facilitates drug diffusion around the site of application and consequently improves efficacy [13,22].

In conclusion, the present study reveals that Ibuprofen-loaded, pH-sensitive niosomes are able to produce consistent and long-lasting antinociceptive effects. The antinociceptive effects of Ibuprofen-loaded niosomes were observed both in acute and chronic animal models of pain and these results, together with those reported in our previous study [21], suggest that an Ibuprofen pH-sensitive nanocarrier formulation could be further developed and used to treat different pain conditions in humans.

Author Contributions: Conceptualization, S.P. and M.C.; Methodology, S.P., M.C. and M.R.; Formal Analysis, P.M. and D.P.; Investigation, F.M., P.M., F.R. and D.P.; Writing-Original Draft Preparation, F.M., S.P., C.M.; Visualization, P.M. and F.R.

Acknowledgments: We are grateful to Laura Ciarlo for comments that improved the manuscript. We also thanks Catia Dos Santos for the linguistic revision of the manuscript and Alessandro Paparatti for the graphical abstract.

References

1. Patel, A.; Bell, M.; O'Connor, C.; Inchley, A.; Wibawa, J.; Lane, M.E. Delivery of ibuprofen to the skin. *Int. J. Pharm.* **2013**, *457*, 9–13. [CrossRef] [PubMed]
2. Vane, J.R.; Botting, R.M. Anti-inflammatory drugs and their mechanism of action. *Inflamm. Res.* **1998**, *47*, 78–87. [CrossRef]
3. Doherty, N.S.; Beaver, T.H.; Chan, K.Y.; Coutant, J.E.; Westrich, G.L. The role of prostaglandins in the nociceptive response induced by intraperitoneal injection of zymosan in mice. *Br. J. Pharmacol.* **1987**, *91*, 39–47. [CrossRef] [PubMed]
4. Brunton, L.L.; Chabner, B.A.; Knollman, B.C. *Goodman & Gilman's the Pharmacological Basis of Therapeutics*, 12th ed.; McGraw-Hill Medical: New York, NY, USA, 2011.
5. Moffat, A.C.; Osselton, M.D.; Widdop, B. *Clarke's Analysis of Drugs and Poisons: In Pharmaceuticals, Body Fluids and Postmortem Material, 2*; Pharmaceutical Press and American Pharmacists' Association: London, UK, 2004; p. 1125.
6. Berner, G.; Engels, B.; Vögtle-Junkert, U. Percutaneous ibuprofen therapy with Trauma-Dolgit gel: Bioequivalence studies. *Drugs Exp. Clin. Res.* **2004**, *XV*, 559–564.
7. Pereira-Leite, C.; Nunes, C.; Reis, S. Interaction of nonsteroidal anti-inflammatory drugs with membranes: In vitro assessment and relevance for their biological actions. *Prog. Lipid Res.* **2013**, *52*, 571–584. [CrossRef] [PubMed]
8. Stoye, I.; SchrDer, K.; Müller-Goymann, C.C. Transformation of a liposomal dispersion containing ibuprofen lysinate and phospholipids into mixed micelles—Physico-chemical characterization and influence on drug permeation through excised human stratum corneum. *Eur. J. Pharm. Biopharm.* **1998**, *46*, 191–200. [CrossRef]
9. Abdullah, G.Z.; Abdulkarim, M.F.; Salman, I.M.; Ameer, O.Z.; Yam, M.F.; Mutee, A.F.; Chitneni, M.; Mahdi, E.S.; Basri, M.; Sattar, M.A.; et al. In vitro permeation and in vivo anti-inflammatory and analgesic properties of nanoscaled emulsions containing ibuprofen for topical delivery. *Int. J. Nanomed.* **2011**, *6*, 387–396. [CrossRef] [PubMed]
10. Santi, P.; Nicoli, S.; Colombo, G.; Bettini, R.; Artusi, M.; Rimondi, S.; Padula, C.; Rizzo, P.; Colombo, P. Post-iontophoresis transport of ibuprofen lysine across rabbit ear skin. *Int. J. Pharm.* **2003**, *266*, 69–75. [CrossRef]
11. Park, E.S.; Chang, S.Y.; Hahn, M.; Chi, S.C. Enhancing effect of polyoxyethylene alkyl ethers on the skin permeation of ibuprofen. *Int. J. Pharm.* **2000**, *209*, 109–119. [CrossRef]
12. Brown, M.B.; Hanpanitcharoen, M.; Martin, G.P. An in vitro investigation into the effect of glycosaminoglycans on the skin partitioning and deposition of NSAIDs. *Int. J. Pharm.* **2001**, *225*, 113–121. [CrossRef]

13. Di Marzio, L.; Marianecci, C.; Petrone, M.; Rinaldi, F.; Carafa, M. Novel pH-sensitive non-ionic surfactant vesicles: Comparison between Tween 21 and Tween 20. *Colloids Surf. B Biointerfaces* **2011**, *82*, 18–24. [CrossRef] [PubMed]
14. Dalmoro, A.; Bochicchio, S.; Nasibullin, SF.; Bertoncin, P.; Lamberti, G.; Barba, A.A.; Moustafine, R.I. Polymer-lipid hybrid nanoparticles as enhanced indomethacin delivery systems. *Eur. J. Pharm. Sci.* **2018**, *121*, 16–28. [CrossRef] [PubMed]
15. Rinaldi, F.; Hanieh, P.N.; Chan, L.K.N.; Angeloni, L.; Passeri, D.; Rossi, M.; Wang, J.T.; Imbriano, A.; Carafa, M.; Marianecci, C. Chitosan Glutamate-Coated Niosomes: A Proposal for Nose-to-Brain Delivery. *Pharmaceutics* **2018**, *10*, 38. [CrossRef] [PubMed]
16. Marianecci, C.; Di Marzio, L.; Rinaldi, F.; Celia, C.; Paolino, D.; Alhaique, F.; Esposito, S.; Carafa, M. Niosomes from 80s to present: The state of the art. *Adv. Colloid Interface* **2014**, *205*, 187–206. [CrossRef] [PubMed]
17. Rajera, R.; Nagpal, K.; Singh, S.K.; Mishra, D.N. Niosomes: A controlled and novel drug delivery system. *Biol. Pharm. Bull.* **2011**, *34*, 945–953. [CrossRef]
18. Edlow, D.W.; Sheldon, W.H. The pH of inflammatory exudates. *Proc. Soc. Exp. Biol. Med.* **1971**, *137*, 1328–1332. [CrossRef]
19. Naghavi, M.; John, R.; Naguib, S.; Siadaty, M.S.; Grasu, R.; Kurian, K.C.; van Winkle, W.B.; Soller, B.; Litovsky, S.; Madjid, M.; et al. pH Heterogeneity of human and rabbit atherosclerotic plaques: A new insight into detection of vulnerable plaque. *Atherosclerosis* **2002**, *164*, 27–35. [CrossRef]
20. Gatenby, R.A.; Gillies, R.J. Why do cancers have high aerobic glycolysis? *Nat. Rev. Cancer* **2004**, *4*, 891–899. [CrossRef]
21. Rinaldi, F.; Del Favero, E.; Rondelli, V.; Pieretti, S.; Bogni, A.; Ponti, J.; Rossi, F.; Di Marzio, L.; Paolino, D.; Marianecci, C.; et al. pH-sensitive niosomes: Effects on cytotoxicity and on inflammation and pain in murine models. *J. Enzym. Inhib. Med. Chem.* **2017**, *32*, 538–546. [CrossRef]
22. Marianecci, C.; Rinaldi, F.; Di Marzio, L.; Mastriota, M.; Pieretti, S.; Celia, C.; Paolino, D.; Iannone, M.; Fresta, M.; Carafa, M. Ammonium glycyrrhizinate-loaded niosomes as a potential nanotherapeutic system for anti-inflammatory activity in murine models. *Int. J. Nanomed.* **2014**, *9*, 635–651. [CrossRef]
23. Carafa, M.; Marianecci, C.; Rinaldi, F.; Santucci, E.; Tampucci, S.; Monti, D. Span and Tween neutral and pH-sensitive vesicles: Characterization and in vitro skin permeation. *J. Liposome Res.* **2009**, *19*, 332–334. [CrossRef] [PubMed]
24. Kilkenny, C.; Browne, W.J.; Cuthill, I.C.; Emerson, M.; Altman, D.G. Improving bioscience research reporting: The ARRIVE guidelines for reporting animal research. *PLoS Biol.* **2010**, *8*, 1000412. [CrossRef] [PubMed]
25. Pieretti, S.; Di Giannuario, A.; Capasso, A.; Sorrentino, L.; Loizzo, A. Effects induced by cysteamine on chemically-induced nociception in mice. *Life Sci.* **1994**, *54*, 1091–1099. [CrossRef]
26. Sakurada, T.; Katsumata, K.; Tan-No, K.; Sakurada, S.; Kisara, K. The capsaicin test in mice for evaluating tachykinin antagonists in the spinal cord. *Neuropharmacology* **1992**, *31*, 1279–1285. [CrossRef]
27. Colucci, M.; Maione, F.; Bonito, M.C.; Piscopo, A.; Di Giannuario, A.; Pieretti, S. New insights of dimethyl sulphoxide effects (DMSO) on experimental in vivo models of nociception and inflammation. *Pharmacol. Res.* **2008**, *57*, 419–425. [CrossRef] [PubMed]
28. Bennett, G.J.; Xie, Y.K. A peripheral mononeuropathy in rat that produces disorders of pain sensation like those seen in man. *Pain* **1988**, *33*, 87–107. [CrossRef]
29. Curtis, M.J.; Bond, R.A.; Spina, D.; Ahluwalia, A.; Alexander, S.P.; Giembycz, M.A.; Gilchrist, A.; Hoyer, D.; Insel, P.A.; Izzo, A.A.; et al. Experimental design and analysis and their reporting: New guidance for publication in BJP. *Br. J. Pharmacol.* **2015**, *172*, 3461–3471. [CrossRef]
30. Bélichard, P.; Landry, M.; Faye, P.; Bachvarov, D.R.; Bouthillier, J.; Pruneau, D.; Marceau, F. Inflammatory hyperalgesia induced by zymosan in the plantar tissue of the rat: Effect of kinin receptor antagonists. *Immunopharmacology* **2000**, *46*, 139–147. [CrossRef]
31. Ren, K.; Dubner, R. Inflammatory Models of Pain and Hyperalgesia. *ILAR J.* **1999**, *40*, 111–118. [CrossRef]
32. Lucio, M.; Lima, J.L.; Reis, S. Drug-membrane interactions: Significance for medicinal chemistry. *Curr. Med. Chem.* **2010**, *17*, 1795–1809. [CrossRef]
33. Gaur, P.K.; Bajpai, M.; Mishra, S.; Verma, A. Development of ibuprofen nanoliposome for transdermal delivery: Physical characterization, in vitro/in vivo studies, and anti-inflammatory activity. *Artif. Cells Nanomed. Biotechnol.* **2016**, *44*, 370–375. [CrossRef] [PubMed]

34. Bozzuto, G.; Molinari, A. Liposomes as nanomedical devices. *Int. J. Nanomed.* **2015**, *10*, 975–999. [CrossRef] [PubMed]
35. Masotti, A.; Vicennati, P.; Alisi, A.; Marianecci, C.; Rinaldi, F.; Carafa, M.; Ortaggi, G. Novel Tween 20 derivatives enable the formation of efficient pH-sensitive drug delivery vehicles for human hepatoblastoma. *Bioorg. Med. Chem. Lett.* **2010**, *20*, 3021–3025. [CrossRef] [PubMed]
36. Verma, S.; Singh, S.K.; Syan, N.; Mathur, P.; Valecha, V. Nanoparticle vesicular system: A versatile tool for drug delivery. *J. Chem. Pharm. Res.* **2010**, *2*, 496–509.
37. Lehner, R.; Wang, X.; Wolf, M.; Hunziker, P. Designing switchable nanosystems for medical application. *J. Control. Release* **2012**, *161*, 307–316. [CrossRef]
38. Das, M.K.; Palei, N.N. Sorbitan ester niosomes for topical delivery of rofecoxib. *Indian J. Exp. Biol.* **2011**, *49*, 438–445.
39. Naresh, R.A.; Raja, G.K.; Pillai, N.; Udupa, N.; Chandrashekar, G. Anti-inflammatory activity of niosome encapsulated diclofenac sodium in arthritic rats. *Indian J. Pharmacol.* **1994**, *26*, 46–48.
40. Shahiwala, A.; Misra, A. Studies in topical application of niosomally entrapped Nimesulide. *J. Pharm. Pharm. Sci.* **2002**, *5*, 220–225.
41. Goh, J.Z.; Tang, S.N.; Zuraini, A.; Zakaria, Z.A.; Kadir, A.A.; Chiong, H.S. Enhanced anti-inflammatory effects of nanoencapsulated diclofenac. *Eur. J. Inflamm.* **2013**, *11*, 855–861. [CrossRef]
42. Sankhyan, A.; Pawar, P. Recent Trends in Niosome as Vesicular Drug Delivery System. *J. Appl. Pharm. Sci.* **2012**, *2*, 20–32. [CrossRef]
43. Goh, J.Z.; Tang, S.N.; Chiong, H.S.; Yong, Y.K.; Zuraini, A.; Hakim, M.N. Evaluation of antinociceptive activity of nanoliposome-encapsulated and free-form diclofenac in rats and mice. *Nanomedicine* **2014**, *10*, 297–303. [CrossRef]
44. Narasimha Reddy, D.; Udupa, N. Formulation and Evaluation of Oral and Transdermal Preparations of Flurbiprofen and Piroxicam Incorporated with Different Carriers. *Drug Dev. Ind. Pharm.* **2008**, *19*, 843–852. [CrossRef]
45. Joshi, S.K.; Hernandez, G.; Mikusa, J.P.; Zhu, C.Z.; Zhong, C.; Salyers, A.; Wismer, C.T.; Chandran, P.; Decker, M.W.; Honore, P. Comparison of antinociceptive actions of standard analgesics in attenuating capsaicin and nerve-injury-induced mechanical hypersensitivity. *Neuroscience* **2006**, *143*, 587–596. [CrossRef]

3

Latest Advances in the Development of Eukaryotic Vaults as Targeted Drug Delivery Systems

Amanda Muñoz-Juan [1,†], Aida Carreño [1], Rosa Mendoza [1,2] and José L. Corchero [1,2,3,*]

1 Institut de Biotecnologia i de Biomedicina, Universitat Autònoma de Barcelona, 08193 Bellaterra, Spain
2 Networking Center on Bioengineering, Biomaterials and Nanomedicine (CIBER-BBN), 28029 Madrid, Spain
3 Department of Genetics and Microbiology, Universitat Autònoma de Barcelona, 08193 Bellaterra, Spain
* Correspondence: jlcorchero@ciber-bbn.es;
† Current address: Institut de Ciència de Materials de Barcelona (ICMAB-CSIC), Campus UAB, 08193 Bellaterra, Spain.

Abstract: The use of smart drug delivery systems (DDSs) is one of the most promising approaches to overcome some of the drawbacks of drug-based therapies, such as improper biodistribution and lack of specific targeting. Some of the most attractive candidates as DDSs are naturally occurring, self-assembling protein nanoparticles, such as viruses, virus-like particles, ferritin cages, bacterial microcompartments, or eukaryotic vaults. Vaults are large ribonucleoprotein nanoparticles present in almost all eukaryotic cells. Expression in different cell factories of recombinant versions of the "major vault protein" (MVP) results in the production of recombinant vaults indistinguishable from native counterparts. Such recombinant vaults can encapsulate virtually any cargo protein, and they can be specifically targeted by engineering the C-terminus of MVP monomer. These properties, together with nanometric size, a lumen large enough to accommodate cargo molecules, biodegradability, biocompatibility and no immunogenicity, has raised the interest in vaults as smart DDSs. In this work we provide an overview of eukaryotic vaults as a new, self-assembling protein-based DDS, focusing in the latest advances in the production and purification of this platform, its application in nanomedicine, and the current preclinical and clinical assays going on based on this nanovehicle.

Keywords: eukaryotic vaults; nanoparticle; drug delivery systems; nanocage; protein self-assembly

1. Introduction

Nanomedicine is a translational science whose objective is to obtain new therapies and diagnostic tools using the new available capabilities of nanotechnology [1]. It is applied in drug delivery, diagnosis, imaging, and therapy fields. The application of nanotechnology in the design of new drug delivery systems (DDSs) is, at this moment, one of the most active fields in nanomedicine research.

Conventional drug administration regimes use large amounts of the active principle, resulting in high costs, undesired side-effects and low therapeutic efficacy because only small amounts of the drug finally reach the target cells or tissues [2,3]. DDSs based on nanoparticles (NPs) have made a remarkable difference in site-specific release of chemotherapeutic agents, due to their physical and chemical characteristics and biological attributes. The use of such nanocarriers improves drug biodistribution, targeting active molecules to diseased cells and tissues while protecting healthy ones.

Several NPs types are being extensively explored, including polymeric micelles [4], solid nanoparticles [5], solid lipid nanoparticles (SLN) [6], nanostructured lipid carriers (NLC) [7], liposomes [8], inorganic nanoparticles [9], dendrimers [10], or magnetic nanoparticles [11]. Among them, biopolymer-based nanoparticles, including protein nanoparticles, are actively explored and used in pharmaceuticals [12,13].

Protein nano-DDSs are protein structures formed by the assembly of multiple copies of one or several different proteins [14]. Nature offers such functional macromolecular structures that can be easily manipulated for nanobiotechnology applications. Such naturally occurring protein cages, as virus capsids and ferritin cages, serve as excellent templates for functional biomaterials with precise architectures, unattainable by synthetic processes. The regular arrangement of protein subunits within protein cage structures allows for the engineering of specific regions and surfaces of the cage, such as the exterior or interior surfaces. The advantages of using proteins to prepare NPs for drug delivery applications include their abundance in natural sources, biocompatibility, biodegradability, easy synthesis process, and cost-effectiveness. In contrast, other particulate systems such as metallic nanoparticles show several drawbacks including potential toxicity, large size, accumulation, or rapid clearance from the body.

Most requirements for designing an ideal nano-DDS (stability, specificity, or controlled release of the drug) can be acquired using proteins in its structure since protein domains with these functions have been described [15]. As an advantage, proteins can be easily produced in different biological systems [16] such as bacteria [14,17], insect cells [18–20], or mammalian cells [21], among others.

In addition, protein-based NPs offer the opportunity for surface modification by standard genetic engineering techniques, or by conjugation of other protein/s and carbohydrate ligands. Protein engineering has been extensively used to redesign structure and function, yielding particles with very narrow size distributions and multiple functionalities. In this context, virus-like particles and other caged protein structures have been explored as nanocarriers for introducing non-native functionalities. This enables targeted delivery to the desired tissue and organ, which further reduces systemic toxicity. Such materials have been developed for applications in the fields of nanotechnology, biotechnology, or drug delivery. The use of protein NPs for such applications could, therefore, prove to be a better alternative to manipulate and improve the pharmacokinetic and pharmacodynamic properties of the various types of drug molecules. Research in this area has been very active for more than two decades, but only in the last years several of these products have been released to the market and are now routinely used in clinics [22].

Protein nano-DDSs can be classified according to the structure resulting from protein interactions in protein nanoboxes, nanoparticles, microspheres, matrices, and fibers. The vast majority of protein nano-DDSs classified as protein boxes have been designed and optimized by nature [23] and have a well-defined structure, divided into external, intermediate, and internal surfaces [24]. Generally, specific ligands of target cells can be bound on the outer surface; the intermediate surface gives stability to the complex; and the internal surface determines which cargo molecules can be introduced [25]. The loaded molecules inside these structures are protected against undesired degradation [23]. Some DDSs, such as viral particles, also have an intrinsic tendency to introduce components into the cell interior [26]. In other cases, they must be modified to incorporate specific peptides and direct them to the target cells. Not being the specific target of this review, these issues (and others) regarding protein-based DDS can be examined in much more detail in previous revisions available in the literature [27,28].

The main interest of protein boxes as nano-DDS is their internal cavity, which will determine the number of molecules that can be internalized. Eukaryotic vaults are protein NPs with a large internal cavity that makes them attractive as a nanocarrier for diverse types of molecules [18,29]. This feature, together with their homogeneity and versatility to be modified and specifically delivered to target cells, make vaults powerful candidates as nano-DDSs.

2. Eukaryotic Vaults

Vaults are ribonuclear-protein cytoplasmic complexes of 13 MDa [19] described for the first time in 1986 [30] as small ovoid bodies similar in structure to the vaults of ecclesiastical buildings ("vaulted ceilings") [31], by which they were named. Their natural function is not completely elucidated, although several functions related to nuclear transport, immune response [32] and multiresistance in cancer cells [33] have been hypothesized. Although it is well known that they participate in these functions, the mechanism through which it intervenes is not defined. Vault structure is highly conserved among different eukaryotic organisms [20,25,33], which indicates the importance of its functions and the putative biocompatibility that it can present as nano-DDSs [33].

2.1. Vaults Structure

The ribonucleoprotein complex is composed of proteins and nucleic acids. The main component is the "major vault protein" (MVP), representing more than 70% of natural vaults [25], while the remaining components are proteins such as poly(ADP-ribose) polymerase (VPARP) and telomerase; and small nontranslated RNA. The recombinant synthesis of MVP monomers is sufficient and allows their spontaneous self-assembling into vaults indistinguishable from natural ones. This has allowed the design, engineering, and production of recombinant vaults [19].

The structure of rat liver vault ribonucleoprotein particles was examined by different staining techniques in conjunction with EM and digestion with hydrolytic enzymes. Quantitative scanning transmission EM demonstrates that each vault particle is a homodimer, composed by two symmetrical halves with a total of 39 copies of MVP in each one [19]. Hydrophobic interactions between MVP domains (the strongest of the structure [18]) direct self-assembling of the vault. Each MVP monomer folds into 12 domains: nine structural repeat domains, a shoulder domain, a cap-helix domain, and a cap-ring domain. Interactions between the 42-turn-long cap-helix domains are key to stabilizing the particle. Freeze-etch revealed that vault can open into flower-like structures, in which eight rectangular petals are joined to a central ring, each by a thin hook. Vaults examined by negative stain and conventional transmission EM (CTEM) confirmed the flower-like structure [34]. The hierarchical self-assembly of MVP monomers into vaults is shown in detail in Figure 1.

The structural arrangement of a single MVP chain into the assembled vault was further analyzed and proven when an ~9 Å X-ray crystal structure of recombinant vaults purified from insect cells was carried out [35]. A further refinement to 3.5 Å resolution using crystallized rat liver vaults verified the previous low resolution structure prediction [36]. Vault structure analysis by X-ray diffraction at 3.5 Å resolution [25] gives dimensions of approximately 67 × 40 × 40 nm as well as an interior volume of 3.87×10^7 Å^3. Vaults show a hollow, barrel-shaped structure with two protruding caps and an invaginated waist, based on hierarchical protein self-assembly [36].

Moreover, studies based on electron cryotomography showed that intracellular vaults are similar in overall size and shape to purified and recombinant vaults previously analyzed [37]. A 2.1 Å resolution structure of the seven N-terminal repeats (R1–7) of MVP has also been determined [38].

Under physiological conditions there is a balance between the closed and open conformations (separate halves) of vaults, allowing the entry of molecules [39]. An acidification of the medium destabilizes the bonds between monomers, with the exception of the strong hydrophobic joints between the head-helix domains, giving rise to a "flower-like" structure [20,40]. Low-pH condition triggers vault conformational change. Closed intact vaults at pH 6.5 dissociate quickly into half-vaults as the solution pH decrease to less than 4.0 [41]. This dissociation triggered at low pH has been proposed as a useful tool for controlled drug delivery within cellular systems given that endosomes and lysosomes are normally maintained at acidic pH. Thus, this phenomenon is being studied in order to achieve a controlled release of cargo drugs [40]. In this line, Esfandiary et al. employed a variety of spectroscopic techniques (i.e., circular dichroism, fluorescence spectroscopy, and light scattering) along with electron microscopy, to characterize the structural stability of vaults over a wide range of pH (3–8) and temperature (10–90 °C). Ten different conformational states of the vaults were identified over the pH and temperature range studied with the most stable region at pH 6–8 below 40°C and least stable at pH 4–6 above 60 °C [42].

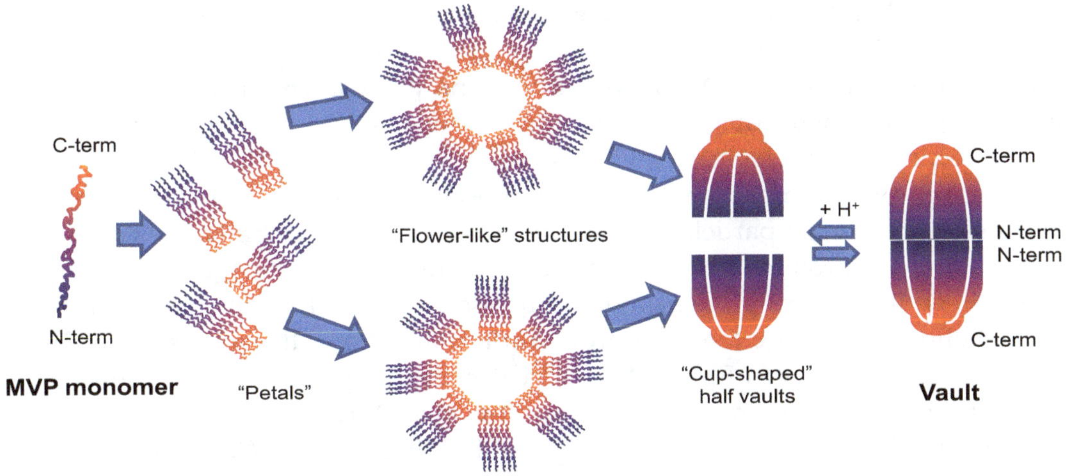

Figure 1. Hierarchical self-assembly of major vault protein (MVP) monomers into closed vaults. Each vault consists in a hollow, barrel-like structure composed of two identical cup-like halves joined at their open ends. Each half vault is in turn composed of a single eight-petaled "flower-like" structure, which is folded into the cup shape. At low pH, the acidic residues at the half-vault interfaces would become neutral, leaving a highly positive charge and inducing the disassembly of the vault particle by charge repulsion. Adapted from [20,36,40,41].

Prior crystal structures of the vault have provided clues of its structure but are non-conclusive due to crystal packing. To addres this concern, a recent study determined vaults near-atomic resolution (~4.8 Å) structures in a solution/noncrystalline environment [43]. Authors obtained vaults by engineering at the N-terminus of rat major vault protein (MVP) an HIV-1 Gag protein segment. The barrel-shaped vaults in solution adopt two conformations, 1 and 2, both with D39 symmetry, and comparison with crystallography results shows a major flexible region at the vault shoulder, suggesting that loops near this region could be utilized as peptide fusion sites for engineering purposes. Also in the line to determine vault structure under physiological conditions, Llauró et al. examined the local stiffness of individual vaults and probed their structural stability with atomic force microscopy (AFM) under physiological conditions, showing that the barrel, the central part of the vault, governs both the stiffness and mechanical strength of these particles [44]. In another study, same authors used AFM to monitor the structural evolution of individual vault particles while changing the pH in real time. The results showed that decreasing the pH of the solution destabilize the barrel region, the central part of vault particles, leading to their aggregation. Additional analyses using Quartz-Crystal Microbalance (QCM) and Differential Scanning Fluorimetry (DSF) confirmed AFM experiments [20]. This confirms that low pH weakens the bonds between adjacent proteins.

As described previously, single MVP self-assembly into final vault was modeled using the cryo-EM technique, showing that N-terminal tags were located at the vault waist facing the inside of the particle with longer tags having greater internal density [45]. On the other hand, vaults assembled from MVP containing C-terminal tags displayed extra density at the top and bottom (caps) of the vault, indicating that whereas the N-terminus begins at the inside of the vault waist, MVP C-terminus is exposed at the vault surface [45,46]. The implications of such findings in the putative applications of vault will be discussed in detail in next sections.

2.2. *Drug Encapsulation within Vaults*

A key issue in order to apply engineered vaults as an efficient DDS was the development of a procedure to encapsulate foreign materials into the vault lumen. The development of such a strategy relies on previous studies of the VPARP protein, an essential component of native vaults that was identified using the yeast two-hybrid method employing MVP as a bait [47]. With this previous knowledge, a strategy was developed to identify a vault targeting sequence. In this line, structural studies of VPARP and MVP interactions revealed the existence of a domain within the VPARP protein (at its C-terminus, aa 1563–1724), called interaction domain (INT) [48–50], which interacts with the inner side of domains 3, 4, and 5 of MVP N-terminal end [51,52]. The fusion of this INT domain at the C-terminus of proteins with therapeutic interest allows their spontaneous encapsulation within vaults without affecting their biological activity, as observed naturally with VPARP. As the INT domain is responsible for binding VPARP to MVP, it was hypothesized to act as a "zip code" directing the protein to the inside of the vault particle (see Figure 2A). This targeting ability was confirmed when the INT domain was fused to proteins with enzymatic or fluorescent activities such as firefly luciferase or a variant of the green fluorescent protein, and coexpressed with MVP in Sf9 insect cells [49], obtaining fluorescently labelled vaults due to cargo protein internalization. INT-tagged proteins copurified with recombinant vaults, and cryo-EM analysis revealed that they were packaged inside the particles into two rings of density, above and below the vault waist. Other proteins with relevant biological activities, such as CCL21 [53], pVI [48], or the antigens MOMP [54] and OVA [55] have been successfully encapsulated by this mechanism. This strategy is depicted in Figure 2. Moreover, this encapsulation process does not not require cotranslation of INT-tagged cargo protein with MVP [39]. INT fusion proteins can be packaged inside recombinant vaults by just mixing them and incubating the mixture on ice for 30 min. This process has been hypothesized to occur via vault "breathing", a process previously characterized for virus particles. As purified vaults are occasionally observed as half vault structures [41,56], a transient half-vault/whole-vault dynamic could also explain INT protein packaging.

As mentioned before, MVP N-terminus faces the vault lumen, offering an excellent opportunity to encapsulate peptides or proteins. In this context, several fusions have been added to MVP cDNA. The added domain did not interfere in the self-assembly of MVP monomers, rendering vaults similar to native ones, and as expected the new domain were found located inside the nanocages (see Figure 2B). Following this strategy, peptides or proteins like green fluorescen protein [49], a cysteine-rich peptide [45], a His-T7 epitope tag [45], a VSVG epitope tag [45], an adenovirus membrane lytic peptide [48] or an epitope of HIV-1 Gag protein [43] have been successfully encapsulated within vaults.

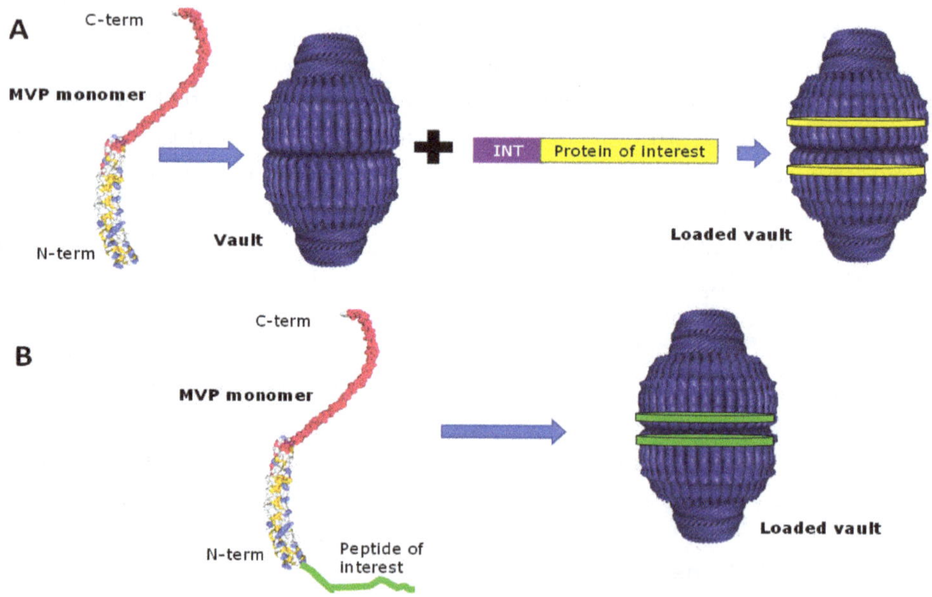

Figure 2. Encapsulation possibilities of recombinant vaults. A. The protein of interest (yellow) is fused to interaction domain (INT) domain (purple). After self-assembly of MVP monomers into vaults, the INT domain will direct loading of cargo protein (shown as two yellow discs) within vaults through specific interaction with MVP monomers. B. The peptide of interest (in green) is expressed as a fusion to N-terminus of MVP monomer. After MVP self-assembly into vaults, cargo peptide will accumulate in the nanoparticle lumen (shown as two green discs). Adapted from [57]. PDB images: 4HL8 Bioassembly 1 and 2.

Compounds not encoded by DNA (a common situation for small molecule drugs) have also been encapsulated within vaults by means of the INT targeting domain [29]. Recombinant INT containing an additional 31 amino acids at the N-terminus including a 6-His tag was used to direct bound species into vaults. This was confirmed with Ni-NTA nanogold, a material with affinity to the 6-His tag. As proof-of-concept, Ni-NTA-nanogold gold clusters were attached to the 6-His tag of three different INT-tagged proteins, forming a Au-INT complex. Then, specific association of gold clusters with the vault was demonstrated by co-immunoprecipitation with agarose beads.

The release rate of proteins encapsulated within vaults by INT-mediated interaction could be slowed down by the substitution of different amino acids of the INT domain by histidines [51]. All these previous results invite to easily visualize that vaults can be in the future an excellent DDS for virtually any peptide or protein with therapeutic potential, just by the simple procedure of fusing them to the INT domain.

Many chemotherapy drugs are small, hydrophobic molecules that are difficult to administer in aqueous solution and to distribute throughout the body. It is evident that such non-protein molecules cannot be fused to the INT domain, but the internal environment of the vault can be modified to favor its encapsulation. In this line, it has been described that a recombinant nanodisk containing "all trans retinoic acid" (ATRA), a potent but toxic therapeutic compound, could be packaged inside vaults [58]. Such nanodisk was obtained by incubating the fusion of a truncated form of the lipoprotein Apo-AI with INT vault binding domain, together with a dispersion of synthetic phospholipids in aqueous buffer, in the presence of the extremely hydrophobic ATRA drug. Finally, all this complex could be encapsulated within vaults thanks to the presence of the INT domain. Moreover, vault protected the hydrophobic nano-DDS, increasing its half-life and allowing the specific release of the drug. To avoid the previous step of the synthesis of another nano-DDS, recombinant MVPs have been designed that create a more hydrophobic interior environment. Thus, an amphipathic α-helix peptide, originally from the NS5A protein of hepatitis C virus, has been covalently bound to the N-terminal end of MVP [18], without hindering vault self-assembly. This modification has allowed the encapsulation of >2000 molecules (such as bryostatin 1, amphotericin B, or ATRA) per single vault. Bryostatin 1 is of particular therapeutic interest because of its ability to potently induce expression of latent HIV. In this line, results showed that vaults loaded with bryostatin 1 released the drug, resulting in the in vitro activation of latent HIV provirus and induction of CD69 biomarker expression following intravenous injection into mice [18]. This strategy can be of great interest to favor the biodistribution of most hydrophobic drugs.

2.3. *Vault Targeting and Internalization*

To address the ability of vaults to be engulfed and internalized in cells, vaults packaged with INT-tagged fluorescent proteins (GFP or mCherry) were added to HeLa cell cultures and their uptake confirmed by confocal microscopy [46]. This uptake, suggested to occur by endocytosis, was not specific or efficient, and thus considered a positive trend in terms of minimizing putative nonspecific incorporation of nano-DDSs in healthy cells. However, loaded vaults need to be targeted and delivered in a specific way to target cells and tissues. For that purpose, MVP C-terminus has been deeply explored. This C-terminal end faces the outside surface of the vault, and thus it can be modified to incorporate targeting peptides to target and promote specific cellular internalization of vaults into desired cells. In the frame of this strategy, the ability to specifically target the vault will rely and depend on the ability to find receptors specifically expressed (or clearly overexpressed in comparison with healthy cells) and the obtention of specific ligands recognizing such specific receptors in the target cell. Then, such ligands should be fused to the vault surface in order to recognize their target. For example, since epidermal growth factor (EGF) is upregulated in numerous cancer cell types, tags have been engineered and tested as fusions to the C-terminus of MVP to facilitate targeting to epithelial cancer cells via the EGF receptor (EGFR): a 33 amino acid Fc-binding peptide (called the Z domain) and the

55 amino acid epidermal growth factor (EGF). The modified vaults bound specifically to cancer cells either directly (EGF modified vaults) or as mediated by a monoclonal antibody (anti-EGFR) bound to recombinant vaults containing the Z domain (see Figure 3A). The EGF modified vaults have the ability to specifically bind cell surface receptors and trigger receptor activation in a manner similar to recombinant human EGF [46]. Thus both specific (peptide-directed) and general (antibody-mediated) methods could be used to target recombinant vault particles to cells, representing an essential advance towards the use of recombinant vaults as targeted DDSs.

Since recombinant vaults will expose one copy of the targeting peptide for each copy of engineered MVP monomer (see Figure 3B), the size of the peptide or protein fused to the C-terminal end of the MVP plays an important role in the stability of the vaults. The fusion of epidermal growth factor (EGF) [46], whose receptor is overexpressed in several cancers has been studied. It was observed that the presence of EGF in all the copies of MVP produces instability, interfering in its structuring, finally rendering insoluble vaults. To solve this problem, vectors were designed with two promoters that allow, on the one hand, the expression of MVP associated with EGF; and on the other, the expression of natural MVP [46]. This reduced the number of EGF present in each vault, allowing its correct structure, solubility, and ability to reach target cells.

The main route of administration of vaults consists of intratumoral injection [53], while the intranasal route has been studied for the use of vaults as vaccines [54]. Oral administration is hampered by the structural changes that vaults may undergo when exposed to acidification [20,40] that occurs in the gastrointestinal tract, and vaults specifically designed to cross the blood–brain barrier has not been developed yet.

Vaults specifically directed to target cells by ligands or antibodies will enter the cell interior by endocytosis [48,53], following the endosomal pathway until its degradation in lysosomes. Its success as nano-DDS depends on its ability to release the therapeutic components to the cytoplasm of the cells and not be degraded in the lysosomes. In order to avoid the degradative pathway and increase the release of the drug to the cytoplasm, the fusion of the lytic domain of the pVI protein of the adenovirus to the N-terminal end of the MVP has been studied [48]. It was demonstrated that pVI-vaults could disrupt the endosomal membrane using three different experimental protocols including enhancement of DNA transfection, codelivery of a cytosolic ribotoxin, and direct visualization by fluorescence. The early exit of the lysosome occurs without causing nonspecific damage to the cell, although it has been observed that a high concentration of this peptide can result in unwanted cellular apoptosis [48]. However, therapeutic effect greatly depends on the efficient release of the cargo protein from the DDS. In this context, it is hypothesized that the release rate of the cargo from the vault lumen is directly related to the interaction between MVP and INT domain. To further explore the release of molecular cargos from the vault nanoparticles, the interactions between isolated INT-interacting MVP domains (iMVP) and wild type INT has been determined and compared to two structurally modified INTs: first, a 15-amino acid deletion at the C terminus (INTΔC15) and, second, a histidine substitution at the interaction surface (INT/DSA/3 H) to impart a pH-sensitive response [51]. The introduction of histidines to His-INT resulted in stronger interaction between His-iMVP and His-INT/DSA/3 H compared to the wild type His-INT at both pH 6.0 and 7.4. This study implies that modulation of molecular release rate from the vault is possible by tuning the proportion of wild type and histidine-substituted INT or by truncation of the INT domain.

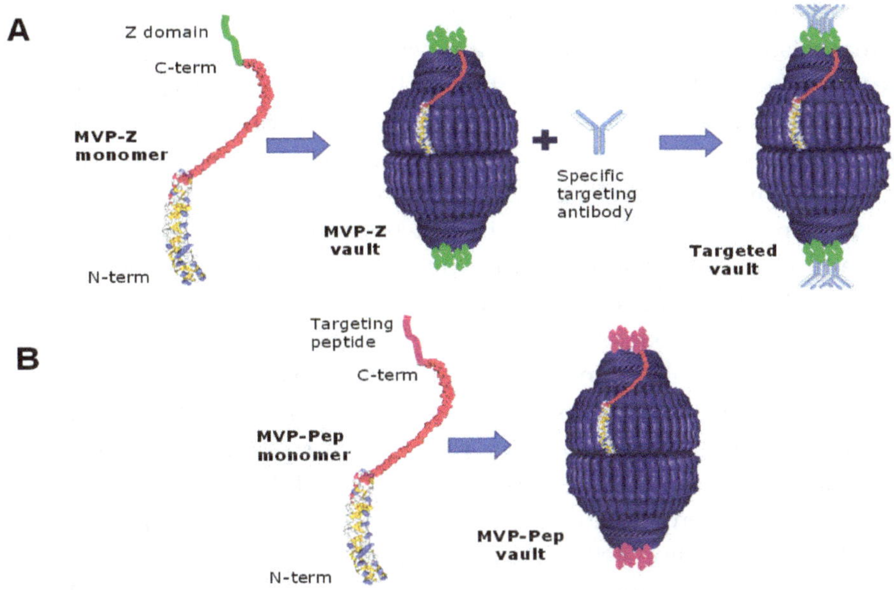

Figure 3. Engineering approaches for targeting vaults. A. The Z domain (in green) is fused to MVP monomer at its C-terminus. After MVP-Z monomer self-assembles into vault, it is incubated with a targeting antibody, that will bind to Z domains through its Fc domain. B. A specific targeting peptide (in purple) is fused to MVP monomer at its C-terminus. After MVP-Pep monomer self-assembles into vault, multiple copies of the targeting peptides will be exposed at the vault's caps. Adapted from [57]. PDB images: 4HL8 Bioassembly 1 and 2.

The above-mentioned strategies are limited by the capability to genetically engineer MVP protein to fuse the desired targeting peptide to it and therefore, to the resulting vault. Recently, a different approach has been proposed based on covalent chemical modifications of MVP residues. As other protein-based supra-macromolecular structures, vaults contain many derivatizable amino acid side chains. The new approach [19] was focused on establishing the comparative selectivity and efficiency of chemically modifying vault lysine and cysteine residues, using Michael additions, nucleophilic substitutions, and disulfide exchange reactions. Given the great number of vault lysine residues and the versatile chemistry of thiols, authors demonstrated a simple, robust technique to efficiently convert these more abundant residues into thiol terminated side chains. Using such chemistry, vaults doubly modified with a fluorescein reporter probe and cell-penetrating octaarginine peptides attached via a redox-sensitive cleavable or noncleavable linker were obtained. Relative to unmodified vaults, the resultant modified vaults showed no adverse particle effects following chemical modification while clearly demonstrating increased cellular uptake into cells of interest. This study provides a chemical foundation for predictable and fast vault modification, as required for the use of engineered vaults in imaging, therapeutic delivery, or basic biological research.

3. Recombinant Vaults Production and Purification

The baculovirus–insect cell system is today one of the most commonly used strategies to produce recombinant proteins. Since insect cells are one of the few eukaryotes lacking endogenous vaults, they have been the standard cell factory to obtain recombinant vaults. The current production of recombinant vault nanoparticles is mainly performed in *Spodoptera frugiperda* (Sf9) insect cells [59], where expression of only the MVP protein can direct the assembly of vault-like particles on polyribosomes [59,60]. However, this approach is complex and costly for industrial scale applications. The construction of a recombinant baculovirus containing a gene of interest requires a tedious and time-consuming (3–6 months) process. After that, routine growing, titration, and maintenance of the baculovirus stocks are also required. Moreover, continuous protein production is hampered by insect cells lysis during infection. Release of intracellular proteins from lysed cells, or removal or inactivation of progeny baculoviruses released by budding off from infected cells, may result in protein degradation by proteases and may also complicate downstream process [61–63].

To date, one significant change in the process has been the proposal of the replacement of the sf9 insect cells for insect larvae, which allows a greater production. Protein expression levels in baculovirus-infected larvae can be very high, reducing costs for large-scale production. In this line, a procedure was reported, based in baculovirus-infected insect larvae as starting material [40]. Nevertheless, due to general unfamiliarity with larval systems and restricted or low access to cell culture facilities to any research laboratory, this approach has not gained widespread popularity in most molecular biology laboratories in North America and Europe.

According to all these drawbacks related to expression systems, there is the need to develop alternative cell factories for recombinant vault production. Among the available organisms, yeast is a promising one for large-scale expression and preparation for human applications. Yeast have been successfully used in the last decades for recombinant protein production [64] and, for the synthesis of protein nanostructures such as virus-like particles [65], are similar in size and structure to vaults. In this context, it has been recently described for the first time the production of vaults in the yeast *Pichia pastoris* [66]. Expression of MVP alone in *P. pastoris* led to the formation of intact vaults, morphologically similar to endogenous vaults isolated from other eukaryotes. Moreover, such yeast vaults retained the ability to interact with INT-fused proteins, revealing *P. pastoris* as a new, promising alternative to insect cells for producing recombinant vaults.

To develop an economically competitive platform based on recombinant vaults, efficient downstream processes also need to be set-up and optimized. The interest of its use as nano-DDS requires the optimization of the process in order to increase the scale and yield [53] of production. The high size of the vault ribonucleoprotein complex complicates its downstream. For its purification, sucrose gradients [59,67], and continuous ultracentrifugation steps [57] have been used in a traditional manner, procedures rather complex and labor intensive. This technique greatly hinders large-scale production [57], both for the time devoted to achieving the needed high purity and the small amount obtained. Recombinant MVP is purified from insect cell extracts in a procedure requiring three ultracentrifugation steps and two additional gradient centrifugations. Sucrose or cesium chloride gradient ultracentrifugation [68,69] is generally considered to be chemically and physically appropriate for purification of different protein-based nanoparticles, including VLPs, but this general approach is labor-intensive, time-consuming, and scale-restricted [70], and can be associated with unexpected batch-to-batch variation. Although several reports have shown that gradient ultracentrifugation could be employed to purify VLPs, it provided only low yield and failed to remove impurities (including recombinant baculoviruses) from the final products [71].

Taking all these facts together, the need for the development of faster and easier downstream procedures for recombinant vaults is clear, and many efforts are being devoted to such purpose. In this line, efforts have been made in the substitution of centrifugation by special chromatographic columns, which significantly reduce the purification time. According to this approach, after removing cell debris, clarified lysate is loaded into an ion exchange column for large particles (Fractogel® EMD TMAE) and then into a gel filtration column, rendering final overall purities higher than 99% [33,40]. More recently, a two-step protocol for vault purification has been described, based on dialysis step and size-exclusion chromatography [72]. In this work, vaults were purified by a first dialysis step using a 1 MDa molecular weight cutoff membrane and a subsequent size-exclusion chromatography (SEC) on a Sepharose CL-6B column, rendering vaults with 90–95% purity and yields of 15 mg protein from 0.7–0.8 g cell samples pelleted from 50 mL of culture medium. Despite all these efforts and advances, vaults purification is still performed basically by the original protocol based on several ultracentrifugations.

In Table 1 it is shown the currently used expression systems and purification procedures for the obtention of recombinant vaults. Apart from those already in use, large scale and reproducible vault particle purification methodologies will be needed, preferably without ultracentrifugation steps. Thus, it is not difficult to foresee that new, improved purification methods will surely appear in the future that will allow a fast, cost-efficient vault purification.

Table 1. Expression systems and purification protocols currently used in the manufacturing of recombinant vaults.

Expression System [Ref.]	Purification Method	Final Yield	Advantages	Disadvantages
Baculovirus infection on sf9 cells [59]	Several saccharose gradient ultra-centrifugations	~10 mg/L	No endogenous vaults	Time-consuming, tedious downstream process
Baculovirus infection on sf21 cells [72]	Dialysis and size-exclusion chromatography	~0.5–1 mg/L	No endogenous vaults Quick, easy and cheap downstream process	Low yields
Baculovirus oral infection on insect larvae [40]	Ion exchange (cationic) and size-exclusion chromatography	Up to several grams	No endogenous vaults High yields	Difficult scale-up Slow production rate
Yeast cells (*Pichia pastoris*) [66]	Sucrose gradient ultracentrifugation and ion exchange (anionic) chromatography	~7–11 mg/L	No endogenous vaults Fast and cost-efficient production	Need scale-up

4. Vaults Applications in Nanomedicine and Clinical Trials

As a naturally occurring nanocage, vault is a promising candidate for DDS to target and deliver therapeutic molecules to damaged cells or tissues. Being highly stable structures in vitro, it is reasonable to hypothesize that vaults will be also stable in the bloodstream. However, putative immunogenic reactions from the body to recombinant vaults could restrict their application in clinical trials, mainly when using repetitive administrations. Several studies indicate that vaults are nonimmunogenic. For example, it was not possible to elicit antibodies in rabbits against purified vaults, and an antigenic response could only be induced when vaults were hemocyanin cross-linked prior to injection into rabbits [30]. In another study, the immunobistocbemical expression of MVP protein in freshly frozen normal human tissues and in 174 cancer specimens of 28 tumor types was analyzed, showing a broad distribution of MVP in both normal and tumoral human tissues [73]. Finally, immunogenicity of recombinant vaults in rats using subcutaneous administration showed no immunoreactivity against the recombinant vaults [57]. All these data suggest that, being ubiquitous throughout the human body, vaults are bio-invisible and nonimmunogenic to the human immune system.

To date, it is the American company Vault Pharma, a spin-off of the research group, that led by Dr. Leonard Rome (Dept. of Biological Chemistry, UCLA) discovered vaults in 1986, which holds intellectual property over vaults and some of their applications by means of several patents and, therefore, which is developing vaults as new DDS, some of them already in clinical trials. Such patents cover aspects including recombinant production, and vaults as carriers for biomolecules (such as cytokines and hydrophobic molecules) delivery. The vault is being explored and used as a tool to modulate the activity of the immune system. Vault Pharma's technology platform uses the vault particle to deliver peptides for unique immune signaling, exploiting the vault natural function as an immunological signal alert progenitor (characterized by vault being rapidly ingested by antigen presenting cells (APCs), specifically macrophages and dendritic cells). It was described that vaults are an early alert signal to the immune system once a cell is lysed and vaults are released to the extracellular space where they are rapidly engulfed by APCs. In this sense, it has been described that dendritic cells efficiently internalize vault nanocapules [54]. Therefore, current clinical trials based on these properties takes advantage of this natural property of vaults to trigger an immune response that is noninflammatory and results in many propitious effects including stimulation of extraordinarily high levels of antigen specific CD4 and CD8 T cells. The projects developed can be classified as oncological immunology and immunological activation to prevent infections.

For the treatment of oncology malignancies, vaults are designed to modulate the immune system, so it can slow or stop tumor development. The most advanced design consists of vaults (not specifically targeted) containing the CCL21 chemokine. This chemokine CCL21 is expressed mainly in the high venules of the lymph nodes and Peyer's patches [53] and act as a chemoattractant of cells of the immune system that express the CCR7 receptor. The strategy, which has shown its effectiveness, consists of directing the cells of the immune system to the tumor zone to stop the growth of the tumor [53]. The encapsulation of chemokine CCL21 occurs by fusion of the INT [53] domain at the C-terminus of CCL21. The MVP monomer is not fused to peptides ligands or specific antibodies, so the intratumoral administration is the only possible to act in a specific way. This explains that the use of the same nano-DDS is being studied to treat different types of cancer. The most advanced clinical trial that uses the strategy mentioned is directed against lung cancer. In the preclinical phase, the effectiveness of intratumoral administration of vaults loaded with CCL21 in mouse models was demonstrated [33,53]. At these localized sites there is an increase in the activity of the T lymphocytes against the tumor cells which results in the inhibition of their growth. Currently, the project is at the beginning of the development phase I. As future perspectives, the fusion of different ligands or antibodies specific for tumor cells to CCL21-vaults would allow intravenous administration and the possibility of reaching difficult-to-access tumors [74].

Other techniques of activation of the immune system have been used to stop the tumor development. Different cytokines (IL7 and CCL19) [75] have been encapsulated in vault nanoparticles and their effect on tumors is being tested. Another route that is being developed is the encapsulation of antigens characteristic of tumors such as NY-ESO [76], acting the vault as if it were a vaccine, activating the immune system to recognize tumor cells and stop their growth.

On the other hand, the approach to control infectious diseases relies in the controlled encapsulation of specific antigens of certain pathogenic microorganisms (Chlamydia, HIV, Influenza, HPV y Burkholderia), allowing an optimal activation of the immune system by the slow release of immunogenic epitopes from the vault. For example, it has been explored the ability (as vaccines for *Chlamydia trachomatis*) of engineered vaults containing an immunogenic epitope of this pathogen, the polymorphic membrane protein G (PmpG), to be internalized into human monocytes and behave as a "natural adjuvant". Such PmpG-1-vaults were able to activate caspase-1 and to stimulate IL-1β secretion, and immunization of mice with PmpG-1-vaults induced PmpG-1 responsive CD4(+) cells upon restimulation with PmpG peptide in vitro [77]. In another approach to fighting Chlamydia infections [54], the immunogenic protein major outer membrane protein (MOMP) of *Chlamydia muridarum* was encapsulated within hollow, vault nanocapsules (MOMP-vaults) that were engineered to bind IgG for enhanced immunity. Intranasal immunization with such constructions induced anti-chlamydial immunity plus a significantly attenuated bacterial burden following challenge infection. Based on all these backgrounds, Vault Pharma is conducting several clinical trials against different infections, being the most advanced of such trials in their preclinical phases and alert the immune system against Chlamydia, HIV and Influenza pathogens. A brief list of such trials is shown in Table 2.

Table 2. Current vaults applications in nanomedicine. Specific applications are classified according to the stage of their respective clinical trials. Source: https://vaultpharma.com/pipeline/.

Vaults Application	Clinical Trial Stage		
	Drug Discovery	Preclinical	Phase I
Oncology immunology	Pancreatic cancer Prostate cancer Head and neck cancer Renal cancer Bladder cancer Colon cancer Breast cancer Graft vs host disease Pulmonary fibrosis Solid tumors	Lung cancer Melanoma Glioblastoma	Lung cancer
Immunological activation for infection prevention	HPV cancer Burkholderia	Chlamydia HIV/AIDS Influenza	

However, transfer of vaults use to the clinic presents different challenges to overcome. First, current protocols for the production and purification of vaults need to be optimized. Each recombinant vault requires the design, construction and maintenance of a baculovirus vector, a tedious and time-consuming process. In this line, new expression systems (mainly insect larva or yeast cells) are emerging as new actors in the field, with promising (but still preliminary) results. Also, downstream processeses (based on tedious and time-consuming ultracentrifugation steps) need to be optimized.

On the other hand, administration routes for vault-based nanomedicines is another issue that has been explored in detail. Oral administration of vaults—the preferred route of administration in the pharmaceutical industry—presents a clear problem due to the structural changes suffered by the vault in acidic environments such as the stomach. Thus, for this case, vaults would need to be strongly engineered and modified to overcome such barrier. To date, the design of vaults to cross the blood–brain barrier has not been developed. However, the natural presence of vaults in the central nervous system [78] has been identified, suggesting that with the right ligand, vaults could cross the blood–brain barrier without causing damage to the central nervous system. Intranasal administration has also been explored for vault-based nanomedicines containing immunogenic proteins, successfully acting as "smart adjuvants" inducing protective immunity at distant mucosal surfaces while avoiding inflammation. Current clinical trials are focused on the treatment of different tumors by vaults loaded with molecules boosting the immune system. In this case, vaults are locally (intratumoral) administered, thus not taking advantage of the possibility to engineer vaults to specifically target them. This may be due to the interest of obtaining a generalized product for different tumors. The use of targeted and engineered vaults will surely expand the portfolio of available therapies for malignancies and other pathologies in the next years. However, and as far as we know, the immunogenicity of recombinant vaults using other administration routes (as intraperitoneal or intravenous) has not been tested yet.

5. Conclusions and Future Perspectives

Vaults are naturally occurring nanoparticles found widely in eukaryotic cells. They can be produced in recombinant expression systems in large quantities by expressing the MVP protein monomer, which spontaneously self-assembles to originate the final barrel structure. Vaults have been proposed as a new nano-DDS able to improve the efficacy and reduce the side effects of current treatments since they show the characteristics of an ideal nano-DDS: biocompatibility, encapsulation capacity of hydrophobic and hydrophilic molecules, controlled release, and specific targeting, among other features. Its large internal cavity allows the encapsulation of large quantities of molecules of interest. Vaults are a versatile system, in which encapsulation of cargo proteins is achieved by the fusion of the INT domain to the C-terminal end of the therapeutic protein. Non-protein cargo molecules can also be charged inside by modifying the internal cavity of the vault. Moreover, modification of MVP C-terminal end by the fusion of appropriate targeting peptides allows vault specific targeting to cells and organs.

Despite the great potential shown by vaults as smart DDSs, research related to these protein-based nanoparticles has not been blooming as expected for such promising DDS. As mentioned before, a single company holds the intellectual property of vaults through numerous patents covering several aspects related to their production and exploitation. Such protection might represent a factor hampering the further study of vaults by other research groups. However, and despite this potentially discouraging fact, other laboratories are also devoting efforts to the study of different aspects of vaults, from more basic and structural characterization, to their application in fields other than cancer or infectious diseases treatment, confirming vaults as one of the most promising protein-based DDS.

Finally, it is worthy to note that vaults appear at present day as a promising tool not only in the nanomedicine field, but also in another biotechnological applications. A preliminary study [79] showed the development of efficient and sustainable vault-based bioremediation approaches for removing multiple contaminants, such as phenol, from drinking water and groundwater, using vaults loaded with the enzyme manganese peroxidase [80]. In this line, vaults have been recently proposed as a highly efficient system to immobilize enzymes ("nanosupported" enzymes with biodegradative or antimicrobial activities) with potential use as portable water treatment technologies [80]. This will surely expand the opportunities and applications of these protein-based, self-assembled nanoparticle named vaults.

Author Contributions: Conceptualization, A.M.-J. and J.L.C.; writing—original draft preparation, A.M.-J., A.C., and R.M.; writing—review and editing, A.M.-J., A.C., and J.L.C.; supervision, J.L.C.

Acknowledgments: We acknowledge financial support to our research in the field of vault nanoparticles as DDS received from Instituto de Salud Carlos III, through "Acciones CIBER". The Networking Research Center on Bioengineering, Biomaterials, and Nanomedicine (CIBER-BBN) is an initiative funded by the VI National R&D&I Plan 2008-2011, Iniciativa Ingenio 2010, Consolider Program, CIBER Actions and financed by the Instituto de Salud Carlos III with assistance from the European Regional Development Fund. The authors also appreciate the support of Spanish Ministry of Economy and Competitiveness (MINECO) and Instituto de Salud Carlos III through the projects "Design of protein-only nanomedicines for the targeted treatment of pancreatic cancer" (PI17/00553) and "Targeted nanotherapy and combined SBRT radiotherapy for selective elimination of cancer stem cells in pancreatic cancer " (PI17/ 00150), Asociación Española contra el cancer (AECC) through the project "Development of an antitumor protein delivery system into ovarian cancer cells using the subcellular vault", and Centro de Investigación Biomédica en Red (CIBER) de Bioingeniería, Biomateriales y Nanomedicina (project PANCREATOR, "Design of protein nanomedicines for targeted therapies in pancreatic cancer"). We also acknowledge the ICTS "NANBIOSIS", more specifically the support from the Protein Production Platform of CIBER-BBN/IBB, at the UAB SepBioES scientific-technical service (http://www.nanbiosis.es/unit/u1-proteinproduction-platform-ppp/).

References

1. Freitas, R.A. What is nanomedicine? *Nanomed. Nanotechnol. Biol. Med.* **2005**, *1*, 2–9. [CrossRef] [PubMed]
2. Burgess, R. *Understanding nanomedicine: An introductory textbook*; Pan Stanford: Singapore, 2012; ISBN 9789814303521.
3. Safari, J.; Zarnegar, Z. Advanced drug delivery systems: Nanotechnology of health design: A review. *J. Saudi Chem. Soc.* **2014**, *18*, 85–99. [CrossRef]
4. Li, W.; Feng, S.; Guo, Y. Tailoring polymeric micelles to optimize delivery to solid tumors. *Nanomedicine* **2012**, *7*, 1235–1252. [CrossRef] [PubMed]
5. Pridgen, E.M.; Alexis, F.; Farokhzad, O.C. Polymeric nanoparticle drug delivery technologies for oral delivery applications. *Expert Opin. Drug Deliv.* **2015**, *12*, 1459–1473. [CrossRef]
6. Mishra, V.; Bansal, K.; Verma, A.; Yadav, N.; Thakur, S.; Sudhakar, K.; Rosenholm, J. Solid Lipid Nanoparticles: Emerging Colloidal Nano Drug Delivery Systems. *Pharmaceutics* **2018**, *10*, 191. [CrossRef] [PubMed]
7. Beloqui, A.; Solinís, M.Á.; Rodríguez-Gascón, A.; Almeida, A.J.; Préat, V. Nanostructured lipid carriers: Promising drug delivery systems for future clinics. *Nanomed. Nanotechnol. Biol. Med.* **2016**, *12*, 143–161. [CrossRef] [PubMed]
8. Leung, A.W.Y.; Amador, C.; Wang, L.C.; Mody, U.V.; Bally, M.B. What Drives Innovation: The Canadian Touch on Liposomal Therapeutics. *Pharmaceutics* **2019**, *11*, 124. [CrossRef] [PubMed]
9. Jiao, M.; Zhang, P.; Meng, J.; Li, Y.; Liu, C.; Luo, X.; Gao, M. Recent advancements in biocompatible inorganic nanoparticles towards biomedical applications. *Biomater. Sci.* **2018**, *6*, 726–745. [CrossRef]
10. Chauhan, A. Dendrimers for Drug Delivery. *Molecules* **2018**, *23*, 938. [CrossRef]
11. Liu, Y.-L.; Chen, D.; Shang, P.; Yin, D.-C. A review of magnet systems for targeted drug delivery. *J. Control. Release* **2019**, *302*, 90–104. [CrossRef]
12. Hainline, K.M.; Fries, C.N.; Collier, J.H. Progress Toward the Clinical Translation of Bioinspired Peptide and Protein Assemblies. *Adv. Healthc. Mater.* **2018**, *7*, 1700930. [CrossRef] [PubMed]
13. DeFrates, K.; Markiewicz, T.; Gallo, P.; Rack, A.; Weyhmiller, A.; Jarmusik, B.; Hu, X. Protein Polymer-Based Nanoparticles: Fabrication and Medical Applications. *Int. J. Mol. Sci.* **2018**, *19*, 1717. [CrossRef] [PubMed]
14. Moon, H.; Lee, J.; Min, J.; Kang, S. Developing Genetically Engineered Encapsulin Protein Cage Nanoparticles as a Targeted Delivery Nanoplatform. *Biomacromolecules* **2014**, *15*, 3794–3801. [CrossRef] [PubMed]
15. Villaverde, A. *Nanoparticles in translational science and medicine*; Academic Press: London, UK, 2011; ISBN 9780124160200.
16. Elzoghby, A.O.; Samy, W.M.; Elgindy, N.A. Protein-based nanocarriers as promising drug and gene delivery systems. *J. Control. Release* **2012**, *161*, 38–49. [CrossRef] [PubMed]

17. Unzueta Elorza, U. De novo design of self-assembling protein nanoparticles towards the gene therapy of colorectal cancer. PhD Thesis, Universitat Autònoma de Barcelona, Bellaterra, Spain, 28 June 2013.
18. Buehler, D.C.; Marsden, M.D.; Shen, S.; Toso, D.B.; Wu, X.; Loo, J.A.; Zhou, Z.H.; Kickhoefer, V.A.; Wender, P.A.; Zack, X.J.A.; et al. Bioengineered Vaults: Self-Assembling Protein Shell-Lipophilic Core Nanoparticles for Drug Delivery. *ACS Nano* **2014**, *8*, 7723–7732. [CrossRef] [PubMed]
19. Benner, N.L.; Zang, X.; Buehler, D.C.; Kickhoefer, V.A.; Rome, M.E.; Rome, L.H.; Wender, P.A. Vault Nanoparticles: Chemical Modifications for Imaging and Enhanced Delivery. *ACS Nano* **2017**, *11*, 872–881. [CrossRef] [PubMed]
20. Llauró, A.; Guerra, P.; Kant, R.; Bothner, B.; Verdaguer, N.; De Pablo, P.J. Decrease in pH destabilizes individual vault nanocages by weakening the inter-protein lateral interaction. *Sci. Rep.* **2016**, *6*, 1–9. [CrossRef]
21. Zheng, C.L.; Sumizawa, T.; Che, X.F.; Tsuyama, S.; Furukawa, T.; Haraguchi, M.; Gao, H.; Gotanda, T.; Jueng, H.C.; Murata, F.; et al. Characterization of MVP and VPARP assembly into vault ribonucleoprotein complexes. *Biochem. Biophys. Res. Commun.* **2004**, *326*, 100–107. [CrossRef]
22. Anselmo, A.C.; Mitragotri, S. Nanoparticles in the clinic. *Bioeng. Transl. Med.* **2016**, *1*, 10–29. [CrossRef]
23. Chen, L.; Bai, G.; Yang, S.; Yang, R.; Zhao, G. Encapsulation of curcumin in recombinant human H-chain ferritin increases its water-solubility and stability. *FRIN* **2014**, *62*, 1147–1153. [CrossRef]
24. Flenniken, M.L.; Liepold, L.O.; Crowley, B.E.; Willits, D.A.; Young, M.J.; Douglas, T. Selective attachment and release of a chemotherapeutic agent from the interior of a protein cage architecture. *Chem. Commun.* **2005**, *2*, 447–449. [CrossRef] [PubMed]
25. Tanaka, H.; Tsukihara, T. Structural studies of large nucleoprotein particles, vaults. *Japan Acad.* **2012**, *88*, 416–433. [CrossRef] [PubMed]
26. Douglas, T.; Young, M. Viruses: Making Friends with Old Foes. *Science.* **2006**, *312*, 873–875. [CrossRef] [PubMed]
27. Lee, L.; Wang, Q. Adaptations of nanoscale viruses and other protein cages for medical applications. *Nanomedicine Nanotechnology, Biol. Med.* **2006**, *2*, 137–149. [CrossRef]
28. Lee, E.J.; Lee, N.K.; Kim, I.-S. Bioengineered protein-based nanocage for drug delivery. *Adv. Drug Deliv. Rev.* **2016**, *106*, 157–171. [CrossRef]
29. Goldsmith, L.E.; Pupols, M.; Kickhoefer, V.A.; Rome, L.H.; Monbouquette, H.G. Utilization of a Protein "Shuttle" To Load Vault Nanocapsules with Gold Probes and Proteins. *ACS Nano* **2009**, *3*, 3175–3183. [CrossRef]
30. Kedersha, N.L.; Rome, L.H. Isolation and Characterization of a Novel Ribonucleoprotein Particle: Large Structures Contain a Single Species of Small RNA. *J. Cell Biol.* **1986**, *103*, 699–709. [CrossRef]
31. Suprenant, K.A. Vault Ribonucleoprotein Particles: Sarcophagi, Gondolas, or Safety Deposit Boxes? *Biochemistry* **2002**, *41*, 14447–14454. [CrossRef]
32. Liu, S.; Hao, Q.; Peng, N.; Yue, X.; Wang, Y.; Chen, Y.; Wu, J.; Zhu, Y. Major vault protein: A virus-induced host factor against viral replication through the induction of type-I interferon. *Hepatology* **2012**, *56*, 57–66. [CrossRef]
33. Yang, J.; Srinivasan, A.; Sun, Y.; Mrazek, J.; Shu, Z.; Kickhoefer, V.A.; Rome, L.H. Vault nanoparticles engineered with the protein transduction domain, TAT48, enhances cellular uptake. *Integr. Biol.* **2013**, *5*, 151–158. [CrossRef]
34. Kedersha, N.L.; Heuser, J.E.; Chugani, D.C.; Rome, L.H. Vaults. III. Vault ribonucleoprotein particles open into flower-like structures with octagonal symmetry. *J. Cell Biol.* **1991**, *112*, 225–235. [CrossRef] [PubMed]
35. Anderson, D.H.; Kickhoefer, V.A.; Sievers, S.A.; Rome, L.H.; Eisenberg, D. Draft Crystal Structure of the Vault Shell at 9-Å Resolution. *PLoS Biol.* **2007**, *5*, e318. [CrossRef] [PubMed]
36. Tanaka, H.; Kato, K.; Yamashita, E.; Sumizawa, T.; Zhou, Y.; Yao, M.; Iwasaki, K.; Yoshimura, M.; Tsukihara, T. The Structure of Rat Liver Vault at 3.5 Angstrom Resolution. *Science.* **2009**, *323*, 384–388. [CrossRef] [PubMed]
37. Woodward, C.L.; Mendonça, L.M.; Jensen, G.J. Direct visualization of vaults within intact cells by electron cryo-tomography. *Cell. Mol. Life Sci.* **2015**, *72*, 3401–3409. [CrossRef] [PubMed]
38. Querol-Audí, J.; Casañas, A.; Usón, I.; Luque, D.; Castón, J.R.; Fita, I.; Verdaguer, N. The mechanism of vault opening from the high resolution structure of the N-terminal repeats of MVP. *EMBO J.* **2009**, *28*, 3450–3457. [CrossRef] [PubMed]
39. Poderycki, M.J.; Kickhoefer, V.A.; Kaddis, C.S.; Raval-Fernandes, S.; Johansson, E.; Zink, J.I.; Loo, J.A.; Rome, L.H. The vault exterior shell is a dynamic structure that allows incorporation of vault-associated proteins into its interior. *Biochemistry* **2006**, *45*, 12184–12193. [CrossRef] [PubMed]

40. Matsumoto, N.M.; Buchman, G.W.; Rome, L.H.; Maynard, H.D. Dual pH- and temperature-responsive protein nanoparticles. *Eur. Polym. J.* **2015**, *69*, 532–539. [CrossRef]
41. Goldsmith, L.E.; Yu, M.; Rome, L.H.; Monbouquette, H.G. Vault Nanocapsule Dissociation into Halves Triggered at Low pH. *Biochemistry* **2007**, *46*, 2865–2875. [CrossRef]
42. Esfandiary, R.; Kickhoefer, V.A.; Rome, L.H.; Joshi, S.B.; Middaugh, C.R. Structural Stability of Vault Particles. *J. Pharm. Sci.* **2009**, *98*, 1376–1386. [CrossRef]
43. Ding, K.; Zhang, X.; Mrazek, J.; Kickhoefer, V.A.; Lai, M.; Ng, H.L.; Yang, O.O.; Rome, L.H.; Zhou, Z.H. Solution Structures of Engineered Vault Particles. *Structure* **2018**, *26*, 619–626. [CrossRef]
44. Llauró, A.; Guerra, P.; Irigoyen, N.; Rodríguez, J.F.; Verdaguer, N.; de Pablo, P.J. Mechanical stability and reversible fracture of vault particles. *Biophys. J.* **2014**, *106*, 687–695. [CrossRef] [PubMed]
45. Mikyas, Y.; Makabi, M.; Raval-Fernandes, S.; Harrington, L.; Kickhoefer, V.A.; Rome, L.H.; Stewart, P.L. Cryoelectron Microscopy Imaging of Recombinant and Tissue Derived Vaults: Localization of the MVP N Termini and VPARP. *J. Mol. Biol.* **2004**, *344*, 91–105. [CrossRef] [PubMed]
46. Kickhoefer, V.A.; Han, M.; Raval-fernandes, S.; Poderycki, M.J.; Moniz, R.J.; Vaccari, D.; Silvestry, M.; Stewart, P.L.; Kelly, K.A.; Rome, L.H. Targeting Vault Nanoparticles to Specific Cell Surface Receptor. *ACS Nano* **2009**, *3*, 27–36. [CrossRef] [PubMed]
47. Kickhoefer, V.A.; Siva, A.C.; Kedersha, N.L.; Inman, E.M.; Ruland, C.; Streuli, M.; Rome, L.H. The 193-Kd Vault Protein, Vparp, Is a Novel Poly(Adp-Ribose) Polymerase. *J. Cell Biol.* **1999**, *146*, 917–928. [CrossRef] [PubMed]
48. Han, M.; Kickhoefer, V.A.; Nemerow, G.R.; Rome, L.H. Targeted Vault Nanoparticles Engineered with an Endosomolytic Peptide Deliver Biomolecules to the Cytoplasm. *ACS Nano* **2011**, *5*, 6128–6137. [CrossRef] [PubMed]
49. Kickhoefer, V.A.; Garcia, Y.; Mikyas, Y.; Johansson, E.; Zhou, J.C.; Raval-Fernandes, S.; Minoofar, P.; Zink, J.I.; Dunn, B.; Stewart, P.L.; et al. Engineering of vault nanocapsules with enzymatic and fluorescent properties. *Proc. Natl. Acad. Sci. U.S.A.* **2005**, *102*, 4348–4352. [CrossRef]
50. Van Zon, A.; Mossink, M.H.; Schoester, M.; Scheffer, G.L.; Scheper, R.J.; Sonneveld, P.; Wiemer, E.A.C. Structural Domains of Vault Proteins: A Role for the Coiled Coil Domain in Vault Assembly. *Biochem. Biophys. Res. Commun.* **2002**, *291*, 535–541. [CrossRef]
51. Yu, K.; Yau, Y.H.; Sinha, A.; Tan, T.; Kickhoefer, V.A.; Rome, L.H.; Lee, H.; Shochat, S.G.; Lim, S. Modulation of the Vault Protein-Protein Interaction for Tuning of Molecular Release. *Sci. Rep.* **2017**, *7*, 1–10. [CrossRef]
52. Kozlov, G.; Vavelyuk, O.; Minailiuc, O.; Banville, D.; Gehring, K.; Ekiel, I. Solution Structure of a Two-repeat Fragment of Major Vault Protein. *J. Mol. Biol.* **2006**, *356*, 444–452. [CrossRef]
53. Kar, U.K.; Srivastava, M.K.; Andersson, Å.; Baratelli, F.; Huang, M.; Kickhoefer, V.A.; Dubinett, S.M.; Rome, L.H.; Sharma, S. Novel ccl21-vault nanocapsule intratumoral delivery inhibits lung cancer growth. *PLoS One* **2011**, *6*, 4–11. [CrossRef]
54. Champion, C.I.; Kickhoefer, V.A.; Liu, G.; Moniz, R.J.; Freed, A.S.; Bergmann, L.L.; Vaccari, D.; Raval-Fernandes, S.; Chan, A.M.; Rome, L.H.; et al. A vault nanoparticle vaccine induces protective mucosal immunity. *PLoS One* **2009**, *4*, e5409. [CrossRef] [PubMed]
55. Kar, U.K.; Jiang, J.; Champion, C.I.; Salehi, S.; Srivastava, M.; Sharma, S.; Rabizadeh, S.; Niazi, K.; Kickhoefer, V.; Rome, L.H.; et al. Vault nanocapsules as adjuvants favor cell-mediated over antibody-mediated immune responses following immunization of mice. *PLoS One* **2012**, *7*, 1–13. [CrossRef] [PubMed]
56. Yang, J.; Kickhoefer, V.A.; Ng, B.C.; Gopal, A.; Bentolila, L.A.; John, S.; Tolbert, S.H.; Rome, L.H. Vaults Are Dynamically Unconstrained Cytoplasmic Nanoparticles Capable of Half Vault Exchange. *ACS Nano* **2010**, *4*, 7229–7240. [CrossRef] [PubMed]
57. Rome, L.H.; Kickhoefer, V.A. Development of the Vault Particle as a Platform Technology. *ACS Nano* **2013**, *7*, 889–902. [CrossRef] [PubMed]
58. Buehler, D.C.; Toso, D.B.; Kickhoefer, V.A.; Zhou, Z.H.; Rome, L.H. Vaults engineered for hydrophobic drug delivery. *Small* **2011**, *7*, 1432–1439. [CrossRef] [PubMed]
59. Stephen, A.G.; Raval-Fernandes, S.; Huynh, T.; Torres, M.; Kickhoefer, V.A.; Rome, L.H. Assembly of Vault-like Particles in Insect Cells Expressing only the Major Vault Protein. *J. Biol. Chem.* **2001**, *276*, 23217–23220. [CrossRef] [PubMed]
60. Mrazek, D.A.; Hornberger, J.C.; Altar, C.A.; Degtiar, I. A Review of the Clinical, Economic, and Societal Burden of Treatment-Resistant Depression: 1996–2013. *Psychiatr. Serv.* **2014**, *65*, 977–987. [CrossRef]

61. Kushnir, N.; Streatfield, S.J.; Yusibov, V. Virus-like particles as a highly efficient vaccine platform: Diversity of targets and production systems and advances in clinical development. *Vaccine* **2012**, *31*, 58–83. [CrossRef]
62. Fernandes, F.; Teixeira, A.P.; Carinhas, N.; Carrondo, M.J.; Alves, P.M. Insect cells as a production platform of complex virus-like particles. *Expert Rev. Vaccines* **2013**, *12*, 225–236. [CrossRef]
63. Vicente, T.; Roldão, A.; Peixoto, C.; Carrondo, M.J.T.; Alves, P.M. Large-scale production and purification of VLP-based vaccines. *J. Invertebr. Pathol.* **2011**, *107*, S42–S48. [CrossRef]
64. Cregg, J.M.; Cereghino, J.L.; Shi, J.; Higgins, D.R. Recombinant Protein Expression in Pichia pastoris. *Mol. Biotechnol.* **2000**, *16*, 23–52. [CrossRef]
65. Lua, L.H.L.; Connors, N.K.; Sainsbury, F.; Chuan, Y.P.; Wibowo, N.; Middelberg, A.P.J. Bioengineering virus-like particles as vaccines. *Biotechnol. Bioeng.* **2014**, *111*, 425–440. [CrossRef] [PubMed]
66. Wang, M.; Kickhoefer, V.A.; Rome, L.H.; Foellmer, O.K.; Mahendra, S. Synthesis and assembly of human vault particles in yeast. *Biotechnol. Bioeng.* **2018**, *115*, 2941–2950. [CrossRef] [PubMed]
67. Rome, L.H.; Kickhoefer, V.A.; Raval-Fernandes, S.; Stewart, P.L. Vault and vault-like carrier molecules. US Patent US7482319B2, 27 January 2009.
68. Deo, V.K.; Tsuji, Y.; Yasuda, T.; Kato, T.; Sakamoto, N.; Suzuki, H.; Park, E.Y. Expression of an RSV-gag virus-like particle in insect cell lines and silkworm larvae. *J. Virol. Methods* **2011**, *177*, 147–152. [CrossRef]
69. Chung, Y.-C.; Huang, J.-H.; Lai, C.-W.; Sheng, H.-C.; Shih, S.-R.; Ho, M.-S.; Hu, Y.-C. Expression, purification and characterization of enterovirus-71 virus-like particles. *World J. Gastroenterol.* **2006**, *12*, 921. [CrossRef] [PubMed]
70. Morenweiser, R. Downstream processing of viral vectors and vaccines. *Gene Ther.* **2005**, *12*, S103–S110. [CrossRef] [PubMed]
71. Huhti, L.; Blazevic, V.; Nurminen, K.; Koho, T.; Hytönen, V.P.; Vesikari, T. A comparison of methods for purification and concentration of norovirus GII-4 capsid virus-like particles. *Arch. Virol.* **2010**, *155*, 1855–1858. [CrossRef]
72. Galbiati, E.; Avvakumova, S.; La Rocca, A.; Pozzi, M.; Messali, S.; Magnaghi, P.; Colombo, M.; Prosperi, D.; Tortora, P. A fast and straightforward procedure for vault nanoparticle purification and the characterization of its endocytic uptake. *Biochim. Biophys. Acta - Gen. Subj.* **2018**, *1862*, 2254–2260. [CrossRef]
73. Izquierdo, M.A.; Scheffer, G.L.; Flens, M.J.; Giaccone, G.; Broxterman, H.J.; Meijer, C.J.; van der Valk, P.; Scheper, R.J. Broad distribution of the multidrug resistance-related vault lung resistance protein in normal human tissues and tumors. *Am. J. Pathol.* **1996**, *148*, 877–887.
74. Sharma, S.; Zhu, L.; Srivastava, M.K.; Harris-White, M.; Huang, M.; Lee, J.M.; Rosen, F.; Lee, G.; Wang, G.; Kickhoefer, V.; et al. CCL21 Chemokine Therapy for Lung Cancer. *Int Trends Immun* **2013**, *1*, 10–15.
75. Vault Pharma An Immunology Biotech Company. Available online: https://vaultpharma.com/ (accessed on 29 April 2019).
76. Endo, M.; De Graaff, M.A.; Ingram, D.R.; Lim, S.; Lev, D.C.; Briaire-De Bruijn, I.H.; Somaiah, N.; Bovée, J.V.M.G.; Lazar, A.J.; Nielsen, T.O. NY-ESO-1 (CTAG1B) expression in mesenchymal tumors. *Mod. Pathol.* **2015**, *28*, 587–595. [CrossRef] [PubMed]
77. Zhu, Y.; Jiang, J.; Said-Sadier, N.; Boxx, G.; Champion, C.; Tetlow, A.; Kickhoefer, V.A.; Rome, L.H.; Ojcius, D.M.; Kelly, K.A. Activation of the NLRP3 inflammasome by vault nanoparticles expressing a chlamydial epitope. *Vaccine* **2015**, *33*, 298–306. [CrossRef] [PubMed]
78. Yang, J.; Nagasawa, D.T.; Spasic, M.; Amolis, M.; Choy, W.; Garcia, H.M.; Prins, R.M.; Liau, L.M.; Yang, I. Endogenous Vaults and Bioengineered Vault Nanoparticles for Treatment of Glioblastomas. *Neurosurg. Clin. N. Am.* **2012**, *23*, 451–458. [CrossRef] [PubMed]
79. Wang, M.; Abad, D.; Kickhoefer, V.A.; Rome, L.H.; Mahendra, S. Vault Nanoparticles Packaged with Enzymes as an Efficient Pollutant Biodegradation Technology. *ACS Nano* **2015**, *9*, 10931–10940. [CrossRef] [PubMed]
80. Wang, M.; Chen, Y.; Kickhoefer, V.A.; Rome, L.H.; Allard, P.; Mahendra, S. A Vault-Encapsulated Enzyme Approach for Efficient Degradation and Detoxification of Bisphenol A and Its Analogues. *ACS Sustain. Chem. Eng.* **2019**, *7*, 5808–5817.

4

Interaction of Poly(L-lysine)/Polysaccharide Complex Nanoparticles with Human Vascular Endothelial Cells

Dominik Weber [1], Bernhard Torger [2], Karsten Richter [3], Michelle Nessling [3], Frank Momburg [1], Beatrice Woltmann [4], Martin Müller [5,6,*] and Reinhard Schwartz-Albiez [1]

1 Deutsches Krebsforschungszentrum (DKFZ), Clinical Cooperation Unit Applied Tumor Immunology, D-69120 Heidelberg, Germany; weberdominik@hotmail.de (D.W.); f.momburg@dkfz-heidelberg.de (F.M.); r.s-albiez@dkfz-heidelberg.de (R.S.-A.)

2 Institute of Plant and Wood Chemistry, Technische Universität Dresden, D-01737 Tharandt, Germany; bernhard.torger@tu-dresden.de

3 Deutsches Krebsforschungszentrum (DKFZ), Central Unit Electron Microscopy, D-69120 Heidelberg, Germany; k.richter@dkfz.de (K.R.); m.nessling@dkfz-heidelberg.de (M.N.)

4 Institute of Physiological Chemistry, Faculty of Medicine Carl Gustav Carus, Technische Universität Dresden, 01307 Dresden, Germany; beatrice.woltmann@mailbox.tu-dresden.de

5 Department Polyelectrolytes and Dispersions, Leibniz-Institut für Polymerforschung Dresden e.V., Hohe Straße 6, D-01069 Dresden, Germany

6 Department of Chemistry and Food Chemistry, Technische Universität Dresden, D-01062 Dresden, Germany

* Correspondence: mamuller@ipfdd.de;

Abstract: Angiogenesis plays an important role in both soft and hard tissue regeneration, which can be modulated by therapeutic drugs. If nanoparticles (NP) are used as vectors for drug delivery, they have to encounter endothelial cells (EC) lining the vascular lumen, if applied intravenously. Herein the interaction of unloaded polyelectrolyte complex nanoparticles (PECNP) composed of cationic poly(L-lysine) (PLL) and various anionic polysaccharides with human vascular endothelial cells (HUVEC) was analyzed. In particular PECNP were tested for their cell adhesive properties, their cellular uptake and intracellular localization considering composition and net charge. PECNP may form a platform for both cell coating and drug delivery. PECNP, composed of PLL in combination with the polysaccharides dextran sulfate (DS), cellulose sulfate (CS) or heparin (HEP), either unlabeled or labeled with fluorescein isothiocyanate (FITC) and either with positive or negative net charge were prepared. PECNP were applied to human umbilical cord vein endothelial cells (HUVEC) in both, the volume phase and immobilized phase at model substrates like tissue culture dishes. The attachment of PECNP to the cell surface, their intracellular uptake, and effects on cell proliferation and growth behavior were determined. Immobilized PECNP reduced attachment of HUVEC, most prominently the systems PLL/HEP and PLL/DS. A small percentage of immobilized PECNP was taken up by cells during adhesion. PECNP in the volume phase showed no effect of the net charge sign and only minor effects of the composition on the binding and uptake of PECNP at HUVEC. PECNP were stored in endosomal vesicles in a cumulative manner without apparent further processing. During mitosis, internalized PECNP were almost equally distributed among the dividing cells. Both, in the volume phase and immobilized at the surface, PECNP composed of PLL/HEP and PLL/DS clearly reduced cell proliferation of HUVEC, however without an apparent cytotoxic effect, while PLL/CS composition showed minor impairment. PECNP have an anti-adhesive effect on HUVEC and are taken up by endothelial cells which may negatively influence the proliferation rate of HUVEC. The negative effects were less obvious with the composition PLL/CS. Since uptake and binding for PLL/HEP was more efficient than for PLL/DS, PECNP of PLL/HEP may be used to deliver growth factors to endothelial cells during vascularization of bone reconstitution material, whereas those of PLL/CS may have an advantage for substituting biomimetic bone scaffold material.

Keywords: poly(L-lysine); cellulose sulfate; dextran sulfate; heparin; polyelectrolyte complex nanoparticle (PECNP); vascular endothelial cells; cell attachment; cellular uptake; proliferation

1. Introduction

Angiogenesis plays an important role in both soft and hard tissue regeneration, which can be modulated by therapeutic drugs. Dispersed nanoparticles (NP) can be used to deliver drugs, growth factors or genes to distinct tissues, or NP immobilized at given implants or bone substitution materials (BSM) can be used to increase their biophysical stability, biocompatibility, and cell adherence [1]. When incorporated into scaffold matrices they may additionally support their mechanical stability and enhance biocompatibility of the implanted scaffold material [2]. For both modes of application, vascular endothelial cells represent the prime cellular target as they are port of entry for drugs from the blood circulation into tissue and are essential for the vascularization of tissue reconstitution material [3]. When used as soluble carriers for e.g., anti-cancer drugs, nanoparticles coated with distinct protein ligands for specific cell surface receptors can be directed to the respective tumor tissue thereby improving the pharmacokinetics and pharmacodynamics of the respective cytotoxic drug [4,5]. In particular, encapsulation of these drugs in nanoparticles may increase their half-life in the blood circulation and enhance their concentration in the tumor tissue [6,7]. In order to reach tumor cells, nanoparticles have to overwhelm barriers of the tumor microenvironment which are represented, as one of the first steps, by the endothelial layer of blood vessels during the extravasation of the drug delivery system.

A possible strategy to enhance migration and settlement of vascular endothelial cells, thereby initiating neo-angiogenesis, could be to integrate modified nanoparticles into scaffolds. For instance, attempts have been described to stabilize and controllably release the endothelial chemokine VEGF (vascular endothelial growth factor) by binding to polysaccharide-conjugated polyelectrolyte complexes [8].

In order to find an effective nanoparticle vehicle for delivery of growth factors, cytotoxic drugsor adhesion proteins to vascular endothelial cells, several factors such as composition, size, and charge of nanoparticles with regard to their endothelial binding, uptake, and possible cytotoxicity have to be analyzed [9,10]. Various nanoparticle systems composed of charged polysaccharides, polypeptides or synthetic polyelectrolytes have been used as drug delivery systems [11–13] and may also support cellular ingrowth into a scaffold material [14–16].

Nanoparticles containing biopolymers such as polysaccharides can support controlled release of drugs and cellular adhesion within scaffold material [17,18]. Heparin based nanoparticles have been shown to improve biocompatibility of nanoparticles in various applications [19].

In our study, we applied polyelectrolyte complex nanoparticles (PECNP), composed of the polycation poly(L-lysine) (PLL) combined with the three anionic polysaccharides dextran sulfate (DS), cellulose sulfate (CS) or heparin (HEP), to human umbilical cord vein endothelial cells in vitro (HUVEC) and investigated their effect on cell binding, uptake, intracellular localization, proliferation, as well as on cellular attachment to surfaces and subsequent migration. We analyzed the influence of the composition, namely the effect of the anionic polysaccharides CS, DS, HEP within PECNP, both in the volume phase and immobilized at a model substrate. As an additional feature we used PECNP with either positive or negative net charge, which can be achieved by mixing polycation and polyanion solutions in defined ratios [11]. The potential of these PECNP with regard to directed sizing (20–500 nm), shaping (spheres, rods), and controlled charge of their surfaces has been outlined previously [11].

Adhesive coatings of PECNP were previously investigated for their loading and retarded release of distinct drugs such as bisphosphonates [12,20] and for the effect of their composition on the viability of human mesenchymal stromal cells (hMSC) [21] in the context of bone healing and remodeling. To go further, their interaction to human vascular endothelial cells (HUVEC) is now addressed in the context of angiogenesis during bone healing.

2. Materials and Methods

2.1. Preparation of Polyelectrolyte Complex Nanoparticles (PECNP)

Polyelectrolyte complex nanoparticles (PECNP) composed of the polycation poly(L-lysine) (PLL, M_W = 50,000 g/mol, (Sigma-Aldrich, Schnelldorf, Germany), in combination with the polyanions cellulose sulfate (CS, degree of substitution d_S = 2.8, M_W = 1,200,000 g/mol, Janssen, Beerse, Belgium), dextran sulfate (DS, d_S = 3.0, M_W = 500,000 g/mol, Carl Roth GmbH, Germany) or heparin (HEP, M_W = 20,000 g/mol, Carl Roth GmbH, Karlsruhe, Germany) and the fluorescein isothiocyanate (FITC) labeled PECNP species were prepared as described in detail elsewhere [11,21,22]. Briefly summarized, 2 mM clear solutions of cationic PLL and anionic CS, DS or HEP were mixed at pH = 7.0 and more or less turbid (milky) dispersions resulted. According to their molar number of charged repeating units (n+: molar number of cationic repeating units; n−: molar number of anionic repeating units) two molar mixing ratios denoted n−/n+ were applied, which were n−/n+ = 0.9 and n−/n+ = 1.1. These two molar mixing ratios resulted in PECNP, which had a slightly positive net charge (PECNP-0.9, n−/n+ = 0.9, cationic excess) or slightly negative net charge (PECNP-1.1, n−/n+ = 1.1, anionic excess), which was proven by zeta-potential measurements (see below). Furthermore, sizes i.e., hydrodynamic radii R_H of these PECNP were determined by dynamic light scattering (see below). The particle sizes of the herein used PECNP can be found in the Table 1.

Table 1. Hydrodynamic radius (R_H), zeta-potential at pH = 7.4, PLL conformation and morphology (dry spin coated state at poly(styrene) (PS) film) of the PECNP samples used in this work. Numbers of individual measurements are given in brackets. The data have been partly already given in [21], whereby slight deviations within the error range might prevail.

PECNP Sample	R_H/nm	Zeta-Potential/mV	PLL Conformation	Morphology
PLL/CS-0.9	106 ± 7 (#9)	+45 + 5 mV	α-helical	granular, spherical
PLL/DS-0.9	69 ± 12 (#14)	+45 + 5 mV	α-helical	-
PLL/HEP-0.9	62 ± 8 (#3)	—	α-helical	-
PLL/CS-1.1	101 ± 10 (#13)	−43 + 5 mV	α-helical	granular, spherical
PLL/DS-1.1	88 ± 17 (#8)	−44 + 5 mV	α-helical	granular, spherical
PLL/HEP-1.1	67 ± 7 (#6)	—	α-helical	granular, spherical

2.2. Dynamic Light Scattering (DLS)

Hydrodynamic radii (R_H) of PECNP were determined by DLS using Jianke Portable Particle Sizer (Jianke Instruments Co. Ltd., Wuhu, China). A scattering angle of 89.3° was applied. Two mL of PECNP dispersions were filled in cuvettes with a circular bottom (D = 10 mm). The autocorrelation function was recorded for 180 s and R_H values were calculated from values of the translational diffusion coefficient D using the Stokes–Einstein equation $R_H = k_BT/(D\, 6\, \pi\eta)$ (Boltzmann constant k_B; temperature T = 298 K; and viscosity η). The ALV-5000/E/EPP-Software (ALV GmbH, Langen, Germany) was used for the computation of DLS parameters applying the "Simple Fit" tool. Intensity weighted size distributions were computed and plotted. Error values of R_H given in Table 1 were related to the standard deviation of (3–14) individual but equally prepared PECNP samples.

2.3. Zeta-Potential

The Zeta-potential measurements on PECNP dispersions in order to determine the net charge of PECNP were performed at neutral pH values (pH = 7.4) using a Zetasizer 3000 (Malvern Instruments Ltd., Worchestershire, UK).

2.4. Cells

HUVEC (human umbilical cord vein endothelial cells, PromoCell, Heidelberg, Germany) were cultivated in endothelial cell basal media full medium (ECBM-FM; PromoCell) consisting of endothelial cell basal media supplemented with 10% fetal bovine serum (FBS) and endothelial cell growth medium supplement (PromoCell). Cells were cultured at 37 °C, 5% CO_2 atmosphere and 95% relative humidity. HUVEC were split before reaching confluence and were used up to cell culture passage 6 for functional assays. HUVEC were detached using the Detach Kit (PromoCell) according to the manufacturers' protocol. In detail, cells were washed with HEPES (4-(2-hydroxyethyl)-1-piperazineethanesulfonic acid) and subsequently with trypsin/EDTA (Ethylenediaminetetraacetic acid) for a few seconds. Cells were then detached by applying fresh trypsin/EDTA to the cells. As soon as cells started to detach the cell culture flask was gently tapped to detach the remaining adherent cells. The enzymatic reaction was stopped using trypsin neutralizing solution (PromoCell). All cells were cultured under sterile conditions at 37 °C, 5% CO_2 atmosphere, and 95% relative humidity. Fresh media exchanges were performed twice a week.

2.5. Growth Pattern of HUVEC on PECNP

PECNP (100 μL/cm^2 of a 2 mM PECNP dispersion) were immobilized on the bottom of an 8-well-μ-slide, ibiTreat (Ibidi, Martinsried, Germany) on a waving platform shaker under sterile conditions overnight at room temperature. HUVEC (4×10^4 cells in 300 μL basal ECBM medium) were seeded into the wells and photographic microscopy images were acquired after 0, 10, and 20 h of incubation using a ZEISS cell observer. (Carl Zeiss, Oberkochen, Germany).

2.6. Cellular Uptake of Immobilized PECNP (Light Microscopy)

Fluorescein isothiocyanate (FITC)-labeled PECNP (52.6 μL/cm^2 of a 2 mM dispersion) were immobilized under motion on a 24-well plate overnight. Then, wells were washed with phosphate buffered saline (PBS), 4×10^4 HUVEC were seeded on the PECNP layer in 1 mL basal ECBM and incubated at 37 °C and 5% CO_2 and 95% relative humidity for 24 h. The media were then replaced with fresh basal ECBM and cells were incubated for another 24 h. For further analysis, cells were detached and transferred to an 8-well-μ-slide–ibiTreat. After 24 h of incubation in ECBM-FM, cells were fixed as indicated below.

For fluorescence microscopic analysis of the cellular uptake of dispersed PECNP, 2.3×10^4 cells were seeded on an 8-well μ-slide–ibiTreat and FITC-labeled PECNP were added to the attached cells for 1 h, 4 h, and 24 h after exchange of culture media to ECBM. The uptake of PECNP was stopped by washing the cells with Ca^{2+}/Mg^{2+}-containing PBS followed by fixation with 4% paraformaldehyde (PFA) in PBS (*v/v*) for 10 min at room temperature. After 3 washing steps in PBS, 4 drops of iTFx Signal Enhancer (Thermo Fisher, Dreieich, Germany) were applied for 30 min to block unspecific binding. HUVEC were then incubated with biotinylated anti-CD31 mouse mAb (PECAM-1, platelet/endothelial cell adhesion molecule 1; Becton&Dickenson (B&D), Heidelberg, Germany) for 30 min followed by a Cy3-coupled streptavidin antibody (Dianova, Hamburg, Germany) for 30 min. Cell nuclei were stained with Hoechst 33342 (Biotium, Fremont, CA, USA) for 10 min. For preservation, fluorescent mounting media (Dako, Hamburg, Germany) was added to the cells. Cells were analyzed using a widefield microscope (Zeiss Cell Observer Z1; Carl Zeiss, Oberkochen, Germany) and a confocal microscope (Leica TCS SP5 II, Wetzlar, Germany).

2.7. Analysis of Cellular Interactions with PECNP (Transmission Electron Microscopy, TEM)

ACLAR film slides (Redding, CA, USA) were placed in 24-well plates and 1×10^5 HUVEC were seeded on top in 1 mL media and incubated for 24 h at 37 °C, 5% CO_2, and 95% relative humidity. A volume of 25 μL of a 2 mM PECNP dispersion was added to the media (final dilution 1:40) for 4 h. Incubation was stopped by the addition of a primary fixative (4% formaldehyde,2% glutaraldehyde and 1 mM $MgCl_2$, in 100 mM sodium phosphate buffer at pH 7.2). Following two post-fixations steps, buffered OsO_4 (1%) and ethanolic uranyl acetate (0.5%), respectively, samples were flat-embedded in epoxy resin (Serva, Heidelberg, Germany) for ultrathin sectioning. Sections were post-stained with uranyl and lead and investigated by TEM (EM912, Carl Zeiss, Oberkochen, Germany).

2.8. Analysis of Cellular Interactions with Fluorescent PECNP (Flow Cytometry)

Detached HUVEC were incubated with PE-conjugated mouse antibodies against CD31 on ice for 30 min in the dark. For setting parameters of live-dead discrimination, HUVECs were incubated in parallel with 4% PFA in another reaction tube. After two washing steps, cells were resuspended in 100 µL of basal culture medium (i.e., ECBM) containing FITC-labeled PECNP (1:40 dilution of a 2 mM stock suspension) and incubated for 1 h. After careful washing, cells were resuspended in a 1:15 dilution of BD-via probe^{TM} (B&D, Heidelberg, Germany) for exclusion of dead cells. Flow cytometric analysis was performed using a BD FACS Canto^{TM} II (BD Biosciences, San Jose, CA, USA), analyzing 50.000 cells/sample, and data were analyzed by the FlowJo^{TM} software (Version 10, Ashland, OR, USA). Background values for PE- and FITC-fluorescence were calculated using unstained cells. In order to analyze PECNP internalization, cells incubated with FITC-labeled PECNP were analyzed for their fluorescence signal intensity. Then, trypan blue was added to the samples and the signal intensity was re-analyzed resulting only in the excitation of the internalized PECNP as the signal of PECNP on the surface was quenched [23]. For analysis of uptake kinetic, HUVEC were incubated with FITC-labeled PECNP for 5, 30, 60, or 120 min. HUVECs were first analyzed for the total amount of cell-associated FITC-label (PECNP signal). Then, 120 µL of a 0.4 mg/mL solution of trypan blue was added to the cells and samples were immediately measured again. Unlabeled HUVEC were used as negative control (threshold value for FITC-signal). Each measurement was performed for 10,000 cells.

2.9. Analysis of Cell Proliferation ([^{3}H]-Thymidine Incorporation Assay)

PECNP in several concentrations (2.5, 5, 10, 50 µL/cm^2 of a 2 mM PECNP stock dispersion, diluted in sterile water) were immobilized on a 96-well tissue culture plate. For this, PECNP were applied to the bottom of the wells of a tissue culture plate under sterile conditions, and incubated overnight under motion on a waving platform shaker at room temperature. HUVEC were seeded in triplicates in media without heparin (Promocell culture media supplement DM2, PromoCell, Heidelberg, Germany) on PECNP-coated 96-well plates at a cell density of 3.5×10^3 cells/well. Cells were allowed to adhere for 2–4 h and then 1 µCi [^{3}H]-thymidine/well was applied. For analyzing the influence of dispersed PECNP on proliferation, HUVEC were seeded into 96-well plates, incubated at 37 °C and 5% CO_2 and 95% relative humidity for 1 h and 10 µL of PECNP solution in the concentrations as indicated above was added to the culture media. Then, 1 µCi [^{3}H]-thymidine was added to the media. All tissue culture plates were incubated under cell culture condition for 24–26 h. The incubation was stopped as cells were detached and frozen. For this, the cell media was carefully removed and 200 µL of a solution of trypsin-EDTA (Detach kit, PromoCell) was applied to the well. The plates were incubated at 37 °C for 5–10 min and the cells were subsequently frozen at −20 °C. An additional thawing–freezing step was applied and the cell debris (including the cellular DNA) was transferred to a printed filter mat A (PerkinElmer, Waltham, MA, USA) using a TomTec harvester (TomTec, Hamden, CT, USA). The dried filters were transferred to a sample bag (PerkinElmer) and the [^{3}H]-thymidine incorporated into DNA was measured using a Betaplate scintillator and a MicroBeta TriLux scintillator counter (both PerkinElmer).

3. Results and Discussion

We analyzed the influence of composition and net charge of biorelated polyelectrolyte complex nanoparticles (PECNP) on human umbilical cord vein endothelial cells (HUVEC) with regard to their effect on cell adhesion, uptake, and cytotoxicity. Biorelated cationic poly(L-lysine) (PLL) was combined with the three biorelated anionic polysaccharides cellulose sulfate (CS), dextran sulfate (DS), and heparin (HEP) resulting in the PECNP of PLL/CS, PLL/DS, and PLL/HEP. The interaction to HUVEC was studied for PECNP in the volume phase as well as bound at model substrates such as tissue culture plates. In the following, first colloidal properties of the used PECNP systems are introduced (Section 3.1), second, results on the interfacial interaction between HUVEC and immobilized PECNP coatings (Section 3.2), and third interaction between HUVEC and PECNP in the volume phase (Section 3.3) are shown. Finally, proliferation of HUVEC in contact to PECNP in both states will be screened (Section 3.4).

3.1. Colloidal Properties of PECNP

Six PECNP systems composed of PLL/CS, PLL/DS, and PLL/HEP with positive and negative net charge, indicated as PLL/polysaccharide-0.9 (n−/n+ = 0.9) or PLL/polysaccharide-1.1 (n−/n+ = 1.1), respectively, were prepared. Their colloidal parameters hydrodynamic radius (R_H), from dynamic light scattering (DLS) measurements, as well as net charge from zeta-potential measurements are summarized in Table 1.

Generally, the R_H values (sizes) of all PECNP ranged between 62–106 nm, where PECNP of PLL/CS (101–106 nm) were considerably larger, and those of PLL/DS (69–88 nm) and PLL/HEP (62–67 nm) smaller. However, given the obvious molecular weight (M_W) differences of the polyanions (see Materials and Methods section) no correlation between M_W (CS > DS > HEP) and PECNP size (CS > DS > HEP) should be drawn within the given error range. Hence for all compositions HUVEC should encounter PECNP with diameters $D_H = 2\ R_H$ between ≈ 120–210 nm. Expectedly, PECNP with slight excess of polycation (n−/n+ = 0.9, PEC-0.9) featured positive, while those with slight excess of polyanion (n−/n+ = 1.1, PEC-1.1) featured anionic net charge at pH = 7.4, which was detected by zeta-potential measurements. The extended zeta-potential courses versus pH are given in the Supplementary Material (SM, Figure SM1a–d) for PLL/CS and PLL/DS (data on PLL/HEP not shown). Obviously, for all compositions the cationic PECNP (n−/n+ = 0.9) showed a drop of positive zeta-potential beginning at around pH = 9, which is due to the deprotonation of PLL primary amino groups having isoelectrical point IEP ≈ 9.5. Whereas, anionic PECNP (n−/n+ = 1.1) kept their negative zeta-potential for the whole pH range at values in the range −50 to −40 mV.

Furthermore, the conformation state of PLL within PECNP was studied both in the volume phase by circular dichroism (CD) spectroscopy and bound to polystyrene (PS) films relevant for the cell culture experiments by attenuated total reflection Fourier transform infrared (ATR-FTIR) spectroscopy. In Figure SM2 CD spectra on 0.002 M dispersions of PLL/CS-1.1, PLL/DS-1.1 and PLL/HEP-1.1 are given, which all show a doublet at 208/225 nm with negative intensity as well as a positive signal at 195 nm, both diagnostic for the α-helical secondary structure (similar data for PLL/CS-0.9, PLL/DS-0.9, and PLL/HEP-0.9 is not shown). Additionally, in the Figure SM3 ATR-FTIR spectra on respective PECNP samples bound to PS films show Amide I and Amide II maxima at 1653 and 1546 cm^{-1}, which are also diagnostic for the α-helical secondary structure of PLL (similar data for PLL/DS-0.9 and PLL/HEP-0.9 is not shown). The PLL conformation state for all six PECNP samples is included in the Table 1.

Finally, scanning force microscopy (SFM) images of spin-coated PECNP at poly(styrene) (PS) films after rinsing in HEPES buffer given in the Figure SM4 of the SM show dense coverage and granular morphology of merged and single PECNP, which is summarized in the Table 1. Interestingly, for PLL/CS-0.9 (Figure SM4a) the presence of both microparticles and nanoparticles can be identified, where the microparticle seems to be composed of nanoparticles ("blackberry model") as was also claimed for complexes between synthetic polyelectrolytes earlier [24].

Conclusively, all three PECNP compositions PLL/CS, PLL/DS, and PLL/HEP for both positive (n−/n+ = 0.9) and negative (n−/n+ = 1.1) net charge did not show substantial differences in their colloidal behavior with respect to size and net charge magnitude and also on the secondary structure as well as morphology level there were no significant differences. Hence in the following in-vitro experiments on the PECNP interaction with HUVEC, argumentation on a chemical level should be justified.

3.2. Cell Growth on Immobilized PECNP Coatings

In order to see what impact these PECNP in immobilized state have on the growth behavior of HUVECs , surfaces of various cell culture dishes and microscopic slides were coated with PECNP, modified by CS, DS, and HEP. Additionally, for fluorescence microscopy and flow cytometric analysis also PECNP labeled with FITC were applied. Light microscopy of immobilized PECNP on slides revealed, that even under constant motion during coating, PECNP did not spread and attach homogeneously on the bottom of 8-well ibiTreat slides, coated with 100 μL/cm^2 of a 0.4 mM dispersion of the respective PECNP, which can be obtained from Figure 1A and 1B. HUVEC seemed to avoid areas coated with high concentrations of PECNP. This was also demonstrated by coating the slides with a higher concentration of PECNP (100 μL/cm^2 of a 2 mM dispersion). Cell attachment in areas with high concentration of PECNP (ring-shaped areas) was less dense as compared to those with lower concentration of PECNP, which is shown in kinetics of cell growth on these slides (Figure 1C). This effect was most prominent for PECNP composed of PLL/HEP and PLL/DS (Figure 1C, black dashed line), which grew in a web-shaped manner. As compared to control cultures without PECNP-coating, cells grew in a looser, reticular pattern on PLL/CS PECNP (Figure 1C, dashed red line).

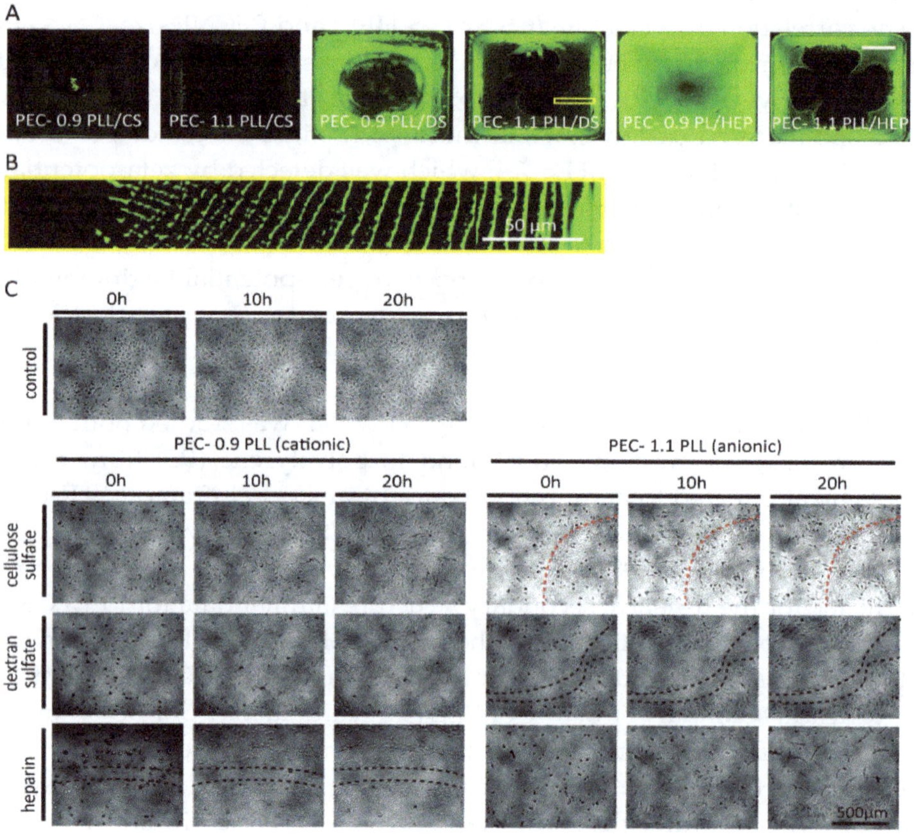

Figure 1. Influence of immobilized polyelectrolyte complex nanoparticles (PECNP) on human umbilical cord vein endothelial cells (HUVEC) seeding. Microscopic images of PECNP distribution on various areas of slide surface (scale bar: 250 μm). Cationic (0.9) or anionic (1.1) PECNP composed of poly(L-lysine) (PLL) and either cellulose sulfate (CS), dextran sulfate (DS) or heparin (HEP) were used. (**A**) PECNP in some cases attached to the surface during the drying process in ring-shaped patterns which entailed areas of high and low PECNP concentration (Scale bar: 250 μm); (**B**) Magnification of PEC-1.1 PLL/DS from A—ring-shaped pattern of dried PECNP; (**C**) PECNP immobilized on Ibidi-slides at high concentrations (100 μL/cm^2 of a 2 mM PECNP dispersion). PECNP distributed inhomogeneously on the surface of the 8-well μ-slide–ibiTreat slides during the drying process. HUVEC cells (4×10^4 cells) were seeded onto the slides and photos were taken at times indicated. Depending on the modification and concentration of PECNP applied, alterations in cell growth and adhesion patterns were observed. Cells avoided areas with higher concentrations of PECNP as outlined by black dashed lines. This effect was most prominent for PECNP composed of PLL/DS-1.1 and of PLL/HEP-0.9. Cells grew in a looser, web-shaped pattern on PECNP of PLL/CS. High concentrations of PLL/CS (red dashed line) had less effect than PLL/DS or PLL/HEP PECNP.

3.3. Cell Growth on Dispersed PECNP in the Volume Phase

3.3.1. Cell Surface Attachment of PECNP

The next issues to be studied were whether and to what extent PECNP in the volume phase attach to the cell surface and are further taken up by HUVECs. The attachment process was quantified by flow cytometric analysis using fluorescein isothiocyanate (FITC)-labeled PECNP in dispersion. For measuring cell surface attachment, HUVEC were incubated with FITC-labeled PECNP on ice for 1 h and the amount of PECNP on the cell surface of live cells was estimated (Figure 2). Apparently, cell surface attachment of PECNP of PLL/HEP, regardless of net charge was slightly better than that of PLL/CS and PLL/DS. An obvious reason for this may be that heparin is an endogenous molecule of mammalian physiology and that heparin may interfere with surface receptors on HUVEC like VEGF-R2 or the hyaluronic acid receptor for endocytosis (HARE) [25]. Thus the charge of interfering particles with, as a rule, slightly negatively charged cell surfaces is less decisive than functional interaction with a specific cell surface receptor for binding efficacy.

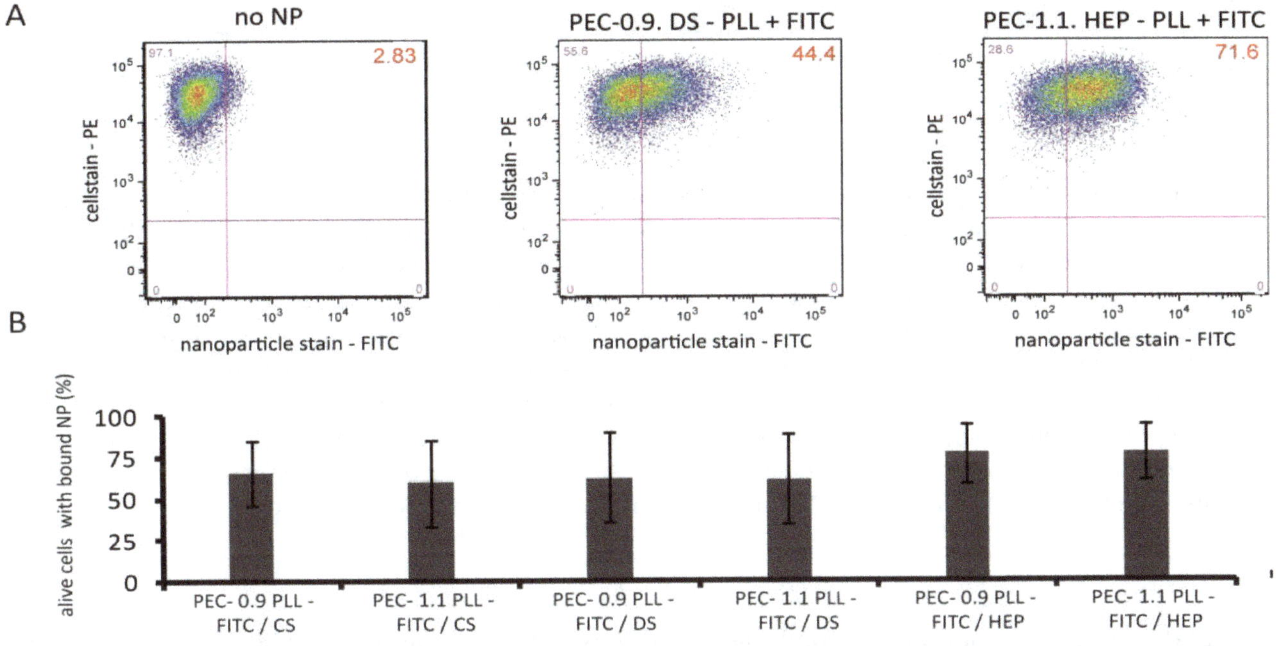

Figure 2. Interaction of polyelectrolyte complex nanoparticles (PECNP) with the cell surface of human umbilical cord vein endothelial cells (HUVEC). HUVEC were incubated on ice for 1 h with fluorescein isothiocyanate (FITC)-labeled PECNP, cells were stained with an anti-CD31 monoclonal antibody conjugated to PE and subjected to flow cytometric analysis. (**A**) Cells were live-gated by VIA-probe and gated according to CD31-PE surface staining (y-axis) and FITC staining (x-axis). As negative control, cells without FITC-labeled PECNP were taken and gates set accordingly. Cells with bound FITC-labeled PECNP were counted in comparison to negative control (percentage of positive cells given for each analysis, right upper quadrant); (**B**) Percentage of cells with surface-bound PECNP compared to control without PECNP set as 100%, mean ± SD, number of experiments: $n = 4$. CS = cellulose sulfate, DS = dextran sulfate, HEP = heparin-containing PECNP.

3.3.2. Cellular Uptake of PECNP

In a next step, the uptake of PECNP was measured in comparison to cell surface attachment in a kinetic experiment (Figure 3). In this experiment, PECNP composed of PLL/CS were picked out and incubated for up to 120 min with HUVECs under cell culture conditions. The cell surface attachment was distinguished from uptake by quenching the FITC signal on the cell surface by trypan blue.

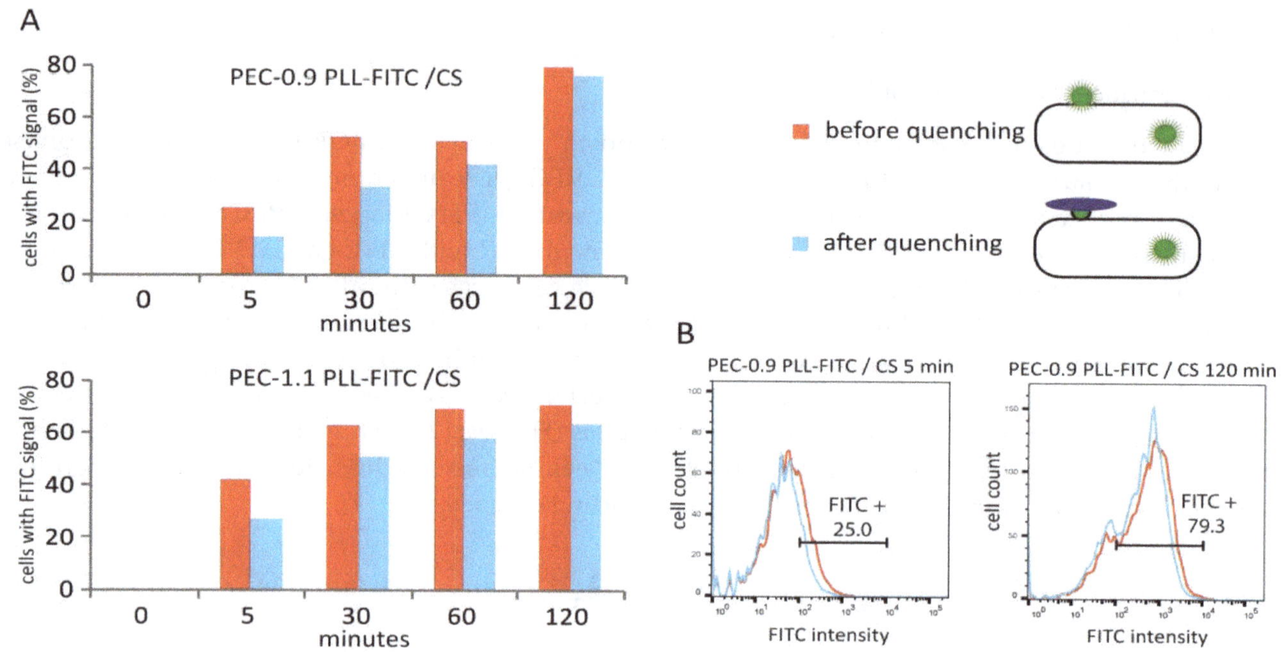

Figure 3. Analysis of polyelectrolyte complex nanoparticles (PECNP) internalization into human umbilical cord vein endothelial cells (HUVEC). FITC-labeled PECNP were incubated with HUVEC for 5 to 120 min, HUVEC were detached and immediately prepared for flow cytometric analysis. Cells were live-gated (VIA-probe) and further gated according to their scatter signals (forward (FSC) vs. sideward scatter signal (SSC)). Cells without PECNP incubation were taken as controls to set the background threshold for PECNP-FITC interaction. Cells were measured and the percentage of cells with bound PECNP in relation to the controls was determined (red bars in (**A**) histograms, red lines in (**B**) flow cytometric diagrams). By the addition of trypan blue, the cell surface attached FITC signal was quenched and flow cytometric analysis was repeated, measuring only the FITC signal within the cells (blue bars in (**A**), blue lines in (**B**) and as exemplified in the upper right scheme).

Uptake of PECNP for all three combinations PLL/CS, PLL/DS and PLL/HEP was also observed in confocal microscopy using both PECNP in the volume phase and immobilized on a model substrate (Figure 4). In a time range of 1 h to 24 h it became apparent, that for all compositions and net charges PECNP were taken up by HUVEC. However, the composition influenced the uptake rate of soluble PECNP. PECNP of PLL/HEP were taken up very early and fast, leading to big clusters already after 1 h incubation. This result was in accordance with our observations shown in Figure 2, where PLL/HEP attached on live cells already after 1 h of incubation. Remarkably, after 24 h of incubation the fluorescence signal of internalized PECNP of PLL/HEP faded in contrast to that of PLL/DS and PLL/DS, which may be due to degradation of the PLL/HEP PECNP by endogenous heparinases of endothelial cells [26] while PLL/CS and PLL/DS PECNP may be non-digestible by endothelial cells. After 24 h incubation, the PECNP signal strength, regardless of net charge and composition, was concentrated to the largest extent in the perinuclear area of the cells. The PECNP were exclusively situated in this endo-lysosomal compartment but none in the cytosol or in the nucleus which was reported for charged polystyrene based nanoparticles [27]. Also, surface-immobilized PECNP were taken up by the cells though to a much smaller extent than of soluble PECNP and within a longer time frame (Figure 4).

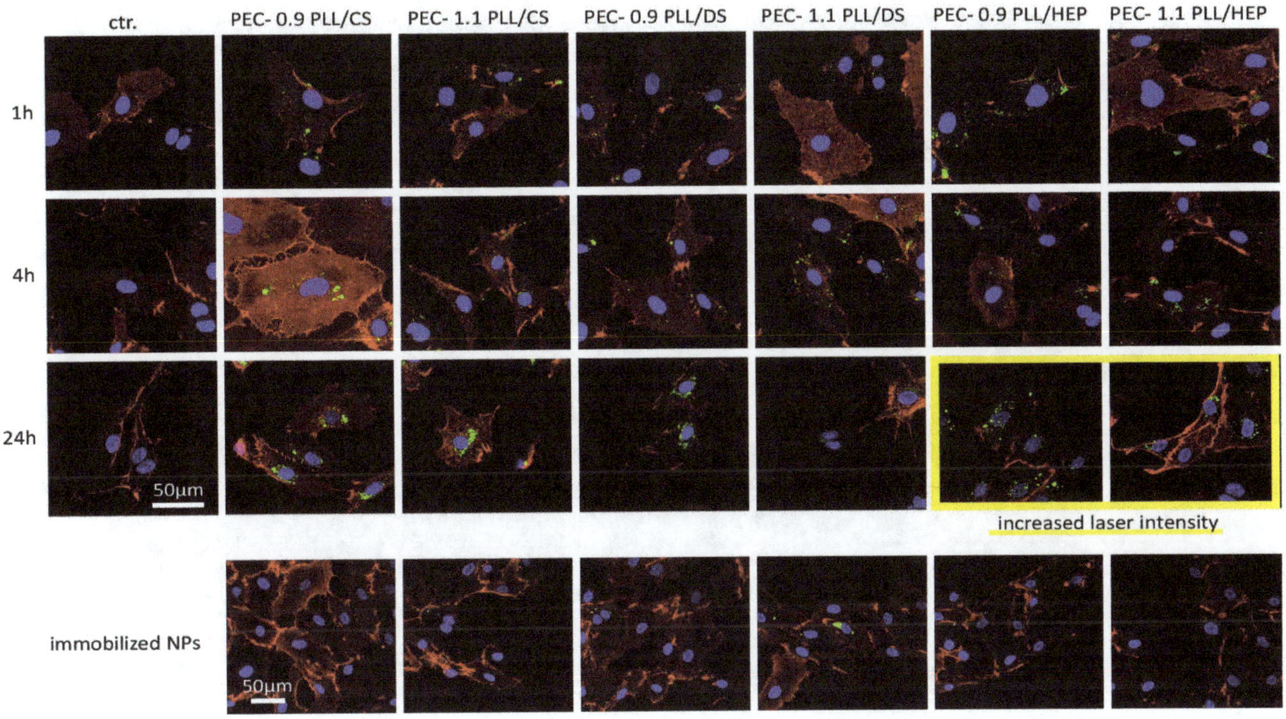

Figure 4. Uptake of polyelectrolyte complex nanoparticles (PECNP) into human umbilical cord vein endothelial cells (HUVEC). HUVEC were investigated for their uptake of PECNP-FITC (fluorescein isothiocyanate), either from the volume phase or from the immobilized state, demonstrated by confocal microscopy. Cells were cultivated either with PECNP in endothelial medium (volume phase) for times indicated or in contact with immobilized PECNP (surface) for 48 h cultivation time (bottom row). After cultivation, cells were detached and transferred to Ibidi slides and stained with Hoechst 33342 (cell nuclei) and an anti-CD31 (PECAM-1) monoclonal antibody conjugated to biotin, followed by incubation with an anti-mouse antibody conjugated to Cy3/streptavidin.

In more detail, transmission electron microscopy (TEM) showed neat attachment of PECNP to the plasma membrane of cells, preferentially in clustered form, and internalized PECNP in vesicles. PECNP in plasma membrane transit had not been seen unambiguously. In particular, none of the many coated vesicles abundant in HUVEC cell periphery ever contained PECNP indicating that internalization is not receptor-mediated in contrast to previously published data on charged nanoparticles which were taken up via the clathrin-mediated pathway [28]. This observation may also be in contrast to another report which describes that differently composed polyelectrolyte nanoparticles have an affinity to caveolae during endothelial cell uptake [29]. No apparent cell surface damage by binding and uptake of PECNP was observed by TEM. The observed vesicles increased with time of incubation, indicating that newly internalized PECNP-containing vesicles fuse with older ones. After long-time incubation, e.g., 72 h, huge vesicles occupied a great portion of the cytoplasmic space. Stuffed with PECNP, they also included stacked membranes, while both components appeared segregated within the same membrane-bound space (Figure 5).

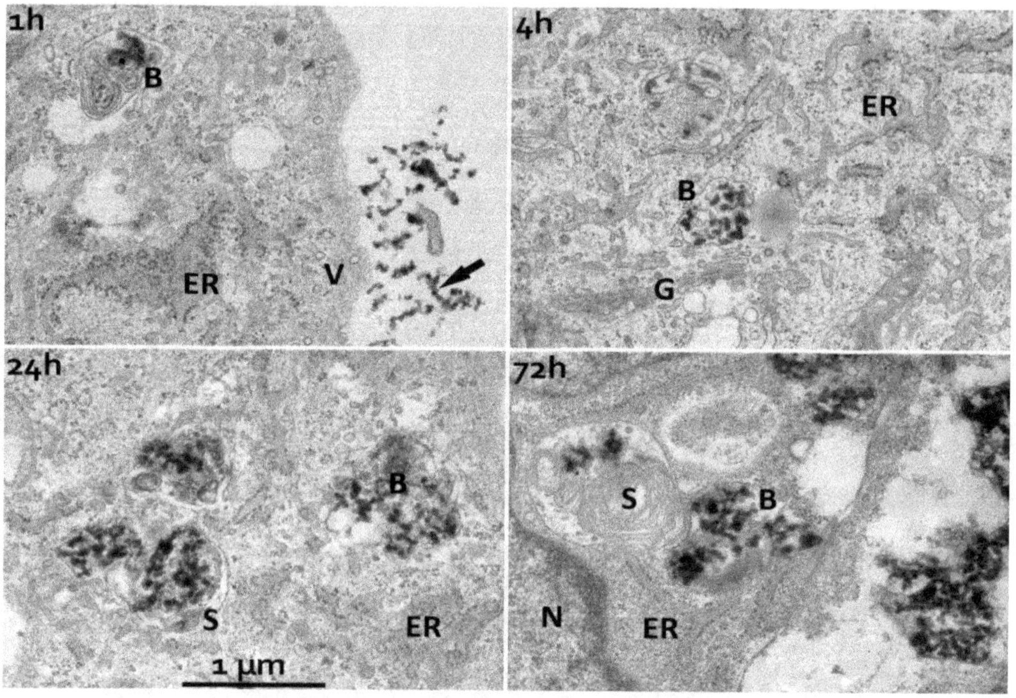

Figure 5. Ultrastructural demonstration of the polyelectrolyte complex nanoparticle PECNP compartment in human umbilical cord vein endothelial cells (HUVEC). HUVEC cell cultures admixed with PECNP composed of positively charged poly(L-lysine)/cellulose sulfate (PLL/CS-0.9) in the volume phase were fixed for TEM measurements after incubation times as indicated (1 h/4 h/24 h/72 h). 1 h/4 h incubation (upper row): disperse clusters of bead-like PECNP are in contact with the cells. Individual beads are compact, of variable shape and of typically 40 nm size. They frequently connect to each other into short chains (arrow). Close contact with the cell surface does not involve particular cell-surface coats. Internalized beads (B), i.e., PECNP, are rarely seen after 1 h incubation, more readily within the 4 h-samples, and always within membrane-enclosed vesicles. These vesicles differ in size from the typical endothelial vesicles of HUVEC. 24 h/72 h incubation (bottom row): vesicles with internalized PECNP grew beyond 1 µm-size. This "nanobead compartment" now occupied an essential volume of the cell cytoplasm. The PECNP-vesicles also feature inclusions of stacked membranes (S) which appear segregated from the bead-clusters. These membrane convolutions get more prominent with increasing time. B: (nano)beads/PECNP; ER: rough endoplasmatic reticulum; N: cell nucleus, G: Golgi apparatus, V: endosomal vesicles, all four images at same magnification.

The observation that PECNP accumulated with time in large endosomal vesicles indicates that lysosomal digest did not efficiently take place. Distinct endothelial proteins, such as PECAM, integrated into vesicles may be crucial for further intracellular processing [30]. Thus, it may be that the PLL/polysaccharide composition of PECNP does not suffice for further intracellular processing of nanoparticles, at least in endothelial cells, but additionally requires specific cell-specific proteins integrated into the PECNP as mentioned above. Also, it has to be considered that incubation with PECNP for several days, which may not occur under physiological conditions, represents an extreme situation and was performed to clearly demonstrate the intracellular localization and showed that lysosomal degradation did not take place. As has been shown by light microscopy and flow cytometry, uptake happened in shorter times (5–120 min).

In contrast to physical measurement of particle size (Table 1), size estimation by TEM revealed somewhat smaller sizes for single PECNP (extracellular: 39 ± 9 nm; intracellular after 4 h incubation: 50 ± 8 nm; intracellular after 24 h incubation: 42 ± 7nm). Interestingly, the incorporated FITC-labeled PECNP were equally distributed during mitosis (Figure 6).

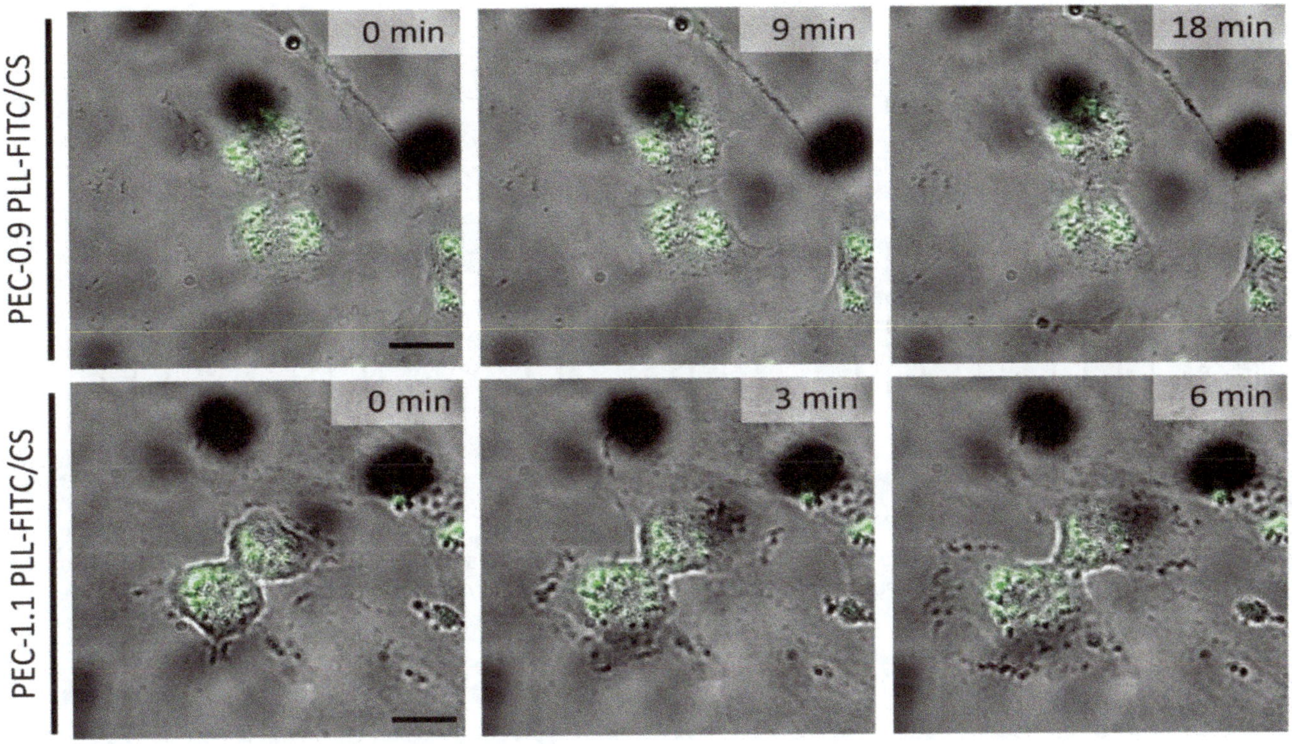

Figure 6. Distribution of internalized polyelectrolyte complex nanoparticles (PECNP) during cell division. Human umbilical cord vein endothelial cells (HUVEC) were incubated with 300 μL each of 50 μM fluorescein isothiocyanate (FITC)-labelled PECNP dispersed in endothelial culture medium for 24 h as described in Materials and Methods. After 3 washing steps, cells carrying PECNP were analyzed in the telophase of cell division by widefield microscopy. Images show separation of cells loaded with PECNP at time points indicated. The number of PECNP within cells apparently was split in approximately equal portions during cell division. PEC: polyelectrolyte complex; PEC-1.1: negatively charged PECNP; PEC-0.9: positively charged PECNP; PLL: (poly-L)lysine; CS: cellulose sulfate; (Scale bar: 20 μm).

3.4. Effect of PECNP on Cell Proliferation in the Volume Phase and Immobilized State

Since PECNP were taken up in large amounts, it was analyzed whether they may influence cell proliferation both in the volume phase and attached on a surface. To this end, the influence of PECNP on proliferation of HUVEC was tested by their [^{3}H]-thymidine uptake during a cultivation time of 24 h (Figure 7). All PECNP samples reduced proliferation in a dose-dependent fashion which was evident both for the immobilized as well as for the volume phase state though the negative influence was stronger for the immobilized PECNP (black bars Figure 7B). PLL/HEP and PLL/DS PECNP had significant anti-proliferative effects at medium and high concentration (20 and 50 μL/cm^2, respectively). Negatively charged PLL/CS PECNP (PEC-1.1), especially in lower concentrations (5 and 10 μ/cm^2), had the lowest anti-proliferative effect. Reflected in reduced proliferation rates after PECNP uptake, the time-dependently high endosomal accumulation of PECNP may have caused stress for the cells. We did not find a significant difference with regard to uptake and intracellular localization between negatively and positively charged nanoparticles as has been reported [26]. However, as estimated by analysis of TEM images it appeared, that positively charged PECNP showed a larger number of vesicles with particles than negatively charged PECNP after 24 and 72 h incubation (data not shown), which may be due to the slightly negatively charged cell membrane. It was suggested that charged nanoparticles of various materials are more cytotoxic than uncharged ones which may however not apply for polysaccharide based nanoparticles as for instance those containing chitosan [10].

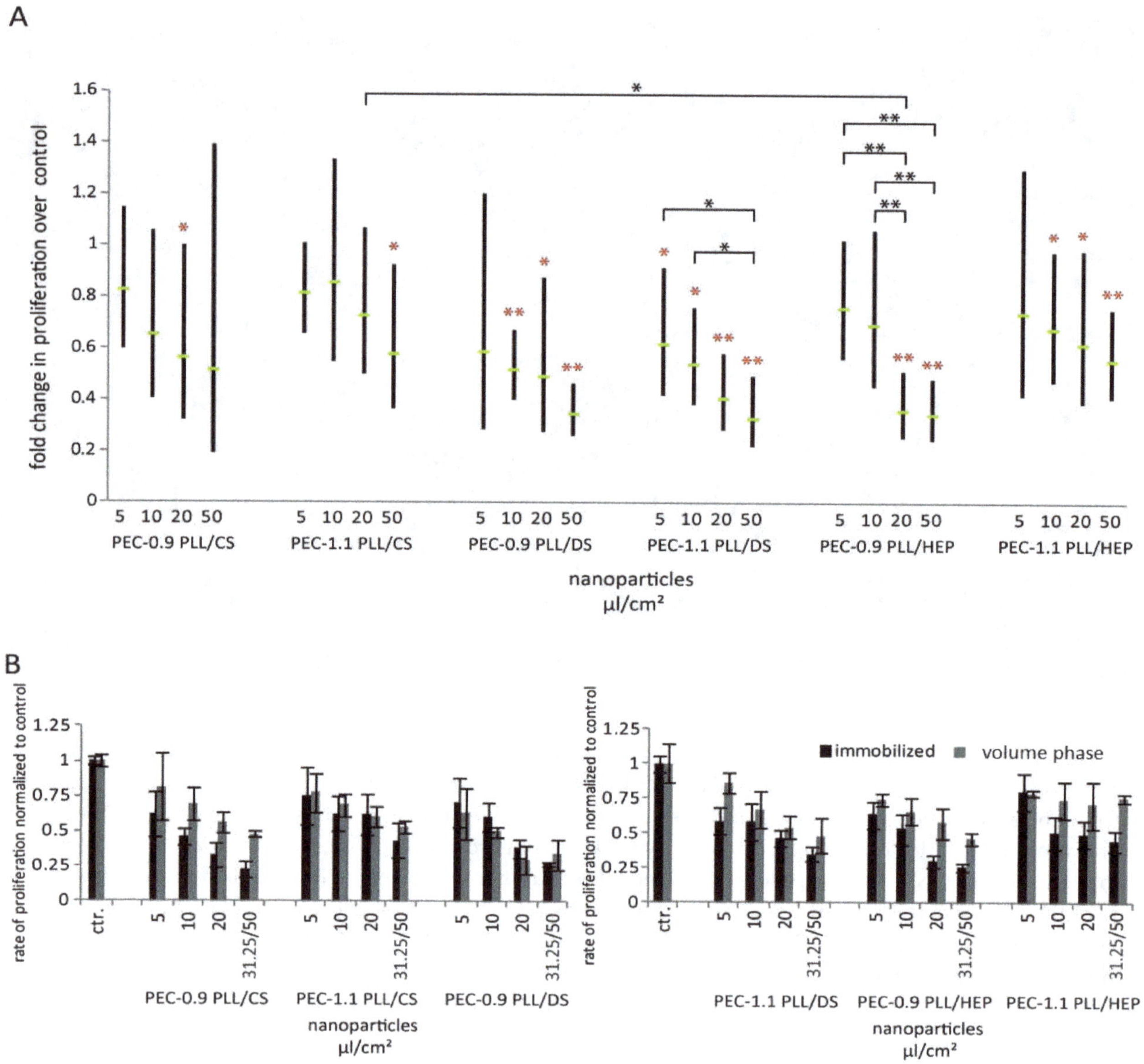

Figure 7. The influence of polyelectrolyte complex nanoparticles PECNP on cell proliferation. The influence of PECNP on proliferation of human umbilical cord vein endothelial cells (HUVEC) was assayed by [3H] thymidine incorporation as described in Materials and Methods. (**A**) Influence on proliferation, shown as fold change for each PECNP preparation compared to untreated (i.e., without PECNP addition) control HUVEC cultures. HUVECs were seeded on culture plates coated with PECNP. Black bars indicate 95% confidence interval (number of experiments: $n = 4$), red * indicate significant changes in proliferation using a two-tailed, paired *t*-test. Horizontal bars and black * indicate significant differences between various concentrations of the same PECNP applied or between various PECNP of same concentration (ANOVA, one way analysis of variance), * $p < 0.05$, ** $p < 0.01$) (**B**) Direct comparison of HUVEC proliferation rates affected by PECNP in the immobilized state (black bars) and in the volume phase (grey bars). Proliferation rates were normalized to those of control cultures (ctr). The highest concentration of PECNP in fluid state was 31 $\mu L/cm^2$, and for immobilized PECNP 50 $\mu L/cm^2$. The other concentrations of PECNP were as indicated. Error bars indicate standard deviation of at least triplicates/assay.

In our study, all PECNP, in the volume phase and in an immobilized state reduced cell proliferation in HUVECs in a concentration-dependent manner albeit to various extents. In another study cytotoxic effects of iron oxide nanoparticles on human endothelial cells were reported [31]. Although in our study the proliferation rate was reduced by addition of PECNP, it has to be stressed that this did not entail a higher cytotoxicity. Flow cytometric analysis of dead versus live cells after application of PECNP did not show a higher propensity for dead cells (data not shown). Also, the fact that mitosis was not influenced by internalized PECNP supports this finding. As the intracellular load of PECNP is apparently bisected after each cell division the non-digestible PECNP will gradually be diminished. In another study uptake of modified polystyrene nanoparticles by mesenchymal stem cells did not affect the viability of these cells [13].

Immobilized PECNP can be used as an integrative part of a scaffold material and hence it is important to know how endothelial cells are able to adhere to and migrate on a PECNP coated surface. Application of PECNP to surfaces of culture dishes or microscopic slides resulted in heterogeneous spreading of nanoparticles. Under these conditions PECNP had generally an anti-adhesive effect. This repulsive effect was lowest with PECNP of PLL/CS, which suggests these nanoparticles are more appropriate for coating of scaffold surfaces. A further advantage for in-vivo application may be that both, HEP and CS have anti-coagulant activities [32,33]. In an earlier study we investigated the interaction between PECNPs and human mesenchymal stromal cells (hMSC) and found, similar to the findings of this study, that net charge did not significantly influence adhesion and uptake, while PECNP composition affected e.g., metabolic activity of hMSC [21]. It has also been shown that PECNP can be applied as drug delivery system when cast as particle films [12,20,34,35]. In our study we found differential effects of PECNP on endothelial cell adhesion. Therefore, when applying PECNP in cast form for surface mediated drug delivery the possible anti-adhesive effect of several PECNP has to be considered and certainly those with lowest anti-adhesive effect have to be preferred for this purpose.

4. Conclusions

Our study showed that PLL/polysaccharide based PECNP attached to the cell surface of vascular endothelial cells and were taken up into the vesicular compartment in a cumulative manner. Among the three PECNP compositions used here, PLL/HEP seemed to be the ideal vehicle for transport of drugs or growth factors to endothelial cells, because (i) attachment and uptake was faster than for the other modifications, (ii) PLL/HEP seemed to be digested in the lysosomal compartment by endogeneous glycosidases and (iii) possibly sulfatases, and (iii) interactions with growth factors, important for vascularization, such as vascular endothelial growth factor (VEGF) and basic fibroblast growth factor (bFGF), have a high binding capacity for heparin, and thus PECNP of PLL/HEP may be helpful for supporting the presentation of these growth factors [36] to vascular endothelial cells and may also reduce release of the growth factors during cellular regeneration for example of bone tissue within scaffolds [14] (iii). On the other side, PECNP of PLL/CS may be better suited for coating surfaces of scaffold material since its anti-adhesive effects and its anti-proliferative impact were much smaller compared to PECNP composed of PLL/HEP or PLL/DS. Depending on the specific requirements for nanoparticle application, mixing of HEP and CS in ternary complexes of PLL/CS/HEP in appropriate fractions may be advantageous to design specific properties for several applications as mentioned here. Finally, the net charge of the PECNP, which can be modulated by the excess of either cationic PLL or one of the three anionic polysaccharides, did not play an essential role in our experimental approach, which is in line with former results on the interaction of PECNP with comparable compositions with human mesenchymal stromal cells (hMSC) [21].

Our study has yielded basic insights into the biocompatibility of PECNP for vascular endothelial cells. In future experiments, using PECNP, the influence of shear stress and stretched conditions has to be taken into account, since it is known that under flow conditions, equivalent to the physiological condition in the blood stream [37], uptake of nanoparticles may be different [38,39]. In an earlier study, by measuring uptake of silica nanoparticles into human endothelial cells it was found, that cytotoxicity was not increased (i) and endocytosis was decreased as compared to maintenance of cells under static conditions (ii) [40]. So far, we were able to show interactions with endothelial cells in the volume phase via the comparatively harsh shear stress conditions of flow cytometry confirming data of other groups [23]. Therefore, adhesion and uptake may be lower under dynamic than under static conditions and thereby anti-proliferative effects may also be diminished in the in-vivo situation. Also, in-vivo studies have to clarify the potential clearance of PECNP from the body with time.

Author Contributions: R.S.A. and M.M. initiated this cooperative research work. D.W. and R.S.A. designed all cell experiments. M.M. and B.T. selected and prepared appropriate PECNP samples. K.R. and M.N. performed TEM analysis. R.S.A. and M.M. drafted and with the help of B.T. and B.W. iteratively refined the manuscript. F.M. assisted with the fluorescent microscopy and cytometric analysis. All authors approved the final manuscript.

References

1. Tautzenberger, A.; Kovtun, A.; Ignatius, A. Nanoparticles and their potential for application in bone. *Int. J. Nanomed.* **2012**, *7*, 4545–4557. [CrossRef] [PubMed]
2. Hartig, S.M.; Greene, R.R.; Dikov, M.M.; Prokop, A.; Davidson, J.M. Multifunctional nanoparticle polyelectrolyte complexes. *Pharm. Res.* **2007**, *24*, 2353–2369. [CrossRef] [PubMed]
3. Baiguera, S.; Ribatti, D. Endothelization approaches for viable engineered tissues. *Angiogenesis* **2013**, *16*, 1–14. [CrossRef] [PubMed]
4. Asai, T. Nanoparticle-mediated delivery of anticancer agents to tumor angiogenic vessels. *Biol. Pharm. Bull.* **2012**, *35*, 1855–1861. [CrossRef] [PubMed]
5. Zhao, G.; Rodriguez, B.L. Molecular targeting of liposomal nanoparticles to tumor microenvironment. *Int. J. Nanomed.* **2013**, *8*, 61–71. [CrossRef] [PubMed]
6. He, C.; Hu, Y.; Yin, L.; Tang, C.; Yin, C. Effects of particle size and surface charge on cellular uptake and biodistribution of polymeric nanoparticles. *Biomaterials* **2010**, *31*, 3657–3666. [CrossRef] [PubMed]
7. Pastorino, F.; Brignole, C.; Loi, M.; Di Paolo, D.; Di Fiore, A.; Perri, P.; Pagnan, G.; Ponzoni, M. Nanocarrier-mediated targeting of tumor and tumor vascular cells improves uptake and penetration of drugs into neuroblastoma. *Front. Oncol.* **2013**, *3*, 190. [CrossRef] [PubMed]
8. Huang, M.; Vitharana, S.N.; Peek, L.J.; Coop, T.; Berkland, C. Polyelectrolyte complexes stabilize and controllably release vascular endothelial growth factor. *Biomacromolecules* **2007**, *8*, 1607–1614. [CrossRef] [PubMed]
9. Alexis, F.; Pridgen, E.; Molnar, L.K.; Farokhzad, O.C. Factors affecting the clearance and biodistribution of polymeric nanoparticles. *Mol. Pharm.* **2008**, *5*, 505–515. [CrossRef] [PubMed]
10. Fröhlich, E. The role of surface charge in cellular uptake and cytotoxicity of medical nanoparticles. *Int. J. Nanomed.* **2012**, *7*, 5577–5591. [CrossRef] [PubMed]
11. Müller, M. Sizing, shaping and pharmaceutical applications of polyelectrolyte complex nanoparticles. *Adv. Polym. Sci.* **2014**, *256*, 197–260.
12. Müller, M.; Torger, B.; Vehlow, D.; Urban, B.; Wehrum, D.; Woltmann, B.; Hempel, U. Drug delivery and cell interaction of adhesive poly(ethylenimine)/sulfated polysaccharide complex particle films. *Biointerphases* **2015**, *10*, 011001. [CrossRef] [PubMed]
13. Baldwin, A.D.; Kiick, K.L. Polysaccharide-modified synthetic polymeric biomaterials. *Biopolymers* **2010**, *94*, 128–140. [CrossRef] [PubMed]
14. Knaack, S.; Lode, A.; Hoyer, B.; Rösen-Wolff, A.; Gabrielyan, A.; Roeder, I.; Gelinsky, M. Heparin modification of a biomimetic bone matrix for controlled release of VEGF. *J. Biomed. Mater. Res. A* **2014**, *102*, 3500–3511. [CrossRef] [PubMed]
15. Nagahata, M.; Nakaoka, R.; Tramoto, A.; Abe, K.; Tsuchiya, T. The response of normal osteoblasts to anionic polysaccharide polyelectrolyte complexes. *Biomaterials* **2005**, *26*, 5138–5144. [CrossRef] [PubMed]
16. Lemarchand, C.; Gref, R.; Passirani, C.; Garcion, E.; Petri, B.; Müller, R.; Costantini, D.; Couvreur, P. Influence of polysaccharide coating on the interactions of nanoparticles with biological systems. *Biomaterials* **2005**, *27*, 108–118. [CrossRef] [PubMed]
17. Rodriguez-Velazquez, E.; Alatorre-Meda, M.; Mano, J.F. Polysaccharide-based nanobiomaterials as controlled release systems for tissue engineering applications. *Curr. Pharm. Des.* **2015**, *21*, 4837–4850. [CrossRef] [PubMed]

18. Kim, D.H.; Termsarasab, U.; Cho, H.J.; Yoon, I.S.; Lee, J.Y.; Moon, H.T.; Kim, D.D. Preparation and characterization of self-assembled nanoparticles based on low-molecular-weight heparin and stearylamine conjugates for controlled delivery of docetaxel. *Int. J. Nanomed.* **2014**, *9*, 5711–5727. [CrossRef] [PubMed]
19. Kemp, M.M.; Linhardt, R.J. Heparin-based nanoparticles. *Wiley Interdiscip. Rev. Nanomed. Nanobiotechnol.* **2010**, *2*, 77–87. [CrossRef] [PubMed]
20. Müller, M.; Keßler, B. Release of pamidronate from poly(ethyleneimine)/cellulose sulphate complex nanoparticle films: An in situ ATR-FTIR study. *J. Pharm. Biomed. Anal.* **2012**, *66*, 183–190. [CrossRef] [PubMed]
21. Woltmann, B.; Torger, B.; Müller, M.; Hempel, U. Interaction between immobilized polyelectrolyte complex nanoparticles and human mesenchymal stromal cells. *Int. J. Nanomed.* **2014**, *9*, 2205–2215.
22. Kokesch-Himmelreich, J.; Woltmann, B.; Torger, B.; Rohnke, M.; Arnhold, S.; Hempel, U.; Müller, M.; Janek, J. Detection of organic nanoparticles in human bone marrow-derived stromal cells using ToF-SIMS and PCA. *Anal. Bioanal. Chem.* **2015**, *407*, 4555–4565. [CrossRef] [PubMed]
23. Hartig, S.M.; Greene, R.R.; Carlesso, G.; Higginbotham, J.N.; Khan, W.N.; Prokop, A.; Davidson, J.M. Kinetic analysis of nanoparticulate polyelectrolyte complex interactions with endothelial cells. *Biomaterials* **2007**, *28*, 3843–3855. [CrossRef] [PubMed]
24. Starchenko, V.; Müller, M.; Lebovka, N. Sizing of PDADMAC/PSS complex aggregates by polyelectrolyte and salt concentration and PSS molecular weight. *J. Phys. Chem. B* **2012**, *116*, 14961–14967. [CrossRef] [PubMed]
25. Pandey, M.S.; Harris, E.N.; Weigel, P.H. HARE-mediated endocytosis of hyaluronan and heparin is targeted by different subsets of three endocytic motifs. *Int. J. Cell Biol.* **2015**, *2015*, 524707. [CrossRef] [PubMed]
26. Hammond, E.; Khurana, A.; Shridhar, V.; Dredge, K. The role of heparanase and sulfatases in the modification of heparan sulfate proteoglycans within the tumor microenvironment and opportunities for novel cancer therapeutics. *Front. Oncol.* **2014**, *4*, 195. [CrossRef] [PubMed]
27. Lorenz, M.R.; Holzapfel, V.; Musyanovych, A.; Nothelfer, K.; Walther, P.; Frank, H.; Landfester, K.; Schrezenmeier, H.; Mailänder, V. Uptakte of functionalized, fluorescent-labeled polymeric particles in different cell lines and stem cells. *Biomaterials* **2006**, *27*, 2820–2828. [CrossRef] [PubMed]
28. Harush-Frenkel, O.; Debotton, N.; Benita, S.; Altschuler, Y. Targeting of nanoparticles to the clathrin-mediated endocytic pathway. *Biochem. Biophys. Res. Commun.* **2007**, *353*, 26–32. [CrossRef] [PubMed]
29. Voigt, J.; Christensen, J.; Shastri, V.P. Differential uptake of nanoparticles by endothelial cells through polyelectrolytes with affinity for caveolae. *Proc. Natl. Acad. Sci. USA* **2014**, *111*, 2942–2947. [CrossRef] [PubMed]
30. Garnacho, C.; Albelda, S.M.; Muzykantov, V.R.; Muro, S. Differential intra-endothelial delivery of polymer nanocarriers targeted to distinct PECAM-1 epitopes. *J. Control. Release* **2008**, *130*, 226–233. [CrossRef] [PubMed]
31. Wu, X.; Tan, Y.; Mao, H.; Zhang, M. Toxic effects of iron oxide nanoparticles on human umbilical vein endothelial cells. *Int. J. Nanomed.* **2010**, *5*, 385–399. [CrossRef]
32. Lane, D.A.; Denton, J.; Flynn, A.M.; Thunberg, L.; Lindahl, U. Anticoagulant activities of heparin oligosaccharides and their neutralization by platelet factor 4. *Biochem. J.* **1984**, *218*, 725–732. [CrossRef] [PubMed]
33. Wagenknecht, W.; Nehls, I.; Philipp, B. Studies on the regioselectivity of cellulose sulfation in an N_2O_4-*N*,*N*-dimethylformamide-cellulose system. *Carbohydr. Res.* **1993**, *240*, 245–252. [CrossRef]
34. Torger, B.; Vehlow, D.; Urban, B.; Salem, S.R.; Appelhans, D.; Müller, M. Cast polyelectrolyte complex particle films of unmodified or maltose-modified poly(ethyleneimine) and cellulose sulphate: Fabrication, film stability and retarded release of zoledronate. *Biointerphases* **2013**, *8*, 25. [CrossRef] [PubMed]
35. Vehlow, D.; Schmidt, R.; Gebert, A.; Siebert, M.; Lips, K.S.; Müller, M. Polyelectrolyte complex based interfacial drug delivery system with controlled loading and improved release performance for bone therapeutics. *Nanomaterials* **2016**, *6*, 53. [CrossRef] [PubMed]
36. Friedel, M.; André, S.; Goldschmidt, H.; Gabius, H.J.; Schwartz-Albiez, R. Galectin-8 enhances adhesion of multiple myeloma cells to vascular endothelium and is an adverse prognostic factor. *Glycobiology* **2016**, *26*, 1048–1058. [CrossRef] [PubMed]

37. Han, J.; Zern, B.J.; Shuvaev, V.V.; Davies, P.F.; Muro, S.; Muzykantov, V. Acute and chronic shear stress differently regulate endothelial internalization of nanocarriers targeted to platelet-endothelial cell adhesion molecule-1. *ACS Nano* **2012**, *6*, 8824–8836. [CrossRef] [PubMed]
38. Han, J.; Shuvaev, V.V.; Davies, P.F.; Eckmann, D.M.; Muro, S.; Muzykantov, V.R. Flow shear stress differentially regulates endothelial uptake of nanocarriers targeted to distinct epitopes of PECAM-1. *J. Control. Release* **2015**, *210*, 39–47. [CrossRef] [PubMed]
39. Freese, C.; Schreiner, D.; Anspach, L.; Bantz, C.; Maskos, M.; Unger, R.E.; Kirkpatrick, C.J. In vitro investigation of silica nanoparticle uptake into human endothelial cells under physiological cyclic stretch. *Part. Fibre Toxicol.* **2014**, *11*, 68. [CrossRef] [PubMed]
40. Folkman, J.; Shing, Y. Control of angiogenesis by heparin and other sulfated polysaccharides. *Adv. Exp. Med. Biol.* **1993**, *313*, 355–364.

5

Stable, Monodisperse and Highly Cell-Permeating Nanocochleates from Natural Soy Lecithin Liposomes

Martina Asprea [1], Francesca Tatini [2], Vieri Piazzini [1], Francesca Rossi [2], Maria Camilla Bergonzi [1] and Anna Rita Bilia [1,*]

[1] Department of Chemistry, University of Florence, Via U. Schiff 6, 50019 Sesto Fiorentino, Florence, Italy; aspreamartina@gmail.com (M.A.); vieri.piazzini@unifi.it (V.P.); mc.bergonzi@unifi.it (M.C.B.)

[2] Institute of Applied Physics "N. Carrara" (IFAC-CNR), Via Madonna del Piano 10, 50019 Sesto Fiorentino, Italy; f.tatini@ifac.cnr.it (F.T.); f.rossi@ifac.cnr.it (F.R.)

* Correspondence: ar.bilia@unifi.it;

Abstract: (1) Background: Andrographolide (AN), the main diterpenoid constituent of *Andrographis paniculata*, has a wide spectrum of biological activities. The aim of this study was the development of nanocochleates (NCs) loaded with AN and based on phosphatidylserine (PS) or phosphatidylcholine (PC), cholesterol and calcium ions in order to overcome AN low water solubility, its instability under alkaline conditions and its rapid metabolism in the intestine. (2) Methods: The AN-loaded NCs (AN–NCs) were physically and chemically characterised. The in vitro gastrointestinal stability and biocompatibility of AN–NCs in J77A.1 macrophage and 3T3 fibroblasts cell lines were also investigated. Finally, the uptake of nanocarriers in macrophage cells was studied. (3) Results: AN–NCs obtained from PC nanoliposomes were suitable nanocarriers in terms of size and homogeneity. They had an extraordinary stability after lyophilisation without the use of lyoprotectants and after storage at room temperature. The encapsulation efficiency was 71%, while approximately 95% of AN was released in PBS after 24 h, with kinetics according to the Hixson–Crowell model. The in vitro gastrointestinal stability and safety of NCs, both in macrophages and 3T3 fibroblasts, were also assessed. Additionally, NCs had extraordinary uptake properties in macrophages. (4) Conclusions: NCs developed in this study could be suitable for both AN oral and parental administration, amplifying its therapeutic value.

Keywords: soy lecithin liposomes; nanocochleates; andrographolide; freeze-drying; gastrointestinal stability; uptake and safety

---

1. Introduction

The design and production of appropriate drug delivery systems, in particular, nanosized ones, offer an advanced approach to optimised bioavailability and/or the stability of drugs, to control drug delivery and to maintain drug stability during transport to the site of action. A successful drug carrier system should possess a long shelf life, optimal drug loading and release properties, and exert a much higher therapeutic efficacy as well as have low side effects [1,2].

Phospholipids are the main amphiphilic components of the cell membrane and currently represent the main constituents of nanovectors because they can self-assembly in aqueous milieu, generating different supramolecular structures such as micelles and vesicles [1,3]. Typically, their variation in head groups, aliphatic chains and alcohols leads to a wide variety of phospholipids, generally classified as glycerophospholipids and sphingomyelins. The most common natural glycerophospholipids are phosphatidylcholine (PC), phosphatidylinositol, phosphatidylserine (PS), phosphatidylglycerol and phosphatidic acid, having diverse acyl moieties, principally myristoyl, palmitoyl, oleoyl and stearoyl.

In particular, glycerophospholipids are the specific constituents of liposomes, which are widely used as drug vectors because of their high biocompatibility, non-toxicity, complete biodegradability, and non-immunogenic effects after both systemic and non-systemic routes of administration [4]. Conversely, the therapeutic use of vesicles has some limitations, principally poor stability and availability under the harsh conditions typically presented in the gastrointestinal tract [1,2,5,6]. A very limited number of studies report on the use of cochleates as an alternative platform to vesicles in order to overcome these limitations. Cochleates were first observed by Verkleij et al. [7] using phosphatidylglycerol liposomes and later by Papahadjopoulos et al. [8], using phosphatidylserine liposomes in the presence of divalent metal cations (Me^{2+}), i.e., Ca^{2+}, Ba^{2+}, Fe^{2+}, Mg^{2+} and Zn^{2+}. Cochleates can be produced as nano- and microstructures and they are extremely biocompatible, with excellent stability due to their unique compact structure. They present an elongated shape and a carpet roll-like morphology always accompanied by narrowly packed bilayers, through the interaction with Me^{2+} as bridging agents between the bilayers (Figure 1). During this arrangement, the close approach of bilayers is dependent on dehydration of the head group of the phospholipid. They roll-up in order to minimise their interaction with water and, consequently, cochleates possess little or no aqueous phase. The relevant differences between cochleates and different liposomes, i.e., small unilamellar vesicle (SUV), large unilamellar vesicle (LUV), multilamellar vesicle (MLV) and multivesicle vesicle (MVV), are reported in Figure 1.

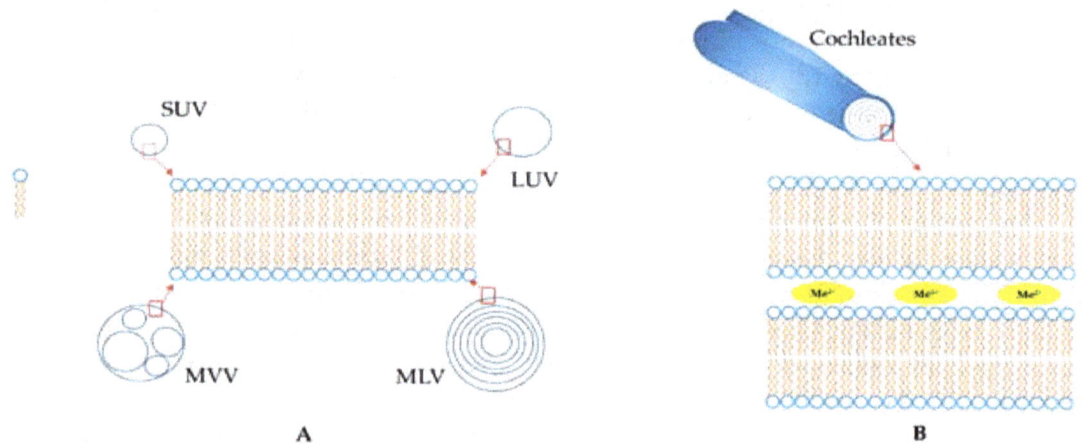

Figure 1. Schematic representation of the structures of liposomes (**A**) and nanocochleates (**B**).

The bilayers in a cochleate are organised very precisely at a very close repeating distance of 54 Angstrom [9] with a water-free interior, which is a rigid, stable, rod-shaped structure. Due to this unique structure, cochleates can be easily lyophilised to a free-flowing powder that can be incorporated in capsules for oral administration or re-dispersed in water for parental administration. Yet what remains very unclear is their mechanism of permeation throughout the biological membranes. It is reported that after oral administration, cochleates cross the epithelium, delivering the loaded drug into the blood vessel [10]. There are two current hypotheses to explain the mechanism of permeation. According to the first assumption, the contact of the calcium-rich membrane of the cochleate with a cell can cause a perturbation and the reordering of the cell membrane. Subsequently, there is fusion between the outer layer of the cochleate and the cell membrane [10]. An alternative hypothesis for the delivery mechanism of cochleates is phagocytosis. In both cases, once within the interior of a cell, a low calcium concentration results in the opening of the cochleate crystal and the release of the entrapped drug [11–13].

Currently, cochleates represent difficult drug delivery systems for clinical use, principally due to the numerous difficulties in producing monodisperse systems because of a tendency to form stable and huge aggregates, which represent a serious drawback at the industrial level. Diverse patents and publications have reported different strategies to overcome these limitations [11], in particular, the use of methylcellulose, casein, or albumin, but proteins may decrease stability and safety due to the change of pharmacokinetic parameters. Methylcellulose is able only in part to disrupt the formed aggregates.

Other natural polysaccharides (including celluloses, gums, and starches) have been recommended as inhibitors of the aggregation processes, but their efficiency still remains ambiguous [11,12]. In recent times, the ability of citric acid to remove Ca^{2+} ions from the external surface of cochleates, leading to the dispersion of the aggregates, has been investigated [13]. Furthermore, a recent approach compared a novel microfluidics-based strategy with the conventional cochleate production methods; however, the formation of aggregates was still present in the samples [14].

The aim of this study was the production of monodisperse and stable nanocochleates (NCs) using two different phospholipids, PC and PS, loaded with a typical small hydrophobic natural product, andrographolide (AN) from the Asiatic medicinal plant *Andrographis paniculata*. Besides the numerous potential activities ranging from anti-inflammatory to neuroprotection, antidiabetic to anti-obesity properties, and antitumor activity to hepatoprotective activity [15], AN has poor water solubility (3.29 ± 0.73 µg at 25 °C) [16], which deeply limits its biodistribution and localisation, resulting in low bioavailability [17]. Additionally, AN is unstable in gastrointestinal media and has a very short biological half-life ($t_{1/2}$ = 1.33 h) after a single oral dose [18]. The stability of developed nanocochleates after lyophilisation and in simulated gastrointestinal fluids was investigated. In addition, the possible hazards and the cellular effects of NCs were determined using J774a.1 murine macrophages and 3T3 fibroblasts. Lastly, studies on uptake using a confocal microscope were carried out in the macrophages cell line.

2. Materials and Methods

2.1. Materials

The phospholipon 90G (soy phosphatidylcholine, PC) was sourced from the Italian agent AVG srl (Milan, Italy) of Lipoid AG (Cologne, Germany). The dioleoyl phosphatidylserine (PS) was a kind gift from Lipoid AG (Cologne, Germany). The following reagents were from Sigma-Aldrich (Milan, Italy): pepsin from porcine gastric mucosa, bile salts, andrographolide (AN), fluorescein isothiocyanate (FITC, purity ≥ 90%, HPLC), lipase from porcin pancreas, sodium hydroxide (NaOH), calcium chloride ($CaCl_2$), cholesterol, phosphate buffered saline (PBS) bioperformance certified, paraformaldehyde (PFA), Dulbecco's Modified Eagle Medium (DMEM), fetal bovine serum (FBS), l-glutamine, penicillin–streptomycin solution, WST-8 kit, acetonitrile (HPLC grade), methanol (HPLC grade), formic acid (analytical grade), hydrochloric acid (HCl) (analytical grade) and dichloromethane (CH_2Cl_2). The water used was from the Milli-Q_{plus} system from Millipore (Milford, CT, USA). The phosphotungstic acid (PTA) was from Electron Microscopy Sciences (Hatfield, PA, USA). The dialysis kit was from Spectrum Laboratories, Inc. (Breda, The Netherlands). The J774a.1 murine macrophages and the 3T3 fibroblasts were purchased from the American Type Culture Collection (ATCC® TIB-67™, Manassas, VA, USA). A LT-4000 reader from Labtech was used to read the absorbance (Bergamo, Italy).

2.2. Preparation of PC- and PS-based Liposomes and NCs

The NCs were obtained from nano-sized liposomes (LPs), which were prepared according to the film hydration method [19]. The liposomes were formulated as follows: the required amounts of phospholipids (60 mg) and cholesterol (20 mg) were dissolved in a dichloromethane/methanol mixture (20 mL of a mixture, 3:2 *v*/*v*). The obtained organic solution was evaporated under vacuum and the lipid film was hydrated by the addition of PBS (10 mL) using a mechanical stirrer (RW20 digital, IKA, Staufen im Breisgau, Germany) for 30 min in a water bath at a constant temperature of 37 °C for PC and 60 °C for PS. The resulting formulations were optimised by ultrasonication (3 min, two cycles of 90 s) in an ice bath to prevent lipid degradation. Subsequently, a gentle centrifugation (1205× *g*, 1 min) was performed to remove possible metallic particles released during the ultrasonication. The NCs were prepared from the nanoliposomes according to the trapping method, described by Asprea et al. [20]. Briefly, a 0.1 M solution of $CaCl_2$ was added drop-by-drop to the liposomal suspension under magnetic stirring (150 rpm, room temperature) until the formulation appeared cloudy, indicating the formation of NCs. The molar ratio between PC and $CaCl_2$ was 1:1, while the molar ratio between PS and $CaCl_2$ was 1:4.

2.3. Characterisation of Nanocarriers: Size, Polydispersity Index and ζ-Potential

The Zsizer Nano series ZS90 (Malvern Instruments, Malvern, UK) outfitted with a JDS Uniphase 22 mW He-Ne laser operating at 632.8 nm, an optical fiber-based detector, a digital LV/LSE-5003 correlator and a temperature controller (Julabo water-bath) set at 25 °C was used for Dynamic Light Scattering (DLS) measurements, including for the particle size, polydispersity index (PdI) and ζ-potential. The cumulant method was used to analyse time correlation functions, obtaining the mean diameter of the nanocarriers (Z-average) and the size distribution using the ALV-60X0 software V.3.X provided by Malvern. The size characterisation technique for the nanoparticles in suspension, based on the measurement of their translational diffusion coefficient, related to the length, L, of their major axis is as

$$D = \frac{kBT}{3\pi\eta L} FD, \tag{1}$$

where η represents the viscosity of the solvent, kB represents the Boltzmann constant and T represents the sample temperature. FD is a geometrical coefficient depending on the shape, but not the size, of the particles [21,22]. In particular, for NCs, the expressions of FD corresponding to these particle shapes are

$$FD = \log\rho + 0.312 + 0.565/\rho - 0.1/\rho^2, \tag{2}$$

ζ-potential values were obtained from the electrophoretic mobility, using the Henry correction to Smoluchowski's equation. The samples were diluted in distilled water and an average of three measurements at the stationary level were taken. A Haake temperature controller kept the temperature constant at 25 °C.

2.4. Morphological and Size Characterisation by Transmission Electron Microscopy (TEM)

A transmission electron microscope (TEM, Jeol Jem 1010, Tokyo, Japan) was used to evaluate the morphology, shape and dimensions of NCs. The NCs dispersion was diluted 10-fold and placed on a carbon film-covered copper grid and stained with a phosphotungstic acid solution 1 g/100 mL in sterile water, before the TEM analysis. The samples were dried for 1 min and then examined under TEM and photographed at an accelerating voltage of 64 kV.

2.5. Stability Study of NCs after Lyophilisation

The lyophilisation process of NCs provides an extended storage period at room temperature and can be carried out without the use of lyoprotectants because of the very low water content. The samples were frozen by a freezer (−23 °C) overnight before lyophilisation. Then, the samples were moved to a freeze-drier. The temperature was set to −23 °C and the pressure was −1.0 bar. The drying time was 24 h. The pressure and the temperature remained unchanged during the process.

The stability of the lyophilised NCs was evaluated after reconstitution of the colloidal system to the original volume with distilled water, using a vortex mixer at room temperature. The samples were stored in sealed glass containers after being placed into a desiccator containing silica gel to absorb water vapor. The samples were also protected from light. The stability of the lyophilised NCs was assessed by checking the size, ζ-potential, polydispersity and morphology every week for 2 months.

2.6. Stability Study of NCs in Gastrointestinal Media

NCs could be used to protect the entrapped compound from the effects of the gastrointestinal fluids. Accordingly, NC formulations were tested for their stability using simulated gastrointestinal conditions. Simulated gastric fluid (SGF) was used to investigate the gastric stability of NCs, as previously reported [23,24]. Briefly, 5 mL of NCs was suspended in 5 mL of SGF (0.32% *w*/*v* pepsin, 2 g of sodium chloride and 7 mL HCl dissolved in 1 L water and pH adjusted to 1.8 using 1 M HCl) and incubated at 37 °C under shaking at a speed of 100 strokes/min. After 2 h, the sample was collected. The size and PdI were analysed by DLS, while the morphology of the colloidal systems was analysed by TEM.

The stability of the samples was also investigated in simulated intestinal fluid (SIF) containing an intestinal enzyme complex (lipase 0.4 mg/mL, bile salts 0.7 mg/mL and pancreatin 0.5 mg/mL) and 750 mM calcium chloride solution at 37 °C, under shaking, with a speed of 100 strokes/min. The pH of the mixture was adjusted to a value of 7.0 with NaOH 0.1 N. After 2 h, the sample was collected and its physical and morphological properties were assessed by size and PDI analysis by DLS and TEM.

2.7. Preparation of Nanocarriers Based on AN and FITC

NCs were obtained from nanoliposomes (SUVs), which were prepared using the film hydration method. The nanoliposomes were formulated as follows: phospholipids (60 mg), cholesterol (20 mg) and AN (20 mg) or FITC (5 mg) were dissolved in dichloromethane/methanol mixture (20 mL of a mixture 3:2 *v*/*v*). The obtained organic solution was evaporated under vacuum to obtain a lipid film, which was hydrated by the addition of PBS (10 mL) using a mechanical stirrer (RW20 digital, IKA, Staufen im Breisgau, Germany) for 30 min in a water bath at a constant temperature of 37 °C for PC and 60 °C for PS. The resulting formulations were reduced in size using an ultrasonication probe for 3 min (two cycles of 90 s). During the sonication, the samples were kept in an ice bath to prevent lipid degradation. After that, a gentle centrifugation (1205× *g*, 1 min) was performed to remove possible metallic particles released during the ultrasonication. The NCs were prepared by the trapping method, according to Asprea et al. [20]. A 0.1 M solution of $CaCl_2$ was added drop-by-drop to the liposomal suspension under magnetic stirring (150 rpm, at room temperature) until the formulation became cloudy, indicating the formation of NCs. The molar ratio between PC and $CaCl_2$ was 1:1, while the molar ratio between PS and $CaCl_2$ was 1:4.

2.8. Determination of Encapsulation Efficiency of AN–NCs by HPLC

After preparation of the NCs, free AN was removed by dialysis using bags with a pore size of 3.5–5 kD, and according to previous studies [25]. The dialysis bag was placed in 1 L of distilled water at room temperature for 1 h under stirring. The physical mixture was used as a control to validate the procedure. The AN-loaded content was quantified by HPLC–DAD analysis using a standard sample of AN, after the treatment of NCs with methanol to destroy the cochleates. HPLC–DAD analyses were performed with a HP 1200 Liquid Chromatograph (Agilent Technologies, Palo Alto, CA, USA), equipped with a Diode Array Detector (DAD), managed by a HP 9000 workstation (Agilent Technologies). The column was a Varian Polaris RP18 (250 mm × 4.6 mm i.d., particle size 5 μm) (Agilent Technologies) maintained at 27 °C. The chromatograms were acquired at 223 nm. The eluents were acetonitrile (A) and formic acid/water at pH 3.2 (B) at a flow rate of 1 mL/min. The following gradient profile was applied: 0–3 min, 10% A, and 90% B; 3–11 min, 10–38% A, and 90–62% B; 11–25 min, 38% A, and 62% B; 25–30 min, 38–50% A, and 62–50% B; and 30–34 min, 50–10% A, and 50–90% B. The post time was 10 min. The injected volume of the samples was 10–20 μL.

The calibration curve was obtained from a dilution series of the AN reference standard solubilised in MeOH, in the range between 56 and 0.56 ng/mL. Linear regression was used to establish the calibration curve. AN was quantified using the peak areas acquired at 223 nm. The correlation coefficient (R^2) was 0.9995. The data are expressed as the mean ± SD of the three experiments.

The encapsulation efficiency (EE%) for each preparation was calculated using the following equation:

$$EE\% = (Wt/Wi) \times 100\%, \quad (3)$$

where *Wt* is the total amount of the loaded AN and *Wi* is the total quantity of AN added initially during the preparation. The encapsulation efficiency was determined in triplicate.

2.9. Determination of Encapsulation Efficiency of FITC–NCs by HPLC

Free FITC was removed by means of dialysis, as previously described. The contents of FITC were determined by the same HPLC instrument used for AN quantification. The column was a Lichrosorb RP18 (4.6 mm × 100 mm i.d., 5 μm) (Agilent Technologies) maintained at 27 °C. The mobile phases were (A) acetonitrile and (B) formic acid/water pH 3.2, at a flow rate of 0.8 mL/min and an injection volume of 10 μL. The following gradient profile was used: 0–5 min, 10–40% A, and 90–60% B; 5–10 min, 40–50% A, and 60–50% B; 10–12 min 50–55% A, and 50–45% B; 12–15 min, 55% A, and 45% B; 15–18 min, 55–90% A, and 45–10% B; and 18–20 min, 10% A, and 90% B. The post time was 5 min. The chromatograms were acquired at 224 nm. The linearity range of responses of FITC dissolved in CH_3OH was determined on five concentration levels from 6.40 ng/mL to 520 ng/mL and the correlation coefficient (R^2) was 0.9994 [26].

The encapsulation efficiency was calculated using the equation described in the previous paragraph. In this case, Wt is the total amount of the loaded FITC and Wi is the total quantity of FITC added initially during the preparation.

2.10. In Vitro Release Study

The in vitro release of AN from the NCs was investigated using the dialysis bag method. In order to simulate the physiological conditions, PBS (pH 7.4) and enzyme-free SGF and SIF were used as dissolution media. A total of 2 mL of AN–NCs suspension was deposited into the dialysis membrane (pore size 3.5 kD) and placed in 200 mL of the release medium. The temperature was set at 37 °C and the system was stirred at 150 rpm. Release into the PBS was monitored for 24 h while in SGF and for 2 h while in SIF, corresponding to the theoretical transit through the gastrointestinal tract; aliquots of one millilitre were withdrawn in duplicate and replaced with fresh dissolution medium. The samples were analysed by HPLC for the quantification of released AN. The percentage of AN released was calculated as follows:

$$\%\text{AN released} = \left(\frac{\text{AN}_\text{r}}{\text{AN}_\text{tot}}\right) \times 100, \tag{4}$$

where AN_r is the amount of AN detected by HPLC analyses and AN_{tot} is the total quantity of AN deposited into the dialysis membrane.

Furthermore, to evaluate the kinetics of drug release from the NCs, different mathematical models were used, i.e., zero order and first order kinetics model, the Higuchi model, the Korsmeyer–Peppas model and the Hixson–Crowell model. The best fitting model was selected according to the best regression coefficient (R^2) value for the release data.

2.11. Cell Viability and Uptake Studies

The albino mouse embryonic 3T3 fibroblast cell line and the murine monocyte/macrophage cell line J774a.1 were used for cell viability and uptake studies [27,28]. The cell lines were maintained in Dulbecco's Modified Eagle's Medium (DMEM, Sigma-Aldrich) supplemented with foetal bovine serum, 100 units/mL penicillin, and 100 μg/mL streptomycin; for the 3T3 cell line, an additional glucose concentration (4.5 g/L) was used. The cells were maintained under standard culture conditions (37 °C, 5% CO_2, 95% air and 100% relative humidity).

The cells were inoculated into 96-well microplates and maintained under standard culture conditions for 24 h to test the cell viability. Thereafter, the medium was replaced with fresh medium containing different concentrations of NCs or LPs. After 24 h, a WST-8 test was performed following the kit protocol as indicated by the manufacturer and as described in [28]. Briefly, 100 μL of DMEM supplemented with 10% WST-8 reagent was incubated in each well for 2 h at 37 °C. The formazan concentration was quantified by an optical absorbance at 450 nm, with a reference wavelength of 630 nm and by subtracting blank values. The data were expressed as a percentage of the optical absorbance with respect to the controls.

The cells were inoculated into a 33-mm petri dish and maintained under standard culture conditions for 24 h for uptake experiments. Subsequently, the medium was replaced with fresh medium containing different concentrations of FITC loaded in NCs or SUVs. After 1 h, the medium was removed and the cells were fixed in 3.6% PFA in PBS for 10 min at room temperature, stained with DAPI and analysed by confocal imaging. Images were acquired by a Leica SP7 confocal microscope and underwent no subsequent manipulation. A minimum of five different fields was acquired from each sample and all samples were performed in triplicate.

3. Results

3.1. Preparation and Characterisation of NCs

The NCs were prepared according to the multi-step preparation reported in Figure 2.

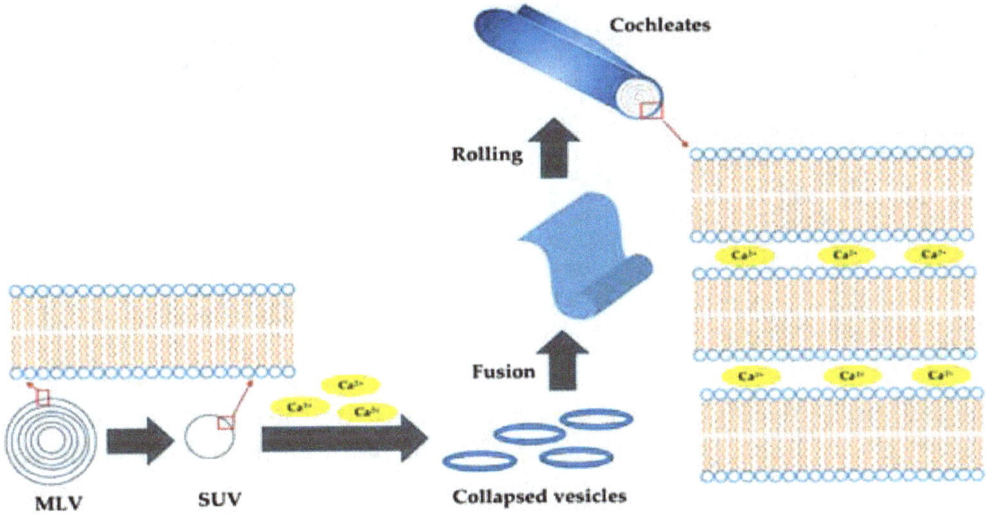

Figure 2. Multi-step preparation process of nanocochleates.

Briefly, as a first step, nanosized LPs were prepared according to the film hydration method using PC or PS and cholesterol, in the gravimetric ratio reported in the experimental part. The lipid film was dispersed in PBS to obtain MLVs. The formation of the SUVs was performed using an ultrasonication probe. In a further step, the SUVs collapsed after the addition of $CaCl_2$ solution when added in the molar ratio 1:1 to PC liposomes (PC–SUVs) and in the molar ratio 4:1 to PS liposomes (PS–SUVs). Then, the collapsed vesicles fused giving large sheets, which rolled-up to give NCs. The calcium ions were essential for the stability of the system, and the aqueous phase in the structure of NCs was very limited, as reported in Figure 2. Both the SUV and NC formulations were characterised in terms of size, homogeneity and ζ-potential by dynamic and electrophoretic light scattering (Table 1).

Table 1. Physical characterisation of empty liposomes and nanocochleates.

Sample	Size (nm)	PdI	ζ-Potential (mV)
PC–SUVs	150 ± 2	0.20 ± 0.02	−29.3 ± 0.9
PC–NCs	150 ± 2	0.24 ± 0.01	−21.6 ± 1.3
PS–SUVs	205 ± 37	0.25 ± 0.03	−37.2 ± 7.1
PS–NCs	207 ± 44	0.55 ± 0.05	−36.4 ± 1.4

PC–SUVs: liposomes made of phosphatidylcholine; PC–NCs: nanocochleates made of phosphatidylcholine; PS–SUVs: liposomes made of phosphatidylserine; PS–NCs nanocochleates made of phosphatidylserine. The data are displayed as the mean ± SD; $n = 3$.

Both PC–SUVs and PC–NCs had a narrow size of ca. 150 nm and they were highly homogeneous as evinced by the PdI (Table 1). Both the liposomes and the NCs based on PC were smaller than those prepared with PS. In particular, the PS–NCs were not homogeneous (Table 1). The dimension of the nanocarriers in the suspension was based on the measurement of their translational diffusion coefficient. This value is related to the length, L, of their major axis as described by Equation (1). The shape of the particles, but not the size, is linked by the geometrical coefficient, FD, which is 1 for spheres. However, it was determined for the NCs using a simplified geometry of long rods, according to Equation (2) [19,20]. All the nanovectors were negatively charged, and, as expected, the ζ-potential was a very low for the nanocarriers based on PS.

The morphological characterisation was completed by the observation of TEM pictures. The size and homogeneity of the liposomes based on PC and PS were confirmed (data not reported). The cigar-like shape of PC–NCs was strongly assessed (Figure 3a). PC–NCs dimensions were comparable with the dimensional distribution results obtained from the DLS analysis. The TEM images of PS–NCs confirmed the presence of polydisperse systems with structures different to NCs (Figure 3b).

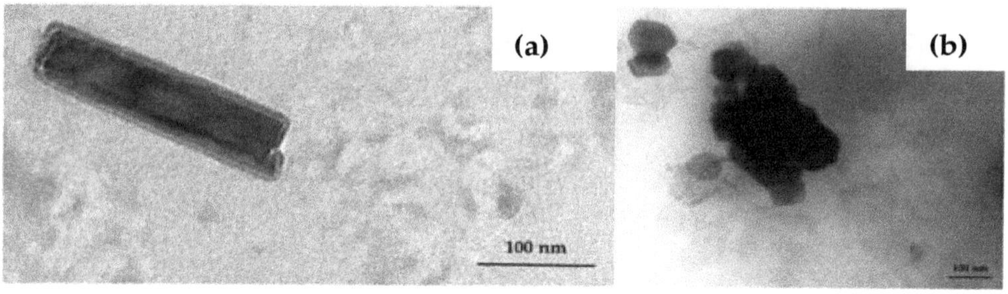

Figure 3. TEM images of PC–NCs (**a**) and PS–NCs (**b**) (scale 100 nm).

3.2. Stability Study of Empty NCs

Firstly, the stability of the NCs was assessed by measuring the changes in terms of the average dimensions, polydispersity and ζ-potential values after the lyophilisation process and resuspension at room temperature with distilled water. The analysis was performed immediately after the lyophilisation process, which did not affect the physical characteristics, when re-suspended in water, as reported in Table 2. All the samples were reconstituted and analysed by DLS, ELS and TEM every week. It was only the PC–NCs that did not experience considerable modification in size, homogeneity and ζ-potential values (Table 2).

Table 2. The particle size, polydispersity index (PdI) and ζ-potential of PC–NCs and PS–NCs as a lyophilised product after two-month storage at 25 °C.

PC–NCs	t_0	After 30 Days	After 60 Days
Size (nm)	150 ± 2	166 ± 5	172 ± 3
PdI	0.24 ± 0.01	0.25 ± 0.02	0.25 ± 0.01
ζ-Potential (mV)	−21.6 ± 1.3	−19.4 ± 1.1	−18.5 ± 1.0
PS–NCs	t_0	**After 30 days**	**After 60 days**
Size (nm)	207 ± 44	292 ± 22	280 ± 25
PdI	0.55 ± 0.05	0.53 ± 0.04	0.55 ± 0.05
ζ-Potential (mV)	−36.4 ± 1.4	−31.4 ± 2.1	−27.2 ± 1.1

PC–NCs: nanocochleates made of phosphatidylcholine; PS–NCs nanocochleates made of phosphatidylserine. The data are displayed as the mean ± SD; $n = 3$.

TEM analyses confirmed the dimensional data obtained by DLS concerning PC–NCs (Figure 4). Instantly after the preparation, PC–NCs had a dimension of 150 nm, while in the following 60 days their size increased by about 20 nm, while their ζ-potential values remained almost constant during this stability study. By contrast, the PS–NCs were not stable and their size increased by about 80 nm during storage. The TEM pictures showed the presence of aggregates (data not reported), confirming the results reported in Table 2.

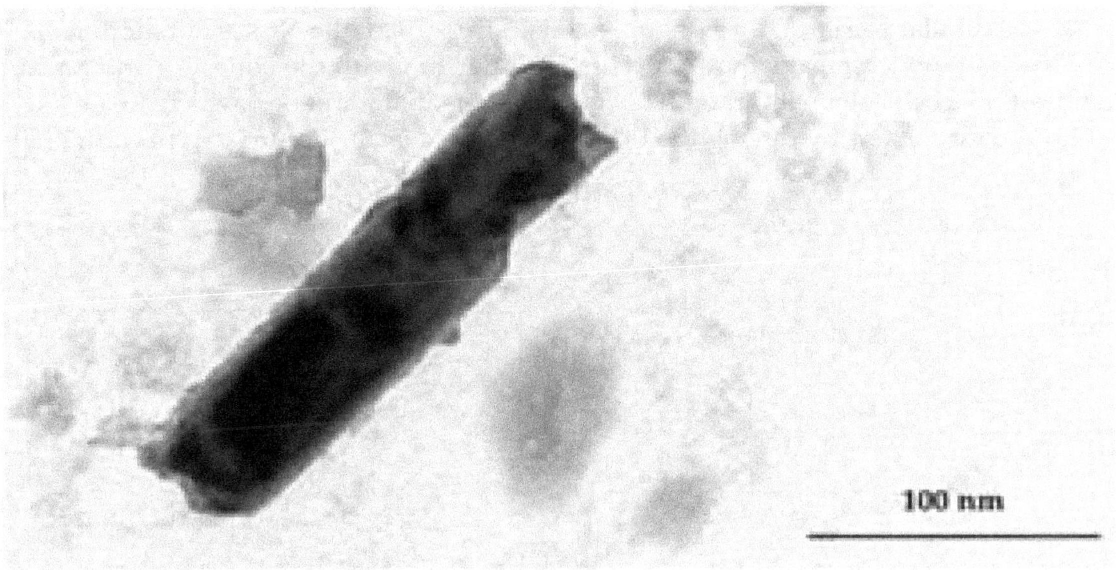

Figure 4. TEM image of PC–NCs re-suspended with distilled water after two months of storage at room temperature in the lyophilised state (scale 100 nm).

3.3. AN–NCs and FITC–NCs Production

As a result of the stability testing of the two NC formulations, PC–NCs were selected as drug delivery systems to be investigated in the present study. AN or FITC was added to the lipid phase and their preparation was carried out using the same scheme reported in Figure 2.

FITC–LPs and FITC–NCs had a good size and homogeneity to test their performance for uptake in the macrophage J774a.1 cell line (Table 3). The average FITC-entrapment efficiency in the SUVs and NCs obtained by HPLC–DAD analyses was 87.5 ± 1.0 and 87.2 ± 0.1%, respectively.

Table 3. Physical and chemical characterisation of AN- and FITC-loaded LPs and NCs.

Sample	Size (nm)	PdI	ζ-Potential (mV)	EE (%)
AN–SUVs	148 ± 2	0.13 ± 0.01	−27.5 ± 2.9	71.1 ± 2.3
AN–NCs	140 ± 1	0.22 ± 0.05	−22.3 ± 3.1	70.6 ± 5.9
FITC–SUVs	180 ± 2	0.20 ± 0.05	−29.2 ± 0.9	87.5 ± 1.0
FITC–NCs	177 ± 1	0.13 ± 0.02	−20.4 ± 2.3	87.2 ± 0.1

AN–SUVs: andrographolide-loaded liposomes; AN–NCs: andrographolide-loaded nanocochleates; FITC–SUVs: fluorescein isothiocyanate-loaded liposomes; FITC–NCs: fluorescein isothiocyanate-loaded nanocochleates. The data are displayed as the mean ± SD; $n = 3$.

The dimensions of the AN–NCs was ca. 150 nm, with a very low PdI, which resulted in suitability for all routes of administration, not only oral [29]. These data were also reflected by the TEM which exhibited NCs as tubular rod structures (Figure 5). The structure of the NCs is not modified in terms of size by AN loading, which means that AN does not interfere with the cohesion and packing of the apolar chains of the cochleate membrane. This is typical of small terpenes, which are able to decrease the size of lipid nanocarriers by forcing the PC structure to increase its surface curvature [30].

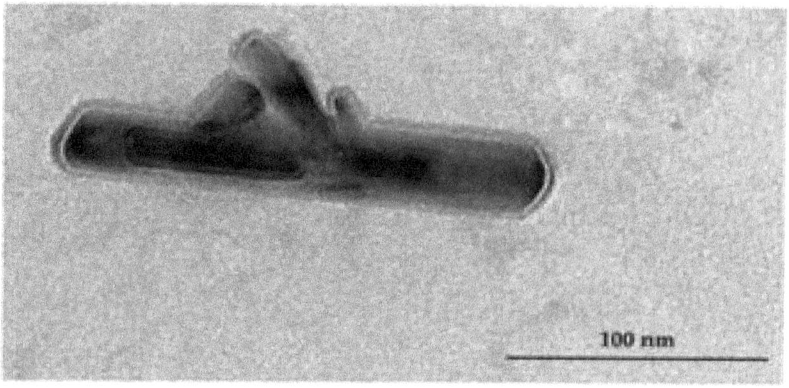

Figure 5. TEM image of AN–NCs (scale 100 nm).

The average AN-entrapment efficiency in both SUVs and NCs was obtained by HPLC–DAD; the results were 71.1 ± 2.3 and 70.6 ± 5.9%, respectively (Table 3).

3.4. Stability of AN–NCs in Gastrointestinal Fluids

It is known that AN is not stable in the presence of gastrointestinal enzymes. Accordingly, one of the aims of this study was the development of a formulation able to protect the incorporated compound from degradation in gastrointestinal fluids. The gastrointestinal fluids may have an influence on the integrity of NCs. The physical stability of AN–NCs was assessed in SGF (pH 2) and in SIF (pH 7). These media did not affect their structure after two hours of incubation. The DLS analyses revealed that the mean diameter of the NCs was not affected by these conditions: after incubation in both gastro-enteric media, their mean size was 143 ± 1 nm with PdI 0.25 ± 0.02.

3.5. In Vitro Release Studies

After demonstrating the physical stability of NCs in gastrointestinal conditions, the in vitro release of AN from NCs was investigated by the dialysis bag diffusion technique. The test was carried out in both SGF (pH 2) and SIF (pH 7) for two hours and in physiological pH conditions (PBS, pH 7.4) for 24 h.

The percentage of AN released in SGF was only 2.31 ± 0.02%, while in SIF, it was 14.75 ± 1.14%. These results suggest that NCs may prevent AN burst release in the gastrointestinal tract, since about 85% of the compound remained entrapped in the NCs.

In PBS, the release of AN from NCs was not immediate, but gradual, unlike in the case of free-AN, indicating that the formulation results in a more prolonged effect (Figure 6).

The AN release from NCs can be described as a biphasic process and the mathematical model of the drug release data was found to best fit the Hixson–Crowell release model: $W_0^{\frac{1}{3}} - W_t^{\frac{1}{3}} = K_s t$; where W_0 is the initial amount of the drug in the pharmaceutical dosage form; W_t is the remaining amount of the drug in the pharmaceutical dosage form, at time t; and K_s is a constant, incorporating the surface–volume relation. The R^2 was 0.9961. This model has been frequently used to describe drug release from several dosage forms with modified release. According to this model, the drug release is described by dissolution, characterised by the surface area and diameter of the particles. Consequently, based on the obtained results, it is possible to hypothesise that this behaviour may be due to the strong affinity of hydrophobic AN to the lipid structure of NCs.

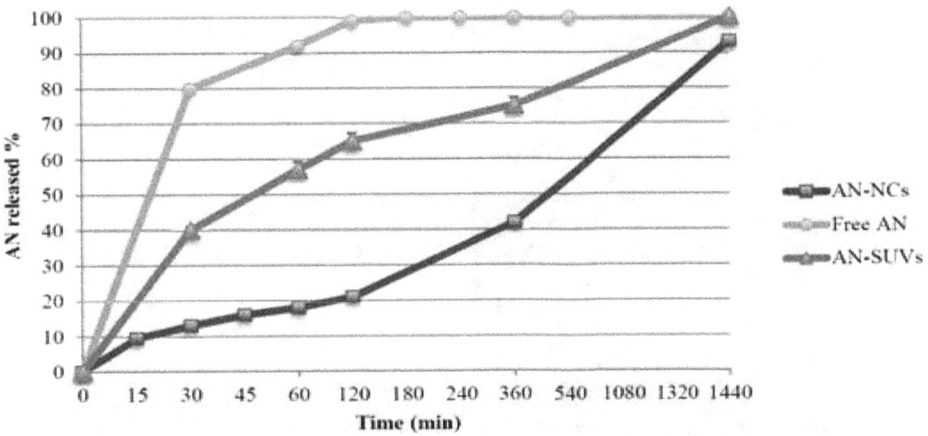

Figure 6. In vitro release profiles of free AN, AN–NCs and AN–SUVs in PBS. AN solution and AN–SUVs were tested to evidence the superiority of AN–NCs on the gradual release of AN. The data are displayed as the mean ± SD; $n = 3$.

3.6. Biocompatibility Studies

The biocompatibility of NCs was tested using two cell lines: macrophage J774a.1 and fibroblasts 3T3. SUVs were used as comparable reference nanovesicles. As a colorimetric, non-radioactive assay, the WST-8 test was selected for assessing cell viability and proliferation because it indicates the mitochondrial activity and hence reflects the cell viability. WST-8, a highly water-soluble tetrazolium salt, is reduced to a soluble purple formazan derivative by trans-plasma membrane electron transport from NADH via an electron mediator. The concentration of formazan was quantified by optical absorbance at 450 nm, with a reference wavelength of 630 nm and by subtracting blank values. The mean value and the standard deviation are the results of nine measurements: the test was performed in three independent experiments and in each experiment, the samples were tested in triplicate. The data were expressed as the percent of optical absorbance with respect to the controls. As indicated in Figure 7, both SUVs and NCs showed no cytotoxicity at the concentration needed for massive uptake, namely, with a dilution of 1:40. Higher concentrations showed a decrease in cell viability, validating the dose–response curve. By contrast, it is remarkable that lower concentrations of the nanovesicles increased the cell metabolism rates, which was probably due to the active uptake process.

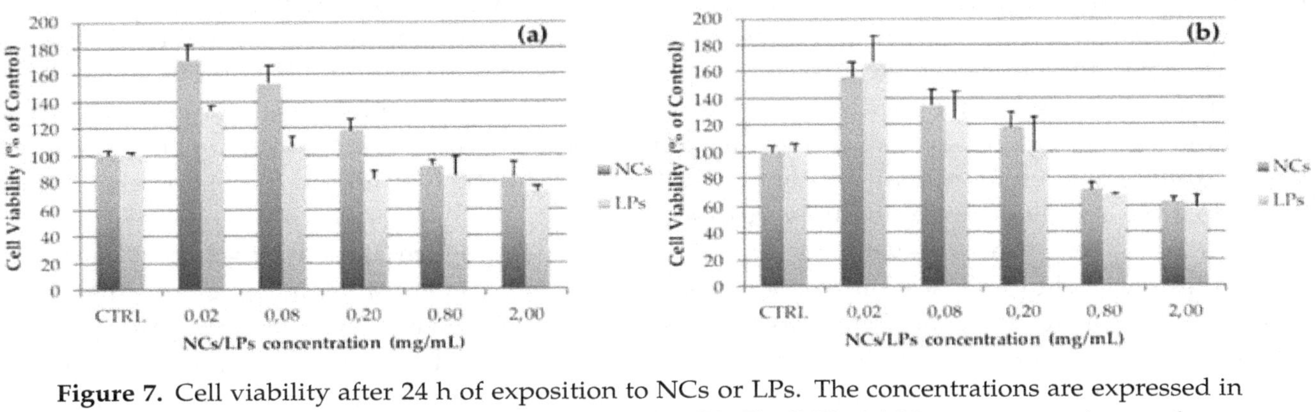

Figure 7. Cell viability after 24 h of exposition to NCs or LPs. The concentrations are expressed in mg/mL. The data represent the percentage of control ± SD. The J774a.1 (**a**) is a monocytes/macrophages cell line; the 3T3 (**b**) is a fibroblasts cell line.

3.7. Cellular Uptake Studies

In Figure 8, the uptake of both NCs and SUVs by macrophage J774a.1 cell line, using nanoparticles loaded with FITC (FITC–NCs and FITC–SUVs), is reported. The uptake was tracked by the green fluorescence of FITC using a confocal microscope (Figure 8).

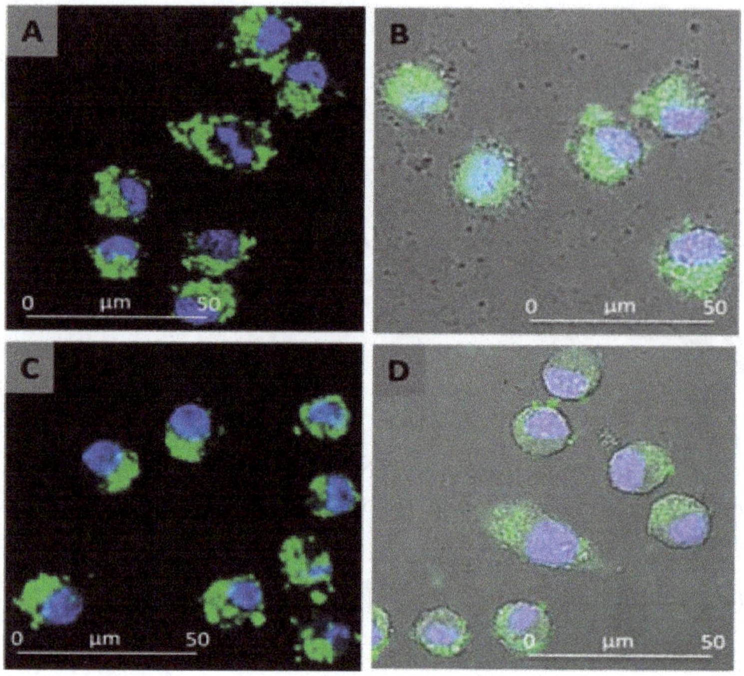

Figure 8. Confocal images of the macrophage uptake of NCs (**a**) and SUVs (**c**). Following nuclear staining with DAPI and FITC encapsulation into NCs and SUVs, the cell nuclei appear in blue and the NCs/SUVs appear in green. The confocal images are also superimposed to Bright Field acquisition (**b**,**d** for NCs and SUVs, respectively) to show the unaltered morphology of the cells and the localisation of intracellular nanocarriers.

As reported in Figure 8, massive uptake takes place but the fluorescence is typically in the cytoplasm without entering the cell nuclei. NCs and SUVs exhibit very similar uptake capability.

4. Discussion

In the present study, the potential of NCs is explored for the delivery of AN, a very promising active natural constituent with various potential therapeutic benefits, but due to the low bioavailability and instability in gastrointestinal media when administered with conventional dosage forms, it has never reached a milestone therapeutic potential. Accordingly, the development of suitable delivery systems for AN represents an urgent issue to formulate effective therapeutic approaches. Lipid-based delivery systems, especially vesicles, have attracted huge efforts as high bio-compatible and biodegradable nanocarriers crossing membrane delivery systems because of their resemblance to the cell membrane. One of the main drawbacks of conventional liposomes for oral administration is their poor stability in the gastrointestinal environment. By contrast, NCs can easily be lyophilised to obtain solid, stable, biocompatible and biodegradable nanovectors [1,2,5,6].

The NCs were simply developed from nanoliposomes (Figure 2), selecting both PS and PC and cholesterol as lipid phases due to their close resemblance to natural membranes and their high compatibility for human use. Ca^{2+} was selected among the diverse divalent cations to generate NCs because it can enhance membrane fusion and phagocytosis. It is well documented that calcium ions induce perturbations of the contact region and thereby promote the membrane fusion [11,31]. Astonishingly, in our studies, only PC and cholesterol generated monodisperse NCs with a tightly packed structure after the addition of Ca^{2+}. As previously reported, PS-based NCs are not stable, producing systems with elevated polydispersity because of a tendency to form stable and huge aggregates, which represents a serious drawback at the industrial level [15]. By contrast, developed PC-based NCs were stable after lyophilisation and re-suspension in distilled water, and after incubation in simulated gastric and intestinal media. In vitro dissolution studies explained an extended release, making AN available over a prolonged period after administration. The PC-based NCs were biocompatible. Even at high concentrations, the cell morphology and vitality were not affected by internalisation. Moreover, high cellular uptake of PC-based NCs was found in macrophages using fluorescent nanovectors. After treatment of the cells with NCs, a bright fluorescent color of the cytoplasm arose due to the FITC and it was clearly distinguished from the nucleus stained with DAPI. Due to the similar uptake performances of SUVs and NCs, it is plausible that the developed NCs fuse with the cell membrane due to the interaction of calcium ions with the membrane containing negatively charged lipids, entering into the cells as nanovesicles [11]. A distinctive geometry, together with peculiar internal interactions, makes NCs ideal as pharmaceutical carriers, which may provide unparalleled protection for the molecular species in order to be carried harmlessly toward its destination. Developed NCs are inexpensive, stable, monodisperse, highly safe, biocompatible, and cell-permeating delivery systems. Moreover, they have high EE%, and suitable drug release properties for oral delivery, but with possible uses in other routes of administration. NCs are characterised by a series of solid-lipid bilayers; the components within the interior of this structure remain intact, even though the outer layers of NCs may be exposed to harsh external environmental conditions or enzymes. This interior structure of NCs is essentially free of water and resistant to penetration by oxygen, which leads to an increased shelf-life of the formulation. NCs can be stored at room temperature or 4 °C, and can be lyophilised to a powder form. Thus, NCs can be used to formulate capsules, pills, tablets, granules, suspensions or emulsions. Due to the ease of the internalisation process, this system could be exploited by employing future in vivo experiments and could be of interest in various therapeutic options.

Author Contributions: The design of the study, A.R.B., M.A. and F.T.; the experimental part, M.A., V.P. and F.T.; data curation, F.T., V.P., M.C.B.; resources, A.R.B., F.R., M.C.B.; writing—original draft preparation, A.R.B., F.T., V.P.; writing—review and editing, A.R.B., F.R.

Acknowledgments: Maria Cristina Salvatici, Electron Microscopy Centre "Laura Bonzi" (Ce.M.E.), ICCOM, CNR, Sesto Fiorentino, Florence, Italy.

References

1. Bilia, A.R.; Piazzini, V.; Guccione, C.; Risaliti, L.; Asprea, M.; Capecchi, G.; Bergonzi, M.C. Improving on Nature: The Role of Nanomedicine in the Development of Clinical Natural Drugs. *Planta Med.* **2017**, *83*, 366–381. [CrossRef]
2. Bilia, A.R.; Piazzini, V.; Risaliti, L.; Vanti, G.; Casamonti, M.; Wang, M.; Bergonzi, M.C. Nanocarriers: A Successful Tool to Increase Solubility, Stability and Optimise Bioefficacy of Natural Constituents. *Curr. Med. Chem.* **2018**. [CrossRef]
3. Sinico, C.; Caddeo, C.; Valenti, D.; Fadda, A.M.; Bilia, A.R.; Vincieri, F.F. Liposomes as carriers for verbascoside: Stability and skin permeation studies. *J. Liposome Res.* **2008**, *18*, 83–90. [CrossRef]
4. Bozzuto, G.; Molinari, A. Liposomes as nanomedical devices. *Int. J. Nanomed.* **2015**, *10*, 975–999. [CrossRef]
5. Nguyen, T.X.; Huang, L.; Gauthier, M.; Yang, G.; Wang, Q. Recent advances in liposome surface modification for oral drug delivery. *Nanomedicine* **2016**, *11*, 1169–1185. [CrossRef]
6. Sankar, V.R.; Reddy, Y.D. Nanocochleate—A new approach in lipid drug delivery. *Int. J. Pharm. Pharm. Sci.* **2010**, *2*, 220–223.
7. Verkleij, A.J.; De Kruyff, B.; Ververgaert, P.H.J.T.; Tocanne, J.F.; Van Deenen, L.L.M. The influence of pH, Ca^{2+} and protein on the thermotropic behaviour of the negatively charged phospholipid, phosphatidylglycerol. *Biochim. Biophys. Acta Biomembr.* **1974**, *339*, 432–437. [CrossRef]
8. Papahadjopoulos, D.; Vail, W.J.; Jacobson, K.; Poste, G. Cochleate lipid cylinders: Formation by fusion of unilamellar lipid vesicles. *Biochim. Biophys. Acta* **1975**, *394*, 483–491. [CrossRef]
9. Zarif, L. Elongated supramolecular assemblies in drug delivery. *J. Control. Release* **2002**, *81*, 7–23. [CrossRef]
10. Syed, U.M.; Woo, A.F.; Plakogiannis, F.; Jin, T.; Zhu, H. Cochleates bridged by drug molecules. *Int. J. Pharm.* **2008**, *363*, 118–125. [CrossRef]

11. Panwar, V.; Mahajan, V.; Panwar, A.S.; Darwhekar, G.N.; Jain, D.K. Nanocochleate as drug delivery vehicle. *Int. J. Pharm. Biol. Sci.* **2011**, *1*, 31–36.
12. Mannino, R.J.; Gould-Fogerite, S.; Krause-Elsmore, S.L.; Delmarre, D.; Lu, R. Novel Encochleation Methods, Cochleates and Methods of Use. U.S. Patent 8,642,073 B2, 4 February 2014.
13. Bozó, T.; Wacha, A.; Mihály, J.; Bóta, A.; Kellermayer, M.S.Z. Dispersion and stabilization of cochleate nanoparticles. *Eur. J. Pharm. Biopharm.* **2017**, *117*, 270–275. [CrossRef] [PubMed]
14. Nagarsekar, K.; Ashtikar, M.; Steiniger, F.; Thamm, J.; Schacher, F.H.; Fahr, A. Micro-spherical cochleate composites: Method development for monodispersed cochleate system. *J. Liposome Res.* **2017**, *27*, 32–40. [CrossRef] [PubMed]
15. Dai, Y.; Chen, S.R.; Chai, L.; Zhao, J.; Wang, Y.; Wang, Y. Overview of Pharmacological Activities of Andrographis paniculata and its Major Compound Andrographolide. *Crit. Rev. Food Sci. Nutr.* **2018**. [CrossRef] [PubMed]
16. Bothiraja, C.; Shinde, M.B.; Rajalakshmi, S.; Pawar, A.P. Evaluation of molecular pharmaceutical and in-vivo properties of spray-dried isolated andrographolide—PVP. *J. Pharm. Pharmacol.* **2009**, *61*, 1465–1472. [CrossRef]
17. Guccione, C.; Oufir, M.; Piazzini, V.; Eigenmann, D.E.; Jähne, E.A.; Zabela, V.; Faleschini, M.T.; Bergonzi, M.C.; Smiesko, M.; Hamburger, M.; et al. Andrographolide-loaded nanoparticles for brain delivery: Formulation, characterisation and in vitro permeability using hCMEC/D3 cell line. *Eur. J. Pharm. Biopharm.* **2017**, *119*, 253–263. [CrossRef] [PubMed]
18. Chellampillai, B.; Pawar, A.P. Improved bioavailability of orally administered andrographolide from pH-sensitive nanoparticles. *Eur. Drug Metab. Pharmacokinet.* **2011**, *35*, 123–129. [CrossRef]
19. Righeschi, C.; Coronnello, M.; Mastrantoni, A.; Isacchi, B.; Bergonzi, M.C.; Mini, E.; Bilia, A.R. Strategy to provide a useful solution to effective delivery of dihydroartemisinin: Development, characterization and in vitro studies of liposomal formulations. *Colloids Surf. B Biointerfaces* **2014**, *116*, 121–127. [CrossRef]
20. Asprea, M.; Leto, I.; Bergonzi, M.C.; Bilia, A.R. Thyme essential oil loaded in nanocochleates: Encapsulation efficiency, in vitro release study and antioxidant activity. *LWT* **2017**, *77*, 497–502. [CrossRef]
21. Arenas-Guerrero, P.; Delgado, A.V.; Donovan, K.J.; Scott, K.; Bellini, T.; Mantegazza, F.; Jiménez, M.A. Determination of the size distribution of non-spherical nanoparticles by electric birefringence-based methods. *Sci. Rep.* **2018**, *8*, 9502–9508. [CrossRef]
22. Tirado, M.; Martınez, C.; de la Torre, J. Comparison of theories for the translational and rotational diffusion coefficients of rod-like macromolecules. Application to short DNA fragments. *J. Chem. Phys.* **1984**, *81*, 2047–2052. [CrossRef]
23. Piazzini, V.; Rosseti, C.; Bigagli, E.; Luceri, C.; Bilia, A.R.; Bergonzi, M.C. Prediction of Permeation and Cellular Transport of *Silybum marianum* Extract Formulated in a Nanoemulsion by Using PAMPA and Caco-2 Cell Models. *Planta Med.* **2017**, *83*, 1184–1193. [CrossRef] [PubMed]
24. Aditya, N.P.; Shim, M.; Lee, I.; Lee, Y.; Im, M.H.; Ko, S. Curcumin and genistein coloaded nanostructured lipid carriers: In vitro digestion and antiprostate cancer activity. *J. Agric. Food Chem.* **2013**, *61*, 1878–1883. [CrossRef] [PubMed]
25. Piazzini, V.; Landucci, E.; Graverini, G.; Pellegrini-Giampietro, D.; Bilia, A.; Bergonzi, M. Stealth and cationic nanoliposomes as drug delivery systems to increase andrographolide BBB permeability. *Pharmaceutics* **2018**, *10*, 128. [CrossRef] [PubMed]
26. Graverini, G.; Piazzini, V.; Landucci, E.; Pantano, D.; Nardiello, P.; Casamenti, F.; Pellegrini-Giampietro, D.E.; Bilia, A.R.; Bergonzi, M.C. Solid lipid nanoparticles for delivery of andrographolide across the blood-brain barrier: In vitro and in vivo evaluation. *Colloids Surf. B Biointerfaces* **2018**, *161*, 302–313. [CrossRef]
27. Borri, C.; Centi, S.; Ratto, F.; Pini, R. Polylysine as a functional biopolymer to couple gold nanorods to tumor-tropic cells. *J. Nanobiotechnol.* **2018**, *16*, 50–58. [CrossRef] [PubMed]
28. Ralph, P.; Nakoinz, I. Phagocytosis and cytolysis by a macrophage tumour and its cloned cell line. *Nature* **1975**, *257*, 393–394. [CrossRef] [PubMed]
29. Bhosale, R.R.; Ghodake, P.P.; Mane, A.N.; Ghadge, A.A. Nanocochleates: A novel carrier for drug transfer. *J. Sci. Ind. Res.* **2013**, *2*, 964–969.
30. Turina, A.V.; Nolan, M.V.; Zygadlo, J.A.; Perillo, M.A. Natural terpenes: Self-assembly and membrane partitioning. *Biophys. Chem.* **2006**, *122*, 101–113. [CrossRef]
31. Papahadjopoulos, D.; Portis, A.; Pangborn, W. Calcium induced lipid phase transitions and membrane fusion. *Ann. N. Y. Acad. Sci.* **1978**, *308*, 50–66. [CrossRef]

6

Novel Formulations of C-Peptide with Long-Acting Therapeutic Potential for Treatment of Diabetic Complications

Natalia Zashikhina [1], Vladimir Sharoyko [2], Mariia Antipchik [1], Irina Tarasenko [1], Yurii Anufrikov [2], Antonina Lavrentieva [3], Tatiana Tennikova [2] and Evgenia Korzhikova-Vlakh [1,*]

1 Institute of Macromolecular Compounds, Russian Academy of Sciences, Saint-Petersburg 199004, Russia; nzashihina@bk.ru (N.Z.); volokitinamariya@yandex.ru (M.A.); itarasenko@list.ru (I.T.)
2 Institute of Chemistry, Saint-Petersburg State University, Saint-Petersburg 198584, Russia; sharoyko@gmail.com (V.S.); anufrikov_yuri@mail.ru (Y.A.); tennikova@mail.ru (T.T.)
3 Institute of Technical Chemistry, Leibniz University, Hannover 30167, Germany; lavrentieva@iftc.uni-hannover.de
* Correspondence: vlakh@mail.ru;

Abstract: The development and application of novel nanospheres based on cationic and anionic random amphiphilic polypeptides with prolonged stability were proposed. The random copolymers, e.g., poly(L-lysine-*co*-D-phenylalanine) (P(Lys-*co*-DPhe)) and poly(L-glutamic acid-*co*-D-phenylalanine) (P(Glu-*co*-DPhe)), with different amount of hydrophilic and hydrophobic monomers were synthesized. The polypeptides obtained were able to self-assemble into nanospheres. Such characteristics as size, PDI and ζ-potential of the nanospheres were determined, as well as their dependence on pH was also studied. Additionally, the investigation of their biodegradability and cytotoxicity was performed. The prolonged stability of nanospheres was achieved via introduction of D-amino acids into the polypeptide structure. The cytotoxicity of nanospheres obtained was tested using HEK-293 cells. It was proved that no cytotoxicity up to the concentration of 500 μg/mL was observed. C-peptide delivery systems were realized in two ways: (1) peptide immobilization on the surface of P(Glu-*co*-DPhe) nanospheres; and (2) peptide encapsulation into P(Lys-*co*-DPhe) systems. The immobilization capacity and the dependence of C-peptide encapsulation efficiency, as well as maximal loading capacity, on initial drug concentration was studied. The kinetic of drug release was studied at model physiological conditions. Novel formulations of a long-acting C-peptide exhibited their effect ex vivo by increasing activity of erythrocyte Na^+/K^+-adenosine triphosphatase.

Keywords: polypeptides; amphiphilic random copolymers; nanoparticles; C-peptide; encapsulation; diabetes

---

1. Introduction

Diabetes is one of the most common socially significant and chronic diseases worldwide. Diabetes and its complications are a major cause of morbidity and mortality. In this regard, the development of new approaches to prevent and treat the diabetic complications is one of the urgent problems of modern pharmacology and biomedical chemistry. In recent years, it has been reported that C-peptide (connecting peptide) can be used for the treatment of diabetic complications and therefore this biologically active peptide has attracted worldwide attention [1,2].

C-peptide, 31-amino acid peptide (EAEDLQVGQVELGGGPGAGSLQPLALEGSLQ), is a byproduct of proinsulin proteolysis in which it connects A and B chains of insulin [2]. The C-peptide provides the correct spatial assembly and packing of proinsulin molecule into the endoplasmic reticulum of insulin-secreting beta cells of pancreatic Langerhans islets. The newly synthesized insulin and C-peptide are stored in equimolar amounts in secretory granules and are released into the systemic blood stream as the blood glucose concentration increases. The role of insulin in the control of carbohydrate-fat metabolism is well known, whereas the role of C-peptide in the regulation of microvascular blood flow has been recognized relatively recently [3,4]. The C-peptide also has an anti-inflammatory effect, it is involved in the repair of lesions of smooth muscle cells; on the models of animals with type 1 diabetes it was shown that the administration of C-peptide normalized the function of nervous and excretory systems [5–7]. A decrease in the concentration of C-peptide or its complete absence is associated with the development and progression of severe complications of diabetes mellitus (strokes, heart attacks, blindness, limb amputation, renal failure) [8]. C-peptide replacement together with the classic insulin therapy may prevent, retard or ameliorate diabetic complications in patients with type-1 diabetes [9].

First results on the C-peptide efficacy were demonstrated in the end of 1990s [10]. It was established that twice a day C-peptide injections to rats with type 1 diabetes during 1.5–3 months at dose 400 μg/kg prevented to a large extent the development of renal, sciatic nerve and aortic vascular disorders and partially restored nerve conduction in muscles. To explore neuroprotective activity of C-peptide on type 1 diabetic neuropathy in rats Zhang et al. tested a range of day doses equal to 10, 100, 500 and 1000 μg/kg during 2 months administration [11]. It was established that 100 μg/kg was enough to prevented the nerve conduction defect.

However, as many other peptide drugs, C-peptide has low stability in vivo and demonstrates also rapid inactivation upon storage. It is known that the half-life of C-peptide in plasma is about 30 min in healthy humans and about 40 min in those with diabetes [12]. Therefore, to maintain plasma concentrations for as long as possible in clinical trials it has been necessary to administer the C-peptide for several times daily. Recently, the positive example on preparation of a long-acting form of C-peptide has been reported by Wahren et al. [13,14]. In the developing medicinal formulation, the authors used well-known approach to increase the resistance of peptide drug via its conjugation with PEG. The treatment of mice with a type 1 diabetic model twice a week for 20 weeks with PEG-C-peptide conjugate at a dose of 0.1–1.3 mg/kg was more efficient comparatively to the control treatment of animals with a native C-peptide. It is important that experiment with native C-peptide required more frequent treatment (twice a day) during the same period and at the same dose [14]. Once-weekly subcutaneous administration of PEG-C-peptide at doses of 0.8 mg and 2.4 mg during 12 months (tested for 250 patients) resulted in marked improvement of VPT (vibration perception threshold) in comparison to placebo injections [15].

Besides the preparation of PEG-peptide conjugates to improve the peptide circulation half-life in vivo and, consequently, to diminish the dose necessary for efficient administration, the application of polymer particles for peptide drug delivery can be also matter of choice [16–18]. Despite the fact that the works devoted to the development of efficient delivery systems of C-peptide were not discovered, several examples on preparation of encapsulated forms of insulin can be found in the current literature [19–23]. The polymer particles of different nature were applied to encapsulate insulin. Microspheres based on Eudragit S-100 copolymer [19], self-assembled chitosan-pectin nano- and microparticles [20], polymersomes based on dextran-*b*-poly(lactic acid-*co*-glycolic acid) [22], microspheres prepared from poly(glycolic acid) [24] were described as successful systems for the development of insulin delivery systems. The efficiency of insulin encapsulation was varied from 32 to 90%. The release explorations in model physiological conditions (PBS, pH 7.4) showed the fast release profiles. For example, insulin release from Eudragit S-100 particles was finished in 8 h and reached almost 100% [19]. In turn, insulin release from dextran-*b*-poly(lactic acid-*co*-glycolic acid) polymersomes took about 9 h to reach the level of 70–85% depending on the polymer composition [22].

The development of novel prospective C-peptide delivery systems undoubtedly represents an actual research goal, firstly, because of high great potential of C-peptide in the treatment of diabetes complications and, secondly, because of absence of commercially available long-acting C-peptide formulations that allow a decrease of administration frequency. Thus, the aim of this study was the creation of the new C-peptide formulations with extended life-time and tissue bioavailability. For this purpose, two different approaches have been suggested and realized: (1) covalent modification of polymer nanosphere's surface with C-peptide; and (2) encapsulation of C-peptide into the developed polymer systems. In our case, synthetic random polypeptides were chosen as the polymers. The interest to synthetic polypeptides is induced by their biocompatibility, biodegradability and the possibility to vary the functional groups in a wide range [25]. The diversity of amino acids allows for the tuning of polymer properties such as hydrophilic/hydrophobic or charge/neutral ones. Since C-peptide is negatively charged molecule we selected P(L-lysine-*co*-D-phenylalanine) (P(Lys-*co*-DPhe) for peptide encapsulation. P(L-glutamic acid-*co*-D-phenylalanine) (P(Glu-*co*-DPhe) nanospheres were chosen for covalent modification with target peptide. An introduction of D-phenylalnine instead of its coding L-isomer into the polypeptide chain should improve the stability of nanospheres regarding to their biodegradation.

It is also known that biological activity of C-peptide belongs to its C-terminal fragment responsible for binding to the cell membrane [26]. Taking this into account, the short C-terminal EGSLQ pentapeptide was additionally synthesized and biological effect of its long-active forms was compared to that observed for the whole length peptide molecule. It is known that C-peptide improvement of human vascular blood flow in type 1 diabetes is mediated through a mechanism involving erythrocyte Na^+/K^+-ATPase activation [27]. In our work, to test the biological activity of different C-peptide forms the method of microcalorimetric titration was used to monitor the activation of Na^+/K^+-adenosine triphosphatase (Na^+/K^+-ATPase) [28].

2. Materials and Methods

2.1. Materials

D-phenylalanine (D-Phe), γ-benzyl-L-glutamic acid (Glu(OBzl), ε-carboxybenzyl-L-lysine (Lys(Z)), triphosgene, α-pinene, *n*-hexylamine (HEXA), trifluoromethanesulfonic acid (TFMSA), trifluoroacetic acid (TFA), *N*-hydroxysuccinimide (NHS), 1-ethyl-3-(3-dimethylaminopropyl) carbodiimide (EDC), PAM-resin (0.75 μmol/g) for solid phase peptide synthesis were delivered from Sigma-Aldrich (Darmstadt, Germany) and used as received. Recombinant insulin C-peptide was purchased from Bachem (Bubendorf, Switzerland). Ouabain specific inhibitor of Na^+/K^+-ATPase was delivered from Sigma-Aldrich (Darmstadt, Germany). Amino acid BOC-derivatives were the products of Iris Biotech (Marktredwitz, Germany). 1,4-dioxane, *n*-hexane, *N,N*-dimethylformamide (DMF), dimethyl sulfoxide (DMSO), tetrahydrofuran (THF), ethyl acetate, methanol, dichloromethane and other solvents were purchased from Vecton Ltd. (St. Petersburg, Russia) and distilled before use. All salts used for buffers preparation were also purchased from Vecton Ltd. and were of ACS reagent grade. The buffer solutions were prepared by dissolving salts in distilled water and additionally purified by filtration through a 0.45-μm membrane microfilter Milex, Millipore Merck (Darmstadt, Germany). Amicon membrane tubes used for ultrafiltration (MWCO 30,000) were the products of Merck (Darmstadt, Germany). The Spectra/Pore® (MWCO: 1000) dialysis bags were purchased from Spectra (Rancho Dominguez, CA, USA).

2.2. Methods

2.2.1. Synthesis and Polymer Characterization

The synthesis of random polypeptides was carried out by ring-opening polymerization (ROP) of α-amino acid *N*-carboxyanhydrides (NCA). NCA monomers of Lys(Z) and Glu(OBzl) (Figure S1 of Supplementary Materials) were prepared as described elsewhere [29]. Dioxane was used as a solvent for Lys(Z) and THF as a solvent for Glu(OBzl) and D-Phe synthesis. Acquired NCAs were purified by recrystallization from ethyl acetate/*n*-hexane. Yields: Lys(Z) NCA—57%, Glu(OBzl) NCA—83%, D-Phe NCA—42%.

The structure and purity of NCAs obtained were proved by ^{1}H NMR at 25 °C in $CDCl_3$. The spectra were recorded at 298 K using a Bruker 400 MHz Avance instrument (Karlsruhe, Germany). Lys(Z) NCA: δ 7.43–7.28 (m, 5H), 6.97 (s, 1H), 5.12 (s, 2H), 4.97 (s, 1H), 4.32–4.23 (t, *J* = 5.2, 1H) (s, 1H), 3.29–3.14 (m, 2H), 2.03–1.90 (m, 1H), 1.90–1.75 (m, 1H), 1.73–1.28 (m, 4H); Glu(OBzl) NCA: 2.05–2.39 (m, 2H), 2.63 (t, 2H), 4.39 (t, 1H), 5.17 (s, 2H), 6.40 (br. s., 1H), 7.39 (m, 5H); D-Phe NCA: 2.94–3.35 (m, 2H), 4.55 (m, 1H), 6.12 (s, 1H), 7.19–7.41 (m, 5H).

P(Lys(Z)-*co*-DPhe) and P(Glu(OBzl)-*co*-DPhe) were synthesized by ROP of corresponding NCAs using hexylamine as initiator. The molar ratio of Glu(OBzl)/Lys(Z) NCA to D-Phe NCA was 1/1, 4/1 and 8/1. The total NCAs/initiator molar ratio was 100/1 for Lys-containing polymers and 50/1 for Glu-based polymers. The synthesis was carried out in 1,4-dioxane or THF using 4 wt.% solution of NCA at 25 °C for 48 h. The product was precipitated with an excess of diethyl ether, the precipitate was washed three times with diethyl ether and then dried. Molecular weight characteristics of P(Lys(Z)-*co*-DPhe) and P(Glu(OBzl)-*co*-DPhe) were determined by size-exclusion chromatography (SEC). SEC was performed with the use of Shimadzu LC-20 Prominence system supplied with refractometric RID 10-A detector (Kyoto, Japan) using 7.8 mm × 300 mm Styragel Column, HMW6E, 15–20 μm bead size (Waters, Milford, MS, USA). The analysis was carried out at 60 °C using 0.1 M LiBr in DMF as eluent. The mobile phase flow rate was 0.3 mL/min. Molecular weights (M_w and M_n) and dispersity (*Đ*) for all synthesized polymers were calculated using GPC LC Solutions software (Shimadzu, Kyoto, Japan) and calibration curve built for poly(methyl methacrylate) standards with M_w range from 17,000 to 250,000 and $Đ \leq 1.14$.

The deprotection of ε-NH_2-groups of P(Lys(Z)-*co*-DPhe) and γ-carboxylic groups of P(Glu(OBzl)-*co*-DPhe) was carried out using TFMSA/TFA mixture in a ratio 1/10 at 25 °C for 3 h. After removing protective groups, the products were precipitated with an excess of diethyl ether, the precipitates were washed three times with diethyl ether, dried and then dispersed in DMF. The suspensions of amphiphilic random copolymers were transferred into dialysis membrane bag MWCO 1000 and dialyzed against water for 48 h.

The contribution of hydrophobic part was determined using HPLC amino acid analysis after total hydrolysis of the samples. The hydrolysis of 3 mg of a sample was carried out in 6 mL of 6 M HCl with 0.0001% phenol in vacuum-sealed ampoule for four days. The solvent was evaporated several times with water to eliminate HCl and to reach finally the neutral pH value. The hydrolysates were analyzed using LCMS-8030 Shimadzu system with triple quadruple mass-spectrometry detection (LC-MS) (all from Shimadzu, Japan) equipped with 2 × 150 mm Luna C18 column packed with 5 μm particles. The isocratic elution mode was applied and 0.1% acetonitrile/HCOOH in a ratio 5/95 wt.% was used as eluent. The mobile phase flow rate was equal to 0.3 mL/min.

2.2.2. Preparation and Characterization of Nanospheres

Polymer nanospheres were prepared by phase inversion during dialysis. For this, polymer sample dissolved in DMSO was placed into dialysis bag with MWCO 1000 which then was deposited into the mixture of DMSO/water = 1/1 (*v*/*v*). After 2 h the solution was replaced with mixture DMSO/water = 1/3 (*v*/*v*) (2 h) and then with water (8 h). Self-assembled nanospheres were freeze-dried with the use of VaCo 5-II lyophilic system (Zirbus, Germany) and stored at 4 °C. Before use, the necessary amount of polymer nanospheres was placed in the medium of choice and redispersed by short-time ultrasonication (30–60 s) by means of ultrasonic probe UP 50H Hielscher Ultrasonics (Teltow, Germany). Average hydrodynamic diameter and polydispersity index (PDI) of polymer nanospheres were measured using dynamic light scattering (DLS) method and Zetasizer Nano-ZS (Malvern Instrument Ltd., Malvern, UK) equipped with a He–Ne laser beam at 633 nm and a detection angle of 173° using the samples with concentration of nanoparticles in the range 0.1–0.5 mg/mL.

ζ-Potential was measured for 0.1 mg/mL colloids in distilled water containing 10^{-3} M NaCl and adjusted with 0.1 M HCl/NaOH to pH 2–12.

The morphological peculiarities were investigated using transmission electron microscopy (TEM) with a Jeol JEM-2100 (Tokyo, Japan) microscope operated at an acceleration voltage of 160 kV. Before analysis, a few drops of a sample were placed onto a copper grid covered with carbon for 30 s. The dried grid was stained negatively with 2% (*w*/*v*) uranyl acetate solution for 30–60 s and used for measurements after 24 h.

2.2.3. Synthesis of C-Terminal Fragment of C-Peptide

C-terminal pentapeptide (27–31 fragment of C-peptide) H-Glu-Gly-Ser-Leu-Gln-OH (EGSLQ) was synthesized via solid phase peptide technique based on application of BOC/OBzl amino acid derivatives. The peptide cleavage from a resin was carried out using TFMSA/TFA system containing 1,2-ethanedithiol and thioanisole as scavengers. The program of synthesis was the same as published earlier [30]. The peptide was purified by size-exclusion chromatography with the use of Sephadex G-75 column (25 × 500 mm) and 6% acetic acid aqueous solution. The RP-HPLC analysis of synthesized product was performed at flow rate 1.0 mL/min using 4.6 × 150 mm Grace Smart C18 column packed with 5 μm particles and 0.1% H_3PO_4/H_2O as buffer A and 0.1% H_3PO_4/AcN as buffer B. A linear gradient of 1 to 30% B in 25 min was applied. MS analysis was performed using MALDI-spectrometer Axima–Resonance Shimadzu (Kiyoto, Japan). The registered molecular ion was found to be $[M + H]^+$ = 533.54, which is consistent with the expected mass of the peptide (532.55 g/mol).

2.2.4. In Vitro Biodegradation Study

Before the biodegradation studies all solutions were filtered through the sterile syringe PES membrane filters with pores of 0.45 μm (Membrane Solutions, Kent, WA, USA). The degradation process of P(Lys-*co*-DPhe) nanospheres was studied in model medium consisting of 0.01 M PBS, pH 7.4, and papain. Briefly, 500 μg of enzyme (papain, ~30 U/mg) were introduced into 1.0 mL of suspension containing 1.0 mg of nanospheres. The experiment was carried out during 35 days. Every several days, the probe of 20 μL of supernatant was sampled for HPLC monitoring of free amino acids (Lys and D-Phe). The commercially available ultra-short monolithic column, namely, CIM-SO3 disk of 3 mm × 12 mm i.d. (BIA Separations, Ajdovscina, Slovenia) was applied as a stationary phase. HPLC experiments were performed with the use of Shimadzu Liquid Chromatographic System LC-20AD (Canby, OR, USA). The data was acquired and processed with LS Solution software (Shimadzu, Kyoto, Japan). UV detection was performed at 210 nm. 0.02 M aqueous Na-acetic buffer, pH 3.7 (eluent A), 0.02 M Na-phosphate buffer, pH 7.0 (eluent B) and 0.0125 M Na-borate buffer, pH 10.0 (eluent C) were used as the components of a mobile phase. The separation was carried out at flow rate 0.5 mL/min following the gradient program: 0–0.5 min—eluent A, 0.5–7 min—eluent B, 7–10 min—eluent C.

2.2.5. Particle Surface Modification with Peptides

The modification of the surface of P(Glu-*co*-DPhe) nanospheres with C-peptide or pentapeptide (C5) was carried out after preliminary activation of the carboxylic groups of glutamic acid. The nanospheres were prepared in 0.01 M Na-borate solution, pH 8.4, and then transferred into 0.01 M MES buffer, pH 5.6, via dialysis using tube membrane (MWCO 30,000). 1.0 mL of suspension with a concentration of 1.0 mg/mL was mixed with a two-fold excess of NHS and EDC required to activate 20% of Glu-units. The activation was carried out at 4 °C for 40 min. The activated nanospheres were washed with 0.01 M PBS (pH 7.4) via ultrafiltration to remove the activating agents and side-products of activation. Then, 200 μg of C-peptide or 50 μg of C5 in 0.01 M PBS were added to the suspension of activated nanospheres and left for 2 h at 22 °C. The excess of the peptide was removed via dialysis using MWCO 30,000 membrane against 0.01 M PBS. The amount of immobilized peptide was calculated as a difference between initial and unbound amounts of peptide. The quantity of unbound peptides was determined by means of HPLC analysis with UV-detection (λ = 210 nm).

CIM DEAE disk of 3 mm × 12 mm i.d. (BIA Separations, Ajdovscina, Slovenia) was applied as stationary phase for this analysis. 0.01 M PBS, pH 7.0 (eluent A) and 0.01 M PBS, pH 7.0, containing 1 M NaCl (eluent B) were used as mobile phases. The flow rate was 0.5 mL/min. Injection volume was 20 μL. The HPLC analysis was carried out under gradient elution: 0–2 min—100% eluent A, 2–17 min—0–100% eluent B. Retention time for C-peptide was 9.8 min and for C5—0.9 min.

Immobilization efficiency (*IE*) was calculated as follows:

$$IE = (m_i - m_s)/m_i \times 100\% \quad (1)$$

where m_i—initial peptide amount (mg), m_s—amount of unreacted peptide in solution (mg).

2.2.6. Encapsulation of C-Peptide

The encapsulation of peptides was carried out via addition of 100 μL of peptide solution with chosen concentration (in a range 0.1–1.0 mg) into suspension of KF1-3 nanospheres immediately after their redispersion in 0.01 M PBS, pH 7.4. After that, the mixture was left at 4 °C for 20 h. Encapsulation of C5 was performed using 100 μL of peptide solution with concentration 1.0 mg/mL. Loading capacity (*LC*) and encapsulation efficiency (*EE*) were calculated using following equations:

$$LC = (m_i - m_s)/m_{NP} \quad (2)$$

$$EE = (m_i - m_s)/m_i \times 100\% \quad (3)$$

where m_i—initial C-peptide amount (mg), m_s—amount of non-encapsulated C-peptide in solution (mg), m_{NP}—amount of nanospheres (mg).

The amount of encapsulated peptides was determined as difference between initial and non-encapsulated peptide amounts. The non-encapsulated peptides were removed from solution via ultrafiltration with the use of tubes supplied with membranes of MWCO 10,000 (used for C-peptide) and 3000 (used for C5). The filtrates were collected and lyophilized and then analyzed as described in Section 2.2.5.

In order to prepare the C-peptide loaded nanospheres with additional coverage with heparin, 1 mL of heparin in PBS with concentration of 1 mg/mL was added to 1 mL of preliminary prepared formulation in PBS with concentration of nanospheres equal to 2 mg/mL. Amount of encapsulated C-peptide in the experiments was varied from 100 to 600 μg.

2.2.7. Drug Release

The release of C-peptide from nanospheres was studied at model physiological conditions, namely 0.01 M PBS, pH 7.4. 1.0 mL of dispersion of nanospheres (conc. 1.0 mg/mL) containing different loaded amount of C-peptide (from 150 to 600 μg/mg of nanospheres) was incubated at 37 °C. After predetermined time intervals, free C-peptide was separated from nanospheres by ultracentrifugation using microtube fitted with a membrane of 30,000 MWCO. The procedure was carried out 4 times with water and the filtered solution was freeze-dried and dissolved in 100 μL of water. The amount of released C-peptide was determined as described in Section 2.2.5.

To determine the stability of colloid system to aggregation as well as drug self-leakage, the suspension of loaded particles in 0.01 M PBS, pH 7.4, was incubated at 4 °C during three months. The supernatant was analyzed by ion-exchange HPLC (Section 2.2.5) to monitor the peptide self-release under storage conditions.

2.2.8. Cell Culture Experiments

HEK-293 (human embryonic kidney) cell line were purchased from German Collection of Microorganisms and Cell Culture (DSMZ). Cells were cultivated in Dulbecco's Modified Eagle Medium (DMEM, Sigma-Aldrich GmbH, Munich, Germany) supplemented with 10% (*v*/*v*) fetal calf serum

(FCS, Biochrom GmbH, Berlin, Germany) and 1% (*v/v*) penicillin/streptomycin (P/S, Biochrom GmbH, Germany) in humidified environment at 37 °C/5% CO_2. The medium was changed 3 times per week and the cells were subcultivated before reaching confluence using trypsin (Biochrom GmbH, Germany).

Eight × 10^3 cells per well were seeded in a 96-well plate (100 µL/well) in DMEM culture medium and cultivated under a humidified atmosphere of 5% CO_2 at 37 °C. After culturing for 24 h, the medium was replaced with the culture medium containing test nanospheres of different concentration (8–500 µg/mL). The viability was determined after 72 h treatment using CTB Assay (Promega, Mannheim, Germany). Culture medium was removed and 200 µL of CTB solution (10% stock solution in basal DMEM medium) were added to each well and incubated for 90 min. The number of viable cells was quantified by measuring fluorescence intensity (λ_{ex} = 544, λ_{em} = 590 nm) using a microplate reader (Fluoroscan Ascent, Thermo Fisher Scientific Inc., Waltham, MA, USA). Relative cell viability (%) was determined by comparing the fluorescence signals with control wells containing untreated cells. Data are presented as average ± SD (n = 4).

2.2.9. Microcalorimetric Ex Vivo Assay of Na^+/K^+-ATPase on Living Erythrocytes

The study was approved by the local ethical committee of Saint-Petersburg State University and was performed in accordance with the relevant guidelines and ethical standards. The volunteers were 25–39 years (males, n = 5) and recruited by the laboratory staff of the Multidisciplinary Clinical Centre of Saint-Petersburg State University. Whole venous blood (10 mL) was collected from healthy volunteers after overnight fasting (12 h) by venepuncture directly into vacutainer tubes (Becton Dickinson, Plymouth, UK) containing heparin. After centrifugation (3000 rpm for 10 min), the plasma, buffy coat, and uppermost layer of erythrocytes were removed by aspiration. The remaining erythrocytes were resuspended and washed three times by inverting the tube to mix in a 10-excess physiological saline NaCl solution (0.9%) and centrifuged for 10 min at 2000 rpm. After the final wash, the hematocrit of the isolated erythrocytes was measured. Finally, living erythrocytes were resuspended in NaCl solution (0.9%) containing 5.5 mM glucose. Human C-peptide and C5 in different preparations were tested at physiological postprandial concentrations of 6 nmol/L.

Microcalorimetric experiments were performed using an isothermal titration calorimeter Nano ITC 2G set at 298.15 K (TA, New Castle, DE, USA). Each experiment consisted of single injection (5 µL) from a 100-µL rotating syringe of a solution containing different formulations of C-peptide or C-terminal pentapeptide (C5) into the microcalorimetric reaction cell (1 mL) charged with 500 µL of suspension of erythrocytes with concentration 1.1 × 10^9 cells per mL. Quite low stirring rate (60 rpm) was necessary to avoid the damage of living erythrocytes. Heat production by the erythrocytes was recorded versus time. The steady state was reached after at least 1 h of incubation. Then, the tested compound was added to the suspension and changes in heat production were recorded. The heat of reaction was corrected for the heat of dilution of the guest solution, determined in the separate experiments. Ouabain (15 mmol/L) specific inhibitor of Na^+/K^+-ATPase was used to verify that heat production effects of C-peptide or C5 peptide and their formulations attributed to Na^+/K^+-ATPase activity. All solutions were degassed prior to titration experiment. Each injection generated a heat burst curve (µJ per second), the area under which was determined by integration using Nano ITC analyze software that gave the measure of the heat of reaction associated with the injection. Each sample was measured for three times.

All experiments were performed at 25 °C. The difference between heat production (µJ) in the steady state before and after the addition of respective test substances corresponds to the erythrocyte Na^+/K^+-ATPase activity normalized to sample volume (mL) and hematocrit (%). Sample volume, C-peptide amount and hematocrit remained constant for each measurement.

3. Results and Discussion

3.1. Polymerization and Polymer Characterization

The synthesis of random copolymers P(Glu-*co*-DPhe) and P(Lys-*co*-DPhe) was carried out using ring-opening polymerization (ROP) of *N*-carboxyanhydrides of L-Glu(OBzl)/L-Lys(Z) and D-Phe (Figure 1). The series of random copolymers were synthesized with different monomer ratios (Table 1). The molecular weight (M_w and M_n) and dispersity ($Đ$) of protected copolymers was determined using size-exclusion chromatography (SEC) (Table 1). All synthesized polymers were characterized with low dispersity ($1.07 \leq Đ \leq 1.29$). $Đ$ values were minimal when the ratio of L-Glu(OBzl)/L-Lys(Z) NCA to D-Phe NCA was 1/1 and maximal for the ratio 8/1.

The preparation of amphiphilic copolymers was achieved after the removal of *Z*- and *Bzl*-protective groups. After deprotection the polymers became to be insoluble in water and demonstrated the tendency to self-assembly. The deprotection was proved by ^1H NMR spectroscopy (Figure S2 of Supplementary Materials).

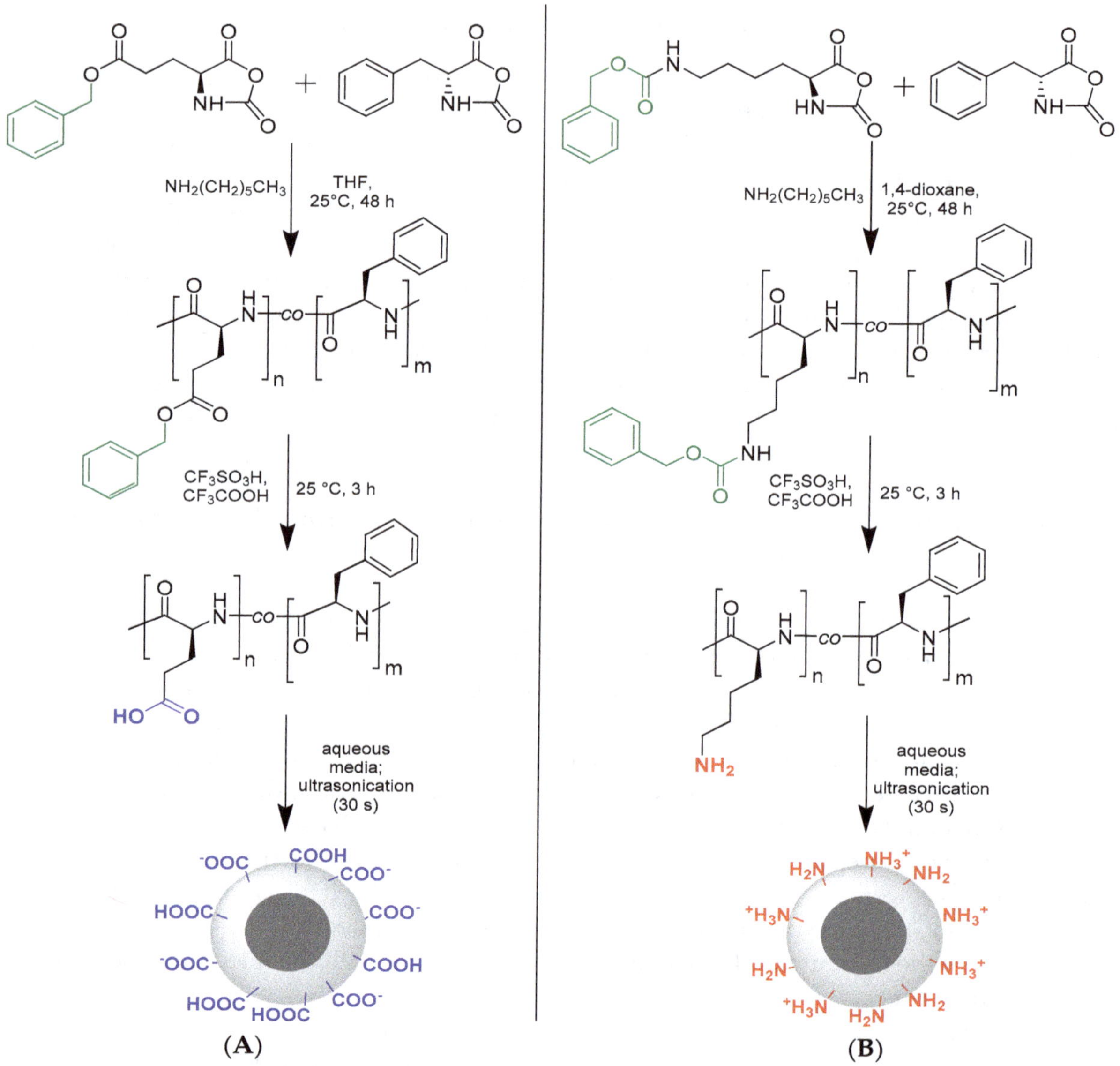

Figure 1. Scheme of polymerization and preparation of self-assembled nanospheres: (**A**) P(Glu-*co*-DPhe); (**B**) P(Lys-*co*-DPhe).

Table 1. Monomer ratios, polymer yields and characteristics of synthesized protected copolymers.

Sample	Initial Ratio of NKAs: [Glu(OBzl)/Lys(Z)]/[D-Phe]	Polymer Characteristics (SEC)			Polymer Yield, %
		M_n	M_w	$Đ$	
		P(Glu(OBzl)$_n$-*co*-DPhe$_m$)			
E(Bzl)F1	1/1	5600	6400	1.15	49
E(Bzl)F2	4/1	6700	8100	1.20	70
E(Bzl)F3	8/1	7100	9200	1.29	72
		P(Lys(Z)$_n$-*co*-DPhe$_m$)			
K(Z)F1	1/1	14,000	15,800	1.07	68
K(Z)F2	4/1	21,500	24,300	1.13	55
K(Z)F3	8/1	24,300	28,000	1.15	71

The composition of synthesized polymers was proved by quantitative HPLC analysis of the samples prepared via total acidic hydrolysis of polypeptides up to free amino acids. The results obtained are presented in Table 2. Additionally, for copolymers based on glutamic acid and phenylalanine the composition was calculated from ^{1}H NMR spectra (Table 2, Figure S2 of Supplementary Materials). Polymer composition established by two methods was in a good agreement. For sample EF1, prepared with initial [Lys(Z) NCA]/[Phe NCA] ratios equal to 1/1, the experimentally found composition was close to the theoretical one. An increase of the ratio of glutamic acid monomer in polymerization mixture was followed by partial diminishing of Glu units in final copolymers. In turn, the polymer compositions for KF1 and KF2 samples were matched well with that of monomer mixture. An increase of [Lys(Z) NCA]/[Phe NCA] to 8/1 was followed by the partial enrichment of final polypeptide with lysine. For copolymers based on lysine and phenylalanine the determination of polymer composition by ^{1}H NMR was impossible because of broadening and overlapping of reference signals.

Table 2. Composition of amphiphilic random polypeptides and polymer yields after deprotection.

Sample	Determined Polymer Composition					
	HPLC			^{1}H NMR		
	n	m	[Glu/Lys]/[Phe] Ratio	n	m	[Glu]/[Phe] Ratio
			P(Glu$_n$-*co*-DPhe$_m$)			
EF1	17	14	1.2	16	15	1.1
EF2	33	11	3.0	37	10	3.7
EF3	38	7	5.4	45	8	5.6
			P(Lys$_n$-*co*-DPhe$_m$)			
KF1	34	34	1.0	-	-	-
KF2	72	17	4.3	-	-	-
KF3	87	9	9.5	-	-	-

3.2. Preparation and Characterization of Nanospheres

There are many different techniques for the preparation of polymer nanoparticles such as solvent evaporation, nanoprecipitation, emulsification/solvent diffusion (ESD), high-pressure homogenization, phase inversion (dialysis), film rehydration, etc. [31]. The approach selection straightly depends on the polymer properties (chemical nature, charge, hydrophilicity/hydrophobicity, swelling, reactivation, pH-dependency, etc.). In our case, the phase inversion (dialysis) method was chosen because of its simplicity and suitability to prepare self-assembled nanosystems [32–34]. The hydrodynamic diameter of nanospheres obtained was determined using dynamic light scattering (DLS) method at different pH.

The hydrodynamic diameter of P(Lys-*co*-DPhe) nanospheres was varied from 110 to 220 nm for the different polymer composition in the pH range from 3 to 11 (Figure 2A). The increase of pH up to

12 induced the immediate aggregation of nanospheres that was a result of the loss of particle surface charge, which was necessary to stabilize the colloid system towards the aggregation (Figure 2B).

The similar tendency was observed for P(Glu-*co*-DPhe) nanospheres but, in this case, the isoelectric point was at pH 3 (Figure 2D). In the range of pH 5–11 the nanospheres were stable. Usually, the colloid system is counted as stable if ζ-potential absolute value is higher than 30 mV [35]. In our case, both kinds of nanospheres met this requirement. For P(Glu-*co*-DPhe), the nanospheres with the smallest hydrodynamic diameter (350–210 nm depending on the polymer composition) were formed in the range of pH from 7 to 11 (Figure 2C). This fact can be explained by better ionization of carboxylic groups at pH higher than 7. The better ionization is followed by the repulsion of like-charged polymer chains that in turn favored to the self-assembly into the smaller-sized nanospheres.

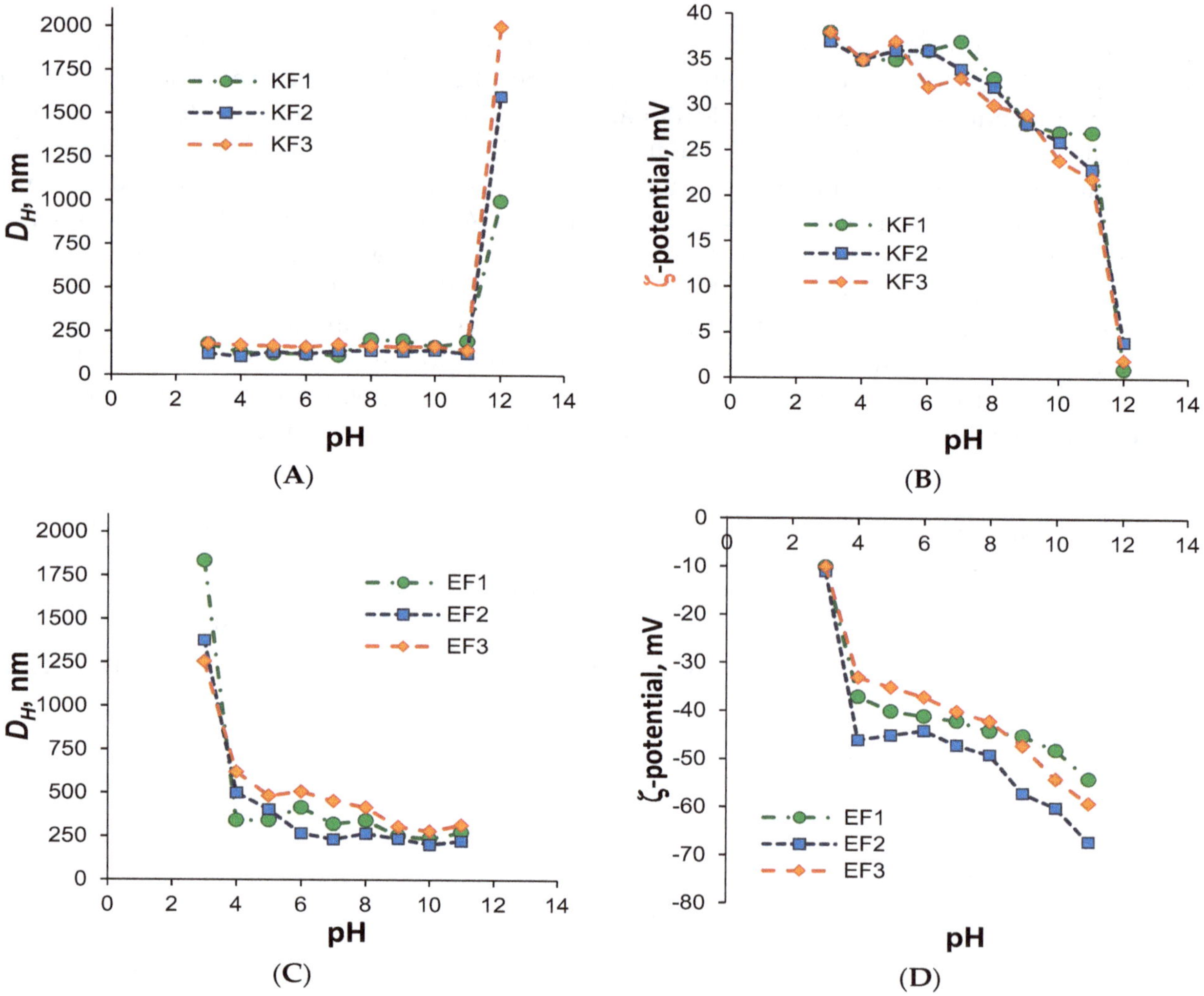

Figure 2. Dependence of hydrodynamic diameter and ζ-potential of polypeptide nanospheres on pH: (**A**,**B**)—P(Lys-*co*-DPhe); (**C**,**D**)—P(Glu-*co*-DPhe).

Additionally, the dependence of average hydrodynamic diameter of nanospheres on the sample dilution was evaluated. The dilution of dispersion with starting concentration of 2 mg/mL in 250 times (up to 0.008 mg/mL) did not follow with the change in D_H of nanoparticles. All colloid systems were stable under incubation in 0.01 M PBS, pH 7.4, during three months without changing their hydrodynamic diameter, aggregation and sedimentation.

The nanospheres prepared in 0.01 M PBS buffer, pH 7.4, were investigated by transmission electron microscopy (TEM) (Figure 3). The size of polymer nanoparticles observed by TEM in a dry state was about 30 ± 5 nm. Such difference between hydrodynamic diameter registered in aqueous media by DLS and diameter of nanospheres determined by TEM in a dry state is known for soft self-assembled materials [36,37]. This effect is related to the volatilization of water during the TEM grid drying before analysis. In aqueous media, the hydrodynamic diameter of nanospheres is provided by the expansion of charged water-soluble-like charged fragments (Lys or Glu) because of their repulsion.

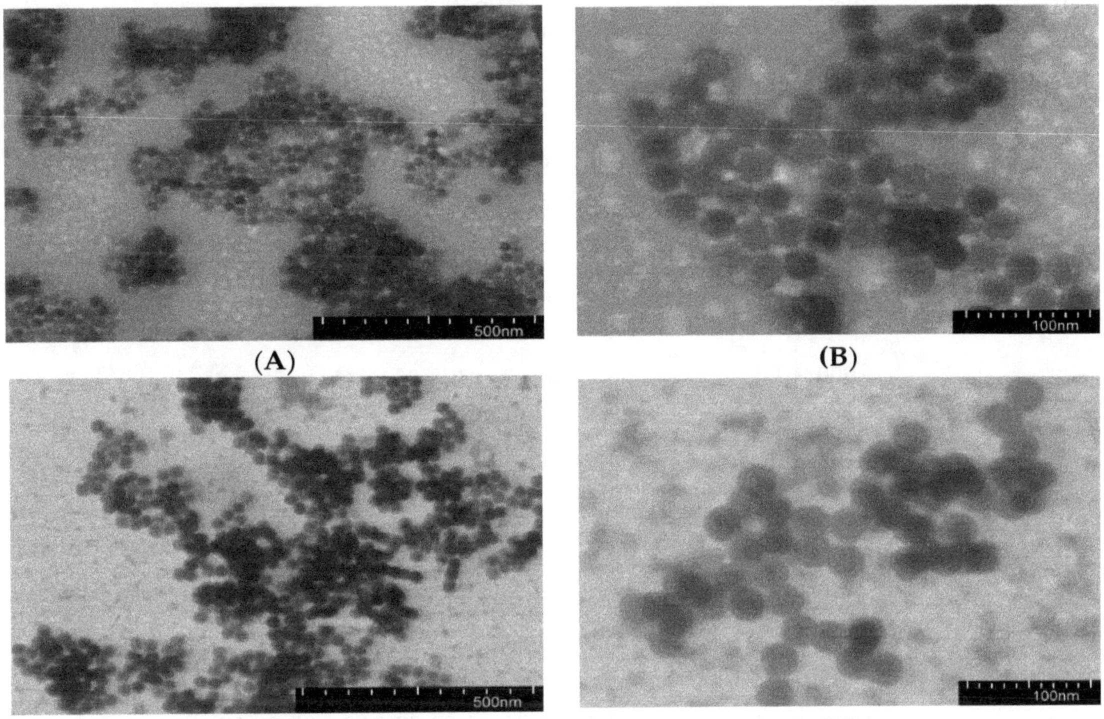

(C) (D)

Figure 3. Transmission electron microscopy (TEM) images of P(Glu-*co*-DPhe) (**A**,**B**) and P(Lys-*co*-DPhe) (**C**,**D**) nanospheres (samples EF2 and KF2).

3.3. *In Vitro Biodegradation Study*

P(Lys-*co*-DPhe) nanospheres were chosen to evaluate the biodegradation process in vitro. The process was performed in 0.01 M PBS, pH 7.4, containing papain as model enzyme. Papain, being a thiol proteinase of plant origin, represents the analogue of lysosomal endopeptidase cathepsin B regarding to its activity towards the bonds formed between different α-amino acids. The biodegradation process was carried out in two ways: (1) as a function of free amino acids accumulation in the reaction mixture during the time and (2) as a function of change in hydrodynamic diameter of particles (Figure 4). According to HPLC data only 14% of L-Lys and 3% of D-Phe were detected for sample KF1 after a month of particle incubation with papain at 37 °C. For sample KF2, 15% of L-Lys and 5% of D-Phe were determined for the same time.

The monitoring of hydrodynamic diameter of nanospheres during a month allowed for detection of decrease in this parameter. In particular, 15% and 17% decrease in D_H was established for KF1 and KF2 samples and 34% for EF1 one. The results obtained were compared to the data on biodegradation of random nanospheres based on copolymer of L-lysine and L-aminoisobutyric acid (P(Lys-*co*-Aib)), containing 29 mol% Aib and developed recently in our group [37]. Aib represents natural but non-coded amino acid, which sometimes is also used to improve the ability to enzymatic degradation [38]. As it can be seen from Figure 4B, the hydrodynamic diameters were drastically diminished of the P(Lys-*co*-Aib)-based nanospheres incubated at the same conditions and for the same time period. The total decrease in D_H corresponded to 87%. Thus, the developed P(Glu-*co*-DPhe) and P(Lys-*co*-DPhe) nanospheres can be counted as biomaterials with increased stability to biodegradation.

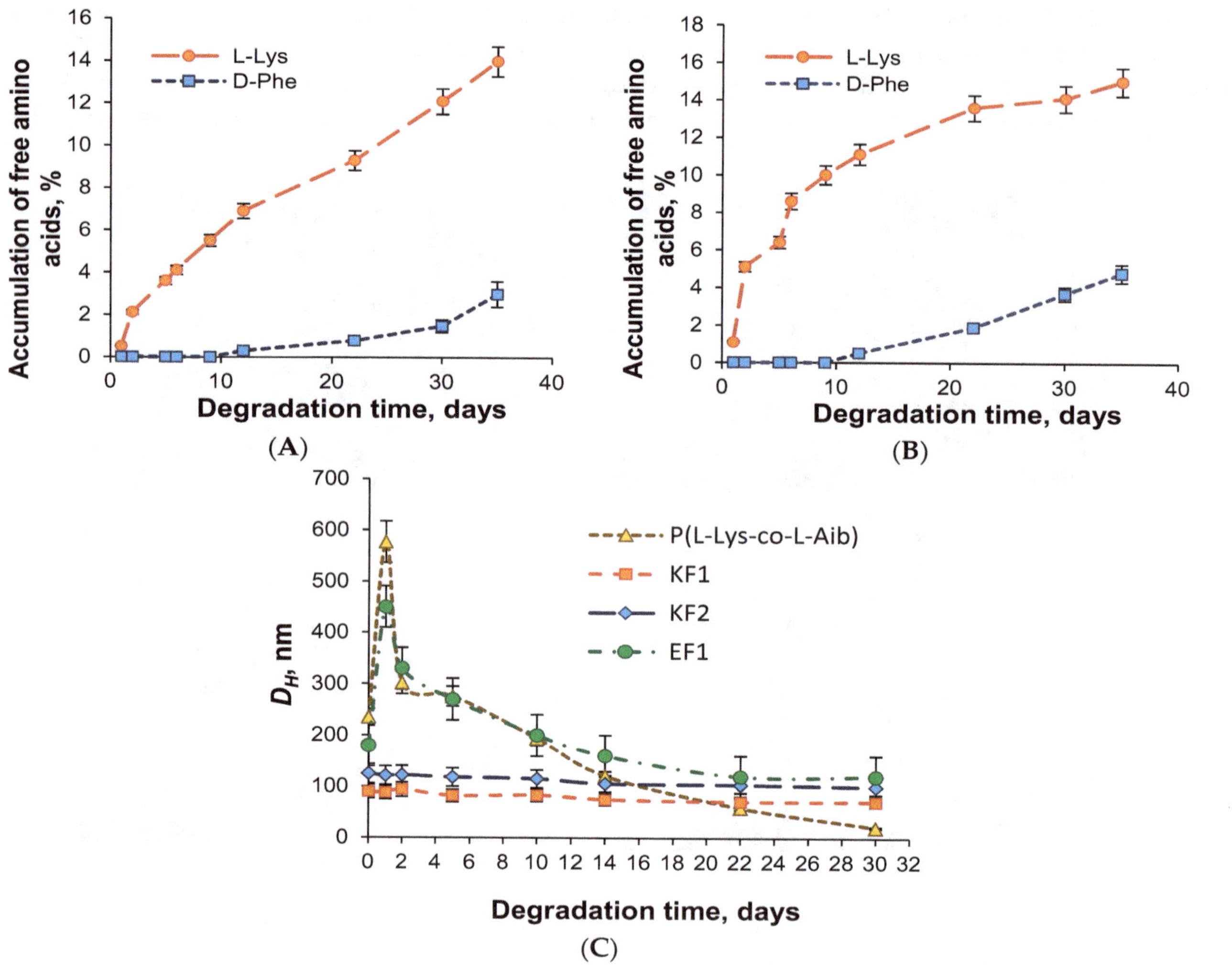

Figure 4. Degradation of P(Lys-*co*-DPhe) nanospheres on time: (**A**,**B**) accumulation of free amino acids during the process for samples KF1 and KF2, respectively (HPLC); (**C**) Decrease of hydrodynamic size on time (DLS). Conditions of biodegradation: incubation was performed in 0.01 M PBS, pH 7.4, and at 37 °C; concentration of nanospheres was 1.0 mg/mL; concentration of papain was 0.5 mg/mL.

3.4. Surface Modification

The presence of chemically reactive functional groups on the surface of poly(amino acid) nanospheres allowed the modification of their surface by different biomolecules including peptides. In present work, for preparation of C-peptide formulation with preserved peptide biological activity and prolonged stability we chose the method of one-point attachment of C-peptide and its short C5 fragment (EGSLQ) via the reaction of α-amino group of N-terminal amino acid with carboxylic group of P(Glu-*co*-DPhe) nanospheres. This approach includes an activation of carboxylic groups with water soluble carbodiimide and *N*-hydroxysuccinimide (NHS) to form activated NHS ester (Figure 5).

The samples EF1, EF2 and EF3 differ in the content of hydrophilic and hydrophobic units were modified with C-peptide (Table 3). For all nanospheres the reaction of covalent immobilization was carried out under the same conditions (2 h at 22 °C) and amount of activated carboxylic groups (20 mol%). It was established that the quantity of the bound C-peptide depended on polymer composition. The highest amount of immobilized C-peptide was determined for the sample EF2 containing intermediate ratio of Glu and Phe units. In this case, 48 μg of C-peptide per mg of nanospheres was attached onto the nanoparticle's surface.

The low immobilization efficiency of C-peptide on the surface of EF1 nanospheres may be related to the lowest amount of Glu units among the tested polymers. In turn, very high content of Glu units in the polymer probably favored to the higher repulsion of highly negative charged nanospheres and like-charged C-peptide.

EF2 nanospheres were selected for the immobilization of C5. It is known that the functional groups of small molecules are characterized with better reactive accessibility comparatively to the more elongated ones. Taking this into account, the initial C5 amount used for immobilization was reduced twice comparatively to C-peptide (from 200 to 100 µg). Despite the fact that immobilization efficiency was only 16%, the molar amount of immobilized C5 was appeared to be higher than this established for C-peptide.

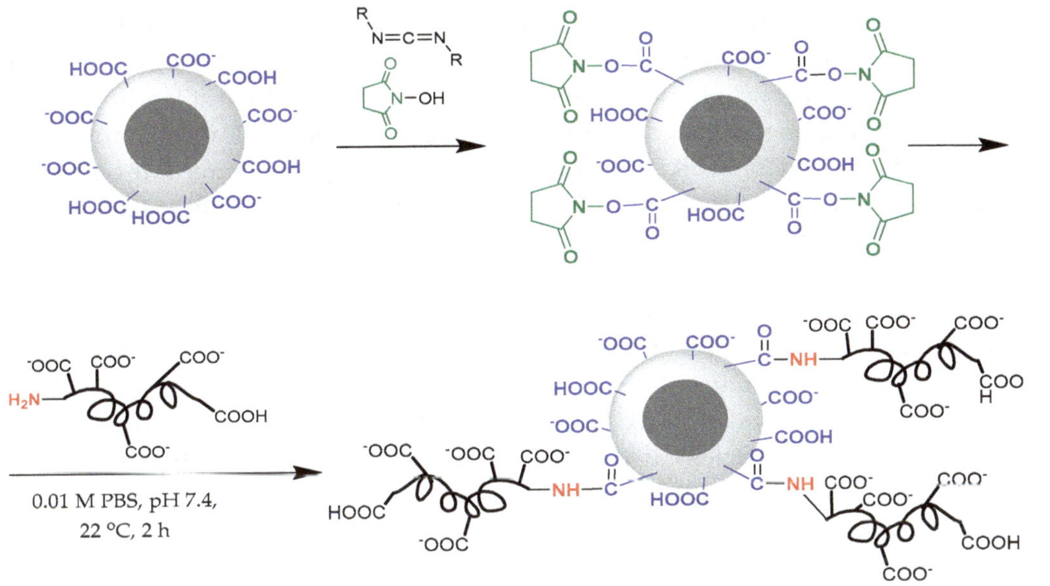

Figure 5. Scheme of covalent modification of P(Glu-*co*-DPhe) particle surface.

Table 3. Characteristics of nanospheres under C-peptide and C5 covalent immobilization. Conditions of immobilization: 0.01 M PBS, pH 7.4; 22 °C; 2 h.

Sample	Amount of Bound Peptide, µg/mg of Nanospheres	Amount of Bound Peptide, nmol/mg of Nanospheres	Immobilization Efficiency, %
		C-peptide	
EF1	20 ± 4	5.5	10 ± 1
EF2	48 ± 5	13.3	24 ± 2
EF3	25 ± 3	6.9	13 ± 2
		C5	
EF2	16 ± 2	30.0	16 ± 2

The developed delivery systems were tested for the storage stability. The samples with concentration of 1 mg/mL were stored at 4 °C during three months. The monitoring of hydrodynamic diameter as well as free C-peptide in 0.01 M PBS, pH 7.4, revealed the high stability of the formulation at low temperatures. In particular, D_H change or aggregation of nanospheres, as well as drug leakage were not detected.

3.5. C-Peptide Encapsulation

Encapsulation of C-peptide into P(Lys-*co*-DPhe) nanospheres represents an alternative approach for the preparation of a long-acting peptide formulation. P(Lys-*co*-DPhe) nanospheres were chosen because of their positive charge, which can provide the ionic interactions with highly negative charged C-peptide (Figure 6).

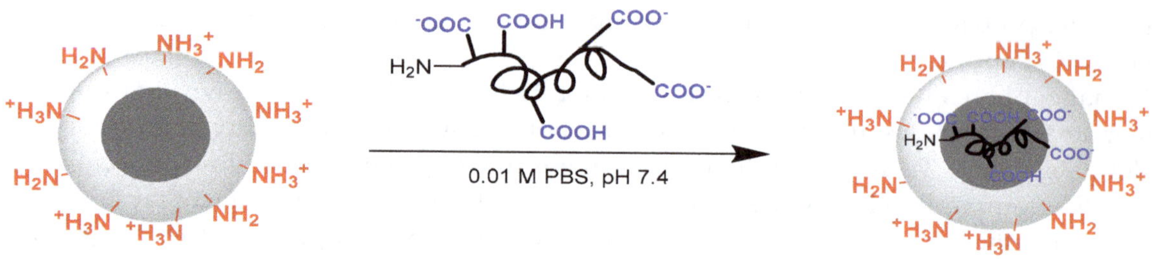

Figure 6. Scheme of encapsulation of C-peptide into the P(Lys-*co*-DPhe) nanospheres.

For the first step, the encapsulation efficiency (EE) and loading content (LC) on the polymer composition were analyzed at constant initial amount of C-peptide (100 µg). All tested polymer nanospheres demonstrated very high loading efficiency (Table 4). The lowest loading efficiency (89.5%) was observed for the nanospheres based on KF1 sample containing the lowest amount of lysine units in the polymer chains. For KF2 and KF3 samples, containing higher content of lysine than KF1, the values of *EE* were very close to 95%. The encapsulation efficiency of C5 into KF3 nanospheres was similar to that established for C-peptide.

Additionally, the hydrodynamic diameter of nanospheres loaded with C-peptide was measured in 0.01 M PBS, pH 7.4, and compared (Table 4). It was found that the D_H values were increased with lysine enrichment in polymer chains. The smallest nanospheres were formed from KF1 polypeptide whereas the largest ones were obtained for KF3 sample. The higher content of hydrophobic monomer favors to compaction of the particles during the polymer self-assembling. In turn, the high number of charged fragments tends to repulse each other and, as a result, the hydrodynamic diameter of self-assembled particles is increased.

Table 4. Dependence of encapsulation efficiency, loading content and hydrodynamic diameter of nanospheres on polymer composition and peptide.

Sample	D_{Ho} *, nm	*EE* **, %	*LC*, µg/mg of Particles	$D_{H\ encaps}$ *, nm	*PDI* $_{encaps}$ *
			C-peptide		
KF1	71 ± 3	89.5 ± 0.6	89.5 ± 0.5	79 ± 8	0.24
KF2	96 ± 3	94.6 ± 1.0	94.6 ± 0.9	130 ± 20	0.16
KF3	150 ± 10	95.0 ± 1.1	95.0 ± 1.0	190 ± 20	0.14
			C5		
KF3	150 ± 10	96.2 ± 0.7	96.2 ± 0.7	178 ± 15	0.13

* measured in 0.01 M PBS, pH 7.4; ** the initial amount of peptide taken for loading was 100 µg.

For the study of the dependences of *LC* and *EE* on initial C-peptide concentration, two samples containing the highest and the lowest amount of hydrophobic amino acid, e.g., KF1 and KF3, were selected. It was established that an increase of initial concentration of C-peptide from 100 µg/mL to 1000 µg/mL followed by nearly linear increase of loading capacity (Figure 7A). The maximum *LC* of C-peptide for KF1 and KF3 nanospheres were equal to 804 ± 6 and 860 ± 5 µg of C-peptide/mg of nanoparticles, respectively. When the initial C-peptide concentration was higher than 1000 µg/mL the aggregation of particles was detected. This fact can be attributed to the partial neutralization of lysine positive charge of the P(Lys-*co*-DPhe) particles with negative charge of C-peptide. It was proved by an intense decrease of ζ-potential from +40 to +20 mV.

In turn, the encapsulation efficiency for KF1 and KF3 particles was just slightly reduced from 89.5% and 95.0%, determined at initial drug concentration of 100 µg/mL, to 80.2% and 86.4% detected for concentration 1000 µg/mL, respectively (Figure 7B).

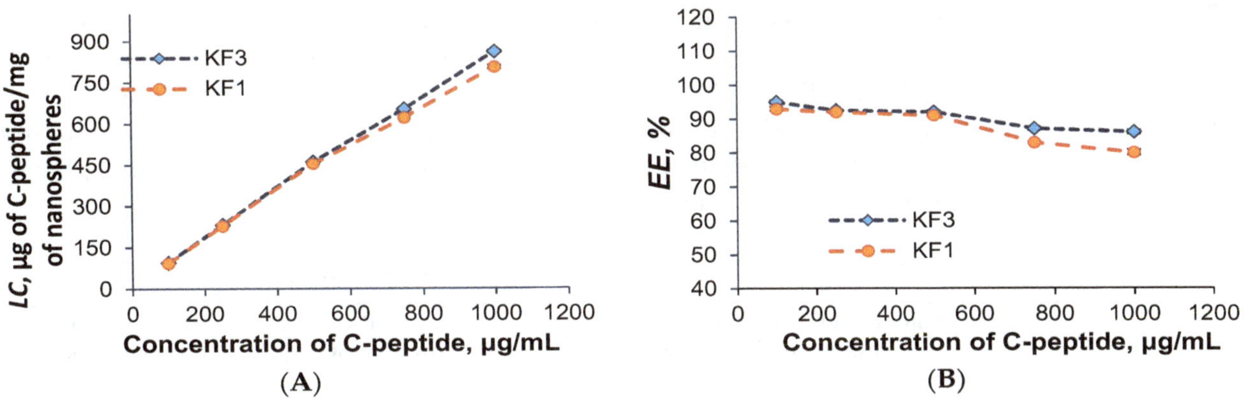

Figure 7. Dependence of loading capacity (LC) (**A**) and encapsulation efficiency (EE) (**B**) on initial concentration of C-peptide.

Since the high drug loading may affect the particle size, the hydrodynamic diameter of KF1 and KF3 nanospheres loaded with the different quantity of C-peptide were analyzed (Figure 8). For nanospheres with the maximal lysine content (KF3) the hydrodynamic diameter did not depend on C-peptide loading amount. On the contrary, the hydrodynamic diameter of KF1 nanospheres, containing the minimal lysine amount, was increased with the growth of drug loading. At maximal value of *LC* equal to 804 µg of C-peptide per mg of polymer nanospheres, ζ-potential of KF1 particles decreased to +30 mV that can be attributed to the partial charge neutralization because of C-peptide loading comparatively to the KF3 nanospheres enriched with lysine units.

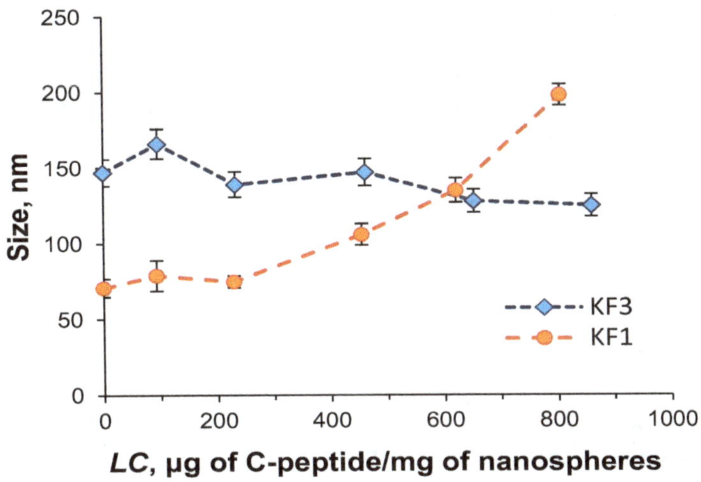

Figure 8. Dependence of nanosphere's hydrodynamic diameter on C-peptide loading content.

As for C-peptide covalently bound to the nanospheres, the encapsulated forms of C-peptide demonstrated also high storage stability towards the preservation of colloid's properties at low temperature (4 °C). During three months the changes in hydrodynamic diameter or precipitation of formulation were not observed. Moreover, the monitoring of free C-peptide in solution revealed the leakage of 8 ± 1% of the drug from KF3 nanospheres with high loading of C-peptide (604 µg/mg). At the same conditions, C-peptide leakage at 37 °C was found to be 30 ± 1%. For KF3 nanospheres with high loading of C-peptide covered with heparin the drug leakage at low temperature was not detected.

3.6. Drug Release

Along with loading content and encapsulation efficiency the drug release kinetics is also one of the important properties of drug delivery systems. For the systems under study, the drug release was studied in 0.01 M PBS, pH 7.4, at 37 °C for KF1 and KF3 nanospheres. The last kind of nanospheres was applied as three formulations with different loaded amount of C-peptide. The summary on tested formulations is presented in Table 5. As it can be seen from Figure 9, during 6 h 57 and 73% of C-peptide were released from KF3 and KF1 nanospheres, respectively. After this time, no further C-peptide release was detected in model conditions. The increase of lysine monomer content in the polymer provided higher retention of peptide inside the nanospheres. Thus, KF3 nanospheres as delivery systems seems to be more preferable.

Table 5. Formulations applied for C-peptide release study.

Sample	Amount of C-Peptide Encapsulated, μg/mg of Nanospheres	Amount of C-Peptide Retained after 14 Days Release, μg/mg of Nanospheres
KF1	581 ± 3	157 ± 4
KF3-HLD	604 ± 4	259 ± 5
KF3-MLD	285 ± 5	225 ± 7
KF3-LLD	147 ± 4	128 ± 3
KF3-HLD + heparin	483 ± 8	335 ± 10

Abbreviations: HLD—high loaded, MLD—middle loaded and LLD—low loaded.

KF3 formulations with lower C-peptide loading demonstrated similar drug release profile (Figure 9) however the amount of released peptide were less than for nanospheres with high drug loading (Table 5).

To diminish the release ratio, the nanospheres with high C-peptide loading (KF3-HLD) were additionally covered with heparin. The covering was evidenced by an inversion of their average ζ-potential value from positive (+35) to negative (−38 mV). The covering of KF3-HLD was followed by substitution of ~20% of surface adsorbed C-peptide with heparin. As it was expected, the heparin envelope prevented the intensive drug leakage and the maximal release ratio did not exceed 31%.

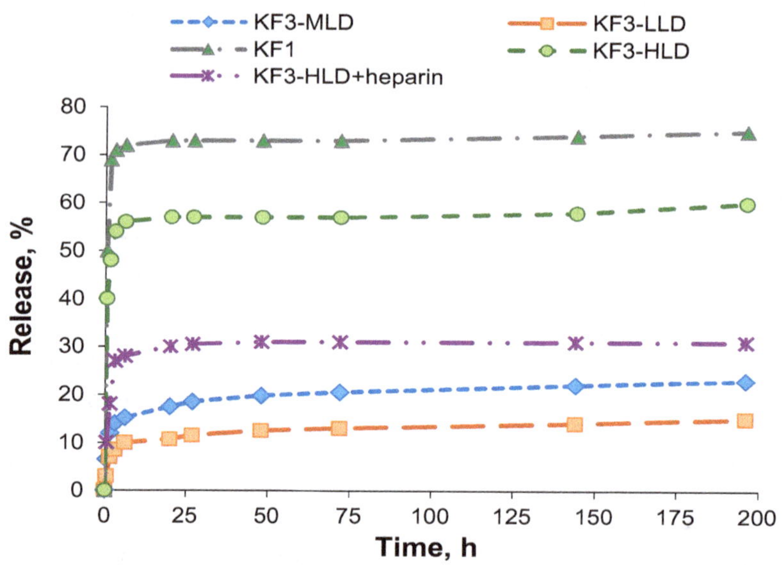

Figure 9. Kinetics of C-peptide release from P(Lys-*co*-DPhe) nanospheres (37 °C, 0.01 M PBS, pH 7.4).

The release observed in model buffer medium can be explained by the leakage of C-peptide, weakly retained due to the ionic interactions, from close to the nanosphere's surface and directly from the surface. The comparable amounts of C-peptide retained inside KF3-HLD and KF3-MLD systems after two weeks of incubation in PBS (Table 5) give reasons for suggestion that retained amounts are deeply buried inside the polymer nanospheres. The release of this portion of C-peptide is possible only as response on some stimuli, for example, due to partial polymer envelope degradation or the nanosphere's disassembly because of interaction with polyanions, proteins, some other peptides, etc. Since the used for the release study buffer medium could not supply any extra stimuli, the further release was suspended. Contrary to the applied model buffer medium the biological fluids can provide many events inducing the second phase of C-peptide release.

However, as it is seen from data presented in Table 5, the highest amount of retained C-peptide (335 μg/mg of nanospheres) was detected for KF3-HLD + heparin formulation. The covering with heparin allows for the safety not only deeply buried C-peptide but also drug distributed near to the surface. Therefore, the covering of loaded nanospheres with heparin favored to C-peptide preservation in the polymer nanospheres. Overall, the covering of polypeptide nanospheres with polysaccharide provides the additional barrier for proteases and can additionally prolong the stability of drug formulation.

Thus, among the developed and tested formulations at least three candidates can be marked out as most potential encapsulated C-peptide delivery systems: (1) KF3-HLD which provides high release rate at the first step and has enough reserve for the second step; (2) KF3-MLD which supplies moderate release ratio at the first step and has enough reserve for the second one; (3) KF3-HLD + heparin which provides moderate release ratio at the first step and has high potential for the second step of release.

3.7. Cell Culture Experiments

The cytotoxicity of prepared nanospheres as well as C-peptide and short C5 peptide was tested with the use of human embryonic kidney cells (HEK-293) (Figure 10). In order to evaluate cell viability, the samples with the best characteristics and properties established in previous experiments were selected. These were KF3, KF3 covered with heparin and EF2 samples. The experiments were carried out during 3 days at concentration of nanospheres from 8 to 500 μg/mL. It was established that KF3 sample was not toxic up to the concentration equal to 32 μg/mL (viability 86%) and then the considerable cell death was detected. The same nanospheres but covered with heparin, as well as EF2 one, demonstrated no cytotoxicity at all tested concentrations (viability ≥ 90%).

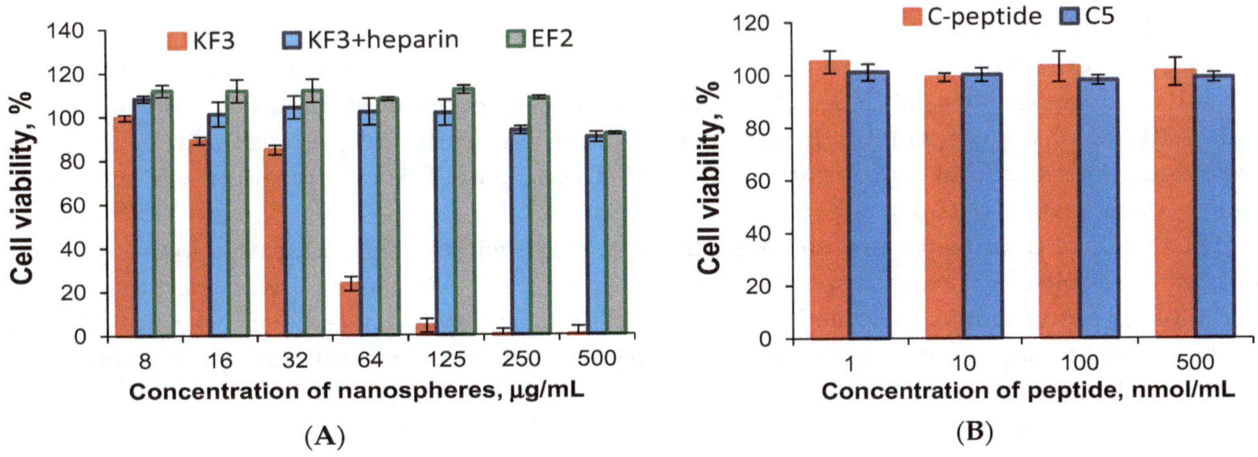

Figure 10. Cell viability (HEK-293) after their incubation for 3 days in presence of different nanospheres (**A**); C-peptide and C5 peptide (**B**).

The study of nanospheres stability in the DMEM+FCS culture medium within three days revealed an increase of particle hydrodynamic diameter (DLS) for KF3 sample (Figure 11). In turn, the negatively charged particles, namely KF3 covered with heparin and EF2, demonstrated stability in protein-containing culture medium. Thus, the cytotoxicity of KF3 may be caused by their high level of aggregation in culture medium [39].

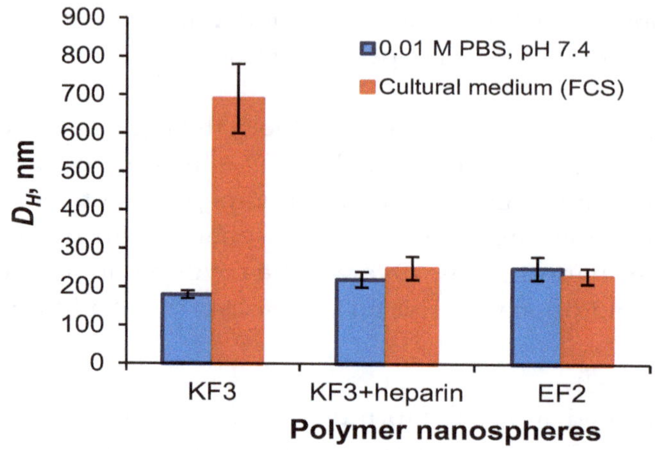

Figure 11. Stability of different nanospheres in culture medium.

3.8. Microcalorimetric Study

Na^+/K^+-adenosine triphosphatase (Na^+/K^+-ATPase) activity is low in various tissues and erythrocytes of Type I diabetic patients [40,41]. This enzyme activity plays a key role in the pathogenesis of diabetic neuropathy and the red cell deformability. Na^+/K^+-ATPase is a ubiquitously expressed transmembrane enzyme that sustains cellular homeostasis by keeping low Na^+ and high K^+ concentrations in cytosol. Cellular homeostasis is pivotal for maintenance of the membrane potential of all types of cells and acts by driving an active Na^+ and K^+ transport through the cellular membrane [42]. It is known that C-peptide improves the human vascular blood flow through a mechanism involving endothelial NO production and erythrocyte Na^+/K^+-ATPase activation [41]. Ohtomo et al. established that C-peptide stimulates Na^+, K^+-ATPase of renal tubule segments due to the activation of a receptor coupled to a pertussis toxin-sensitive G-protein with subsequent activation of Ca^{2+}-dependent intracellular signaling pathways [43,44].

In our case, the biological effects of C-peptide and C5 formulations were studied using isothermal titration microcalorimetry method. The heat released via the Na^+/K^+-adenosine triphosphatase during ATP hydrolysis represents a signal of steady-state enzymatic activity. For this purpose, living erythrocytes were incubated with and without different formulations of C-peptide and C5 (ex vivo study). It was previously established that a concentration-dependent stimulation is observed in the range 1–10 nM of C-peptide [40]. In our case, C-peptide in different preparations were tested at physiological postprandial concentrations of 6 nM. To compare, C5 concentration was chosen to be equal to concentration of C-peptide.

The results of calorimetric titration of erythrocyte suspension by tested formulations of C-peptide are shown in Table 6. Ouabain is specific inhibitor of Na^+/K^+-ATPase, so it was used to prove that observed heat production is attributed to Na^+/K^+-ATPase activity in presence of C-peptide. As it was expected, no heat release was observed under incubation of erythrocytes with C-peptide in presence of ouabain. Both C-peptide and its C-terminal fragment C5 stimulated Na^+/K^+ ATPase in erythrocytes but in the case of C5 activation effect was slightly higher. The high activity of C-terminal pentapeptide fragment of C-peptide was proved earlier both ex vivo and in vivo. Using rat C-peptide Ohtomo et al. has shown that Na^+/K^+-ATPase activity of C-terminal pentapeptide (EVARQ) was found to 103% of the intact molecule's activity [43]. Nordquist et al. showed that administration of the rat C-peptide fragment EVARQ has similar effects on glomerular filtration rate and blood glucose levels as the intact C-peptide molecule in rats [26].

In our case, the biological effect of tested C-peptide formulations was different. For encapsulated systems the drug loading, and consequently the release rate, influenced on measured heat release. The highest value of ΔH was detected when C-peptide loading was high (604 μg/mg of nanospheres). The observed high effect can be a sum of both C-peptide burst release and Na^+/K^+-ATPase activation by the released C-peptide. In turn, the application of low-loaded nanospheres (147 ± 4 µg/mg of nanospheres) that demonstrated a very slow release of C-peptide, gave much lower heat production. This result can be attributed to a much less amount of free C-peptide involved in Na^+/K^+-ATPase activation. A comparable result was also observed for nanospheres with a low loading of C5 (143 ± 3 µg/mg of nanospheres).

Table 6. Results of isothermal titration microcalorimetry experiments.

#	Experimental Condition	ΔH, µJ Normalized to Control
1	C-peptide + ouabain	0 *
2	C-peptide	−102 ± 7 *
3	C5	−136 ± 9 *
4	C-peptide encapsulated in KF3 nanospheres (HLD)	−265 ± 19 **
5	C-peptide encapsulated in KF3 nanospheres (LLD)	−65 ± 5 **
6	C-peptide immobilized on the surface of EF2 nanospheres	−213 ± 16 ***
7	C5 encapsulated in KF3 nanospheres (LLD)	−54 ± 6 **
8	C5 immobilized on the surface of EF2 nanospheres	−15 ± 4 ***

* 0.9% NaCl was used as a control; ** KF3 nanoparticles in 0.9% NaCl was used as a control; *** EF2 nanoparticles in 0.9% NaCl was used as a control.

The covalent immobilization of C-peptide and C5 on the particle surface was carried out in the same way to provide the one-point attachment of peptide through its N-terminus. Firstly, such immobilization ensures the peptide sequence remains untouched and secondly, the accessibility to C-terminus, which is important for biological activity. The formed amide bond between peptide and polymer side-chain is stable in the peptidase-free media and, therefore, no release is possible in PBS. Thus, the heat release measured for immobilized forms of peptides is responsible for Na^+/K^+-ATPase activation with C-peptide/C5 located at surface of nanospheres. As it can be seen from data presented in Table 6, the activity of immobilized C-peptide was much higher than this determined for bound C5. The poor activity of C5 is conditioned by steric hindrances in interaction of short peptide located at the particle's surface with erythrocytes. Contrary to C5, the accessibility of more elongated and better in solution exposed peptide is much higher. Thus, for this kind of formulation, the application of C-peptide-bearing nanospheres rather than that of C5 appears to be a worthy prospect.

4. Conclusions

In this work, the random amphiphilic polypeptides with prolonged stability to biodegradation were synthesized and characterized. For both anionic and cationic polymers, the pH of self-assembly did not influence the hydrodynamic size of nanospheres in a wide range of pH. All self-assembled nanospheres were stable in 0.01 M PBS at 4 °C (storage stability) at least three months. In culture medium-containing proteins, the anionic nanospheres were stable but the cationic ones were aggregated. This instability in the culture medium seems to be one of the main reasons of the cytotoxicity of the P(L-Lys-*co*-D-Phe) nanospheres. In turn, the stable in culture medium anionic particles did not demonstrate any cytotoxicity up to the concentration of 500 µg/mL. The successful application of the developed nanospheres for C-peptide and its short fragment C5 encapsulation and immobilization was demonstrated. Both formulations were stable under storage conditions for three months in regards of their size and C-peptide content. The developed novel formulations of C-peptide demonstrated high biological effects by stimulating Na^+/K^+-ATPase activity in erythrocytes and some can be considered for further examination in experimental animals.

Author Contributions: Investigation, N.Z., V.S., M.A., I.T. and Y.A.; Methodology, A.L.; Formal analysis and writing—original draft preparation, N.Z.; Methodology and writing—review and editing, T.T.; Conceptualization, methodology, data curation, supervision, writing—original draft preparation, review and editing, E.K.-V.

Acknowledgments: N.Z. acknowledges the G-RISC program for personal student scholarship for one-month traineeship in Germany. Thermogravimetric and Calorimetric Research Centre Saint-Petersburg State University acknowledged for Microcalorimetric experiments.

References

1. Sima, A.A.F. *Diabetes & C-Peptide: Scientific and Clinical Aspects*; Springer: New York, NY, USA, 2012; pp. 1–169.
2. Luzi, L.; Zerbini, G.; Caumo, A. C-peptide: A redundant relative of insulin? *Diabetologia* **2007**, *50*, 500–502. [CrossRef] [PubMed]
3. Li, Y.; Zhao, D.D.; Li, Y.; Meng, L.; Enwer, G. Serum C-peptide as a key contributor to lipid-related residual cardiovascular risk in the elderly. *Arch. Gerontol. Geriatr.* **2017**, *73*, 263–268. [CrossRef] [PubMed]
4. Shpakov, A.O. Mechanisms of Action and Therapeutic Potential of Proinsulin C-peptide. *J. Evol. Biochem. Physiol.* **2017**, *53*, 180–190. [CrossRef]
5. Haidet, J.; Cifarelli, V.; Trucco, M.; Luppi, P. C-peptide reduces pro-inflammatory cytokine secretion in LPS-stimulated U937 monocytes in condition of hyperglycemia. *Inflamm. Res.* **2012**, *61*, 27–35. [CrossRef] [PubMed]
6. Leighton, E.; Sainsbury, C.A.; Jones, G.C. A Practical Review of C-Peptide Testing in Diabetes. *Diabetes Ther.* **2017**, *8*, 475–487. [CrossRef] [PubMed]
7. Walcher, D.; Babiak, C.; Poletek, P.; Rosenkranz, S.; Bach, H.; Betz, S.; Durst, R.; Grub, M.; Hombach, V.; Strong, J.; et al. C-peptide induces vascular smooth muscle cell proliferation: Involvementof SRC-kinase, phosphatidylinositol 3-kinase, and extracellular signal-regulated kinase 1/2. *Circ. Res.* **2006**, *99*, 1181–1187. [CrossRef] [PubMed]
8. Lachin, J.M.; McGee, P.; Palmer, J.P. Impact of C-Peptide Preservation on Metabolic and Clinical Outcomes in the Diabetes Control and Complications Trial. *Diabetes* **2014**, *63*, 739–748. [CrossRef] [PubMed]
9. Hansen, A.; Johansson, L.; Wahren, J.; von Bibra, H. C-peptide exerts beneficial effects on myocardial blood flow andfunction in patients with type 1 diabetes. *Diabetes* **2002**, *51*, 3077–3082. [CrossRef]
10. Ido, Y.; Vindigni, A.; Chang, K.; Stramm, L.; Chance, R.; Heath, W.F.; DiMarchi, R.D.; Di Cera, E.; Williamson, J.R. Prevention of vascular and neural dysfunction in diabetic rats by C-peptide. *Science* **1997**, *277*, 563–566. [CrossRef] [PubMed]
11. Zhang, W.; Yorek, M.; Pierson, C.R.; Murakawa, Y.; Breidenbach, A.; Sima, A.A.F. Human C-peptide dose dependently prevents early neuropathy in the BB/Wor-rat. *Int. J. Exp. Diabetes Res.* **2001**, *2*, 187–193. [CrossRef] [PubMed]
12. Faber, O.K.; Hagen, C.; Binder, C. Kinetics of human connecting peptide in normal and diabetic subjects. *J. Clin. Investig.* **1978**, *62*, 197–203. [CrossRef] [PubMed]
13. Foyt, H.; Daniels, M.; Milad, M.; Wahre, J. Pharmacokinetics, safety, and tolerability of a long-acting C-peptide (CBX129801) in patients with type 1 diabetes. *Diabetologia* **2012**, *55*, S455.
14. Jolivalt, C.G.; Rodriguez, M.; Wahren, J.; Calcutt, N.A. Efficacy of a long-acting C-peptide analogue against peripheral neuropathy in streptozotocin-diabetic mice. *Diabetes Obes. Metab.* **2016**, *3*, 147–153. [CrossRef] [PubMed]
15. Wahren, J.; Foyt, H.; Daniels, M.; Arezzo, J.C. Long-acting C-peptide and neuropathy in type 1 diabetes: A 12-month clinical trial. *Diabetes Care* **2016**, *39*, 596–602. [CrossRef] [PubMed]
16. Xie, J.; Yang, C.; Liu, Q.; Li, J.; Liang, R.; Shen, C.; Zhang, Y.; Wang, K.; Liu, L.; Shezad, K.; et al. Encapsulation of Hydrophilic and Hydrophobic Peptides into Hollow Mesoporous Silica Nanoparticles for Enhancement of Antitumor Immune Response. *Small* **2017**, *13*, 1701741. [CrossRef] [PubMed]
17. Li, Y.; Na, R.; Wang, X.; Liu, H.; Zhao, L.; Sun, X.; Ma, G.; Cui, F. Fabrication of antimicrobial peptide-loaded PLGA/Chitosan composite microspheres for long-Acting bacterial resistance. *Molecules* **2017**, *22*, 1637.

18. Tang, R.; Wang, X.; Zhang, H.; Liang, X.; Feng, X.; Zhu, X.; Lu, X.; Wu, F.; Liu, Z. Promoting early neovascularization of SIS-repaired abdominal wall by controlled release of bioactive VEGF. *RSC Adv.* **2018**, *8*, 4548–4560. [CrossRef]
19. Agrawal, G.R.; Wakte, P.; Shelke, S. Formulation, physicochemical characterization and in vitro evaluation of human insulin-loaded microspheres as potential oral carrier. *Prog. Biomater.* **2017**, *6*, 125–136. [CrossRef]
20. Maciel, V.B.V.; Yoshida, C.M.P.; Pereira, S.M.S.S.; Goycoolea, F.M.; Franco, T.T. Electrostatic self-assembled chitosan-pectin nano- and microparticles for insulin delivery. *Molecules* **2017**, *22*, 1707. [CrossRef]
21. Bloch, K.; Vanichkin, A.; Gil-Ad, I.; Vardi, P.; Weizman, A. Insulin delivery to the brain using intracranial implantation of alginate-encapsulated pancreatic islets. *J. Tissue Eng. Regen. Med.* **2017**, *11*, 3263–3272. [CrossRef]
22. Alibolandi, M.; Alabdollah, F.; Sadeghi, F.; Mohammadi, M.; Abnous, K.; Ramezani, M.; Hadizadeh, F. Dextran-b-poly (lactide-co-glycolide) polymersome for oral delivery of insulin: In vitro and in vivo evaluation. *J. Control. Release* **2016**, *227*, 58–70. [CrossRef] [PubMed]
23. Saravanan, S.S.; Malathi, M.S.; Sesh, P.S.L.; Selvasubramanian, S.S.; Balasubramanian, B.S.; Pandiyan, P.V. Hydrophilic poly (ethylene glycol) capped poly (lactic-co-glycolic) acid nanoparticles for subcutaneous delivery of insulin in diabetic rats. *Int. J. Biol. Macromol.* **2017**, *95*, 1190–1198.
24. Gupta, R.; Mohanty, S. Controlled release of insulin from folic acid-insulin complex nanoparticles. *Colloids Surf. B Biointerfaces* **2017**, *154*, 48–54. [CrossRef] [PubMed]
25. Habibi, N.; Kamaly, N.; Memic, A.; Shafiee, H. Self-assembled peptide-based nanostructures: Smart nanomaterials toward targeted drug delivery. *Nano Today* **2016**, *11*, 41–60. [CrossRef] [PubMed]
26. Nordquist, L.; Palm, F.; Andresen, B.T. Renal and vascular benefits of C-peptide: Molecular mechanisms of C-peptide action. *Biologics* **2008**, *2*, 441–452. [CrossRef]
27. De La Tour, D.; Raccah, D.; Jannot, M.; Coste, T.; Rougerie, C.; Vague, P. Erythrocyte Na/K ATPase activity and diabetes: Relationship with C-peptide level. *Diabetologia* **1998**, *41*, 1080–1084. [CrossRef]
28. Djemli-Shipkolye, A.; Gallice, P.; Coste, T.; Jannot, M.F.; Tsimaratos, M.; Raccah, D.; Vague, P. The effects ex vivo and in vitro of insulin and C-peptide on Na/K adenosine triphosphatase activity in red blood cell membranes of type 1 diabetic patients. *Metabolism* **2000**, *49*, 868–872. [CrossRef]
29. Wilder, R.; Mobashery, S. The use of triphosgene in preparation of N-carboxy-alpha-amino acid anhydrides. *J. Org. Chem.* **1992**, *57*, 2755–2756. [CrossRef]
30. Vlakh, E.; Novikov, A.; Vlasov, G.; Tennikova, T. Solid phase peptide synthesis on epoxy-bearing methacrylate monoliths. *J. Pept. Sci.* **2004**, *10*, 719–730. [CrossRef]
31. Amoabediny, G.; Haghiralsadat, F.; Naderinezhad, S.; Helder, M.N.; Akhoundi Kharanaghi, E.; Mohammadnejad Arough, J.; Zandieh-Doulabi, B. Overview of preparation methods of polymeric and lipid-based (niosome, solid lipid, liposome) nanoparticles: A comprehensive review. *Int. J. Polym. Mater. Polym. Biomater.* **2018**, *67*, 383–400. [CrossRef]
32. Sasaki, Y.; Kohri, M.; Kojima, T.; Taniguchi, T.; Kishikawa, K. Preparation of polymer nanoparticles via phase inversion temperature Method using amphiphilic block polymer synthesized by atom transfer radical polymerization. *Trans. Mater. Soc. Jpn.* **2014**, *39*, 125–128. [CrossRef]
33. Zhu, Y.; Yi, C.; Hu, Q.; Wei, W.; Liu, X. Effect of chain microstructure on self-assembly and emulsification of amphiphilic poly(acrylic acid)-polystyrene copolymers. *Phys. Chem. Chem. Phys.* **2016**, *18*, 26236–26244. [CrossRef] [PubMed]
34. Yang, T.; Li, W.; Duan, X.; Zhu, L.; Fan, L.; Qiao, Y.; Wu, H. Preparation of two types of polymeric micelles based on poly(β-l-malic acid) for antitumor drug delivery. *PLoS ONE* **2016**, *11*, e0162607. [CrossRef] [PubMed]
35. Prokop, A.; Iwasaki, Y.; Harada, A. (Eds.) *Intracellular Delivery II: Fundamentals and Applications*; Springer: Heidelberg, Germany, 2014; p. 479.
36. Marsden, H.R.; Gabrielli, L.; Kros, A. Rapid preparation of polymersomes by a water addition/solvent evaporation method. *Polym. Chem.* **2010**, *1*, 1512–1518. [CrossRef]
37. Tarasenko, I.; Zashikhina, N.; Guryanov, I.; Volokitina, M.; Biondi, B.; Fiorucci, S.; Formaggio, F.; Tennikova, T.; Korzhikova-Vlakh, E. Amphiphilic polypeptides with prolonged enzymatic stability for the preparation of self-assembled nanobiomaterials. *RSC Adv.* **2018**, *8*, 34603–34613. [CrossRef]

38. Zikou, S.; Koukkou, A.-I.; Mastora, P.; Sakarellos-Daitsiotis, M.; Sakarellos, C.; Drainas, C.; Panou-Pomonis, E. Design and synthesis of cationic Aib-containing antimicrobial peptides: Conformational and biological studies. *J. Pept. Sci.* **2007**, *13*, 481–486. [CrossRef]
39. Guo, Q.; Zhang, T.; An, J.; Wu, Z.; Zhao, Y.; Dai, X.; Zhang, X.; Li, C. Block versus Random Amphiphilic Glycopolymer Nanopaticles as Glucose-Responsive Vehicles. *Biomacromolecules* **2015**, *16*, 3345–3356. [CrossRef] [PubMed]
40. Johansson, J.; Ekberg, K.; Shafqat, J.; Henriksson, M.; Chibalin, A.; Wahren, J.; Jörnvall, H. Molecular effects of proinsulin C-peptide. *Biochem. Biophys. Res. Commun.* **2002**, *295*, 1035–1040. [CrossRef]
41. Forst, T.; Kunt, T. Effects of C-peptide on microvascular blood flow and blood hemorheology. *Exp. Diabesity Res.* **2004**, *5*, 51–64. [CrossRef]
42. Jørgensen, P. Sodium and potassium ion pump in kidney tubules. *Physiol. Rev.* **1980**, *60*, 864–917. [CrossRef] [PubMed]
43. Ohtomo, Y.; Bergman, T.; Johansson, B.L.; Jörnvall, H.; Wahren, J. Differential effects of proinsulin C-peptide fragments on Na+, K+- ATPase activity of renal tubule segments. *Diabetologia* **1998**, *41*, 287–291. [CrossRef] [PubMed]
44. Forst, T.; De la Tour, D.D.; Kunt, T.; Pfutzner, A.; Goitom, K.; Pohlmann, T.; Schneider, S.; Johansson, B.L.; Wahren, J.; Lobig, M.; et al. Effects of proinsulin C-peptide on nitric oxide, microvascular blood flow and erythrocyte Na+,K+-atpase activity in diabetes mellitus type I. *Clin. Sci.* **2000**, *98*, 283–290. [CrossRef] [PubMed]

7

Transferrin Functionalized Liposomes Loading Dopamine HCl: Development and Permeability Studies across an *In Vitro* Model of Human Blood–Brain Barrier

Antonio Lopalco [1], Annalisa Cutrignelli [1,*], Nunzio Denora [1,2], Angela Lopedota [1], Massimo Franco [1] and Valentino Laquintana [1]

1 Department of Pharmacy–Drug Sciences, University of Bari "Aldo Moro", 4 E. Orabona st, 70125 Bari, Italy; antonio.lopalco@uniba.it (A.L.); nunzio.denora@uniba.it (N.D.); angelaassunta.lopedota@uniba.it (A.L.); massimo.franco@uniba.it (M.F.); valentino.laquintana@uniba.it (V.L.)

2 Institute for Physical and Chemical Processes (IPCF)-CNR, SS Bari, 4 E. Orabona st, 70125 Bari, Italy

* Correspondence: annalisa.cutrignelli@uniba.it;

Abstract: The transport of dopamine across the blood brain barrier represents a challenge for the management of Parkinson's disease. The employment of central nervous system targeted ligands functionalized nanocarriers could be a valid tactic to overcome this obstacle and avoid undesirable side effects. In this work, transferrin functionalized dopamine-loaded liposomes were made by a modified dehydration–rehydration technique from hydrogenated soy phosphatidylcoline, cholesterol and 1,2-stearoyl-*sn*-glycero-3-phosphoethanolamine-*N*-[carboxy(poly(ethylene glycol)-2000)]. The physical features of the prepared liposomes were established with successive determination of their endothelial permeability across an *in vitro* model of the blood-brain barrier, constituted by human cerebral microvascular endothelial cells (hCMEC/D3). Functionalized dopamine-loaded liposomes with encapsulation efficiency more than 35% were made with sizes in a range around 180 nm, polydispersity indices of 0.2, and positive zeta potential values (+7.5 mV). Their stability and drug release kinetics were also evaluated. The apparent permeability (P_e) values of encapsulated dopamine in functionalized and unfunctionalized liposomes showed that transferrin functionalized nanocarriers could represent appealing non-toxic candidates for brain delivery, thus improving benefits and decreasing complications to patients subjected to L-dopa chronical treatment.

Keywords: dopamine; liposomes; drug delivery; transferrin; hCMEC/D3 cells; blood brain barrier

1. Introduction

The delivery of active pharmaceutical ingredients to the central nervous system (CNS) represents the most important challenge for the management of the symptoms of Parkinson's disease (PD) and other neurodegenerative disorders, because of the various defensive barriers surrounding the brain [1,2]. It is well established that many CNS-active molecules, such as dopamine (DA), do not penetrate across the blood–brain barrier (BBB) to enter the CNS, because of their high polarity, ionized state at physiological pH and/or the deficiency of endogenous cellular membrane transporters located within the brain endothelium, which forms the blood vessel walls [3–5]. Only small molecules with adequate hydrophilic/lipophilic balance and molecular weight can be absorbed passively into the CNS, if not substrates for the ABC (ATP-binding cassette) transporters efflux pumps. Different methodologies have been developed to raise the delivery of therapeutics for CNS diseases, including the development of CNS-targeted pro-drugs or co-drugs [6–9] and functionalized nanocarriers with uptake-facilitating ligands [10–12].

Until today, the most successful therapy for the management of PD is represented by L-dopa (LD), a bioprecursor of DA, that crosses the BBB through the active transport mechanism for amino acids and, once in the brain, is metabolized and transformed to DA by the enzyme dopa decarboxylase [13–15]. Even though LD improves the PD manifestations in the early phases of the disorder, an excessive peripheral LD bioconversion into DA from within the peripheral nervous system produces several unwanted secondary effects. In detail, clinical and preclinical investigations have shown that LD long-term use is associated with anomalous spontaneous movements, psychiatric complications and DA- or LD-induced neurotoxicity [16–18].

In this context, to overcome these disadvantages, a promising strategic delivery system to enhance BBB penetration by DA is the use of nanocarriers such as liposomes (LPs) decorated with uptake-facilitating ligands (Figure 1). In particular, the active targeting approach could be reached using LPs decorated with transferrin (β-1 glycopeptide) (Tf), a hydrophilic carrier that regulates the extracellular iron level in human fluid by binding and sequestering it. In fact, Tf receptor, a dimeric transmembrane glycoprotein, certainly represents a successful target molecule since it as well as being overexpressed in different malignant cells that require high levels of iron for their growth is also localized on the endothelia surface of brain capillaries that comprise the BBB [19–21]. Numerous researchers used the targeting to Tf receptor for improving the BBB transport of drugs [22,23].

In this study, we have encapsulated the hydrophilic drug dopamine hychloride (DA·HCl) into Tf functionalized and unfunctionalized LPs (DA·HCl-LPs). These nanocarriers were made by a dehydration-rehydration technique and their particle sizes, polydispersity index, zeta potential and encapsulation efficiency values were determined. Their stability and drug-release behavior were also evaluated. An additional goal in this work was to study the permeability of the functionalized and unfunctionalized DA·HCl-LPs across an *in vitro* model of the BBB, constituted by human cerebral microvascular endothelial cells (hCMEC/D3), using a well-established procedure.

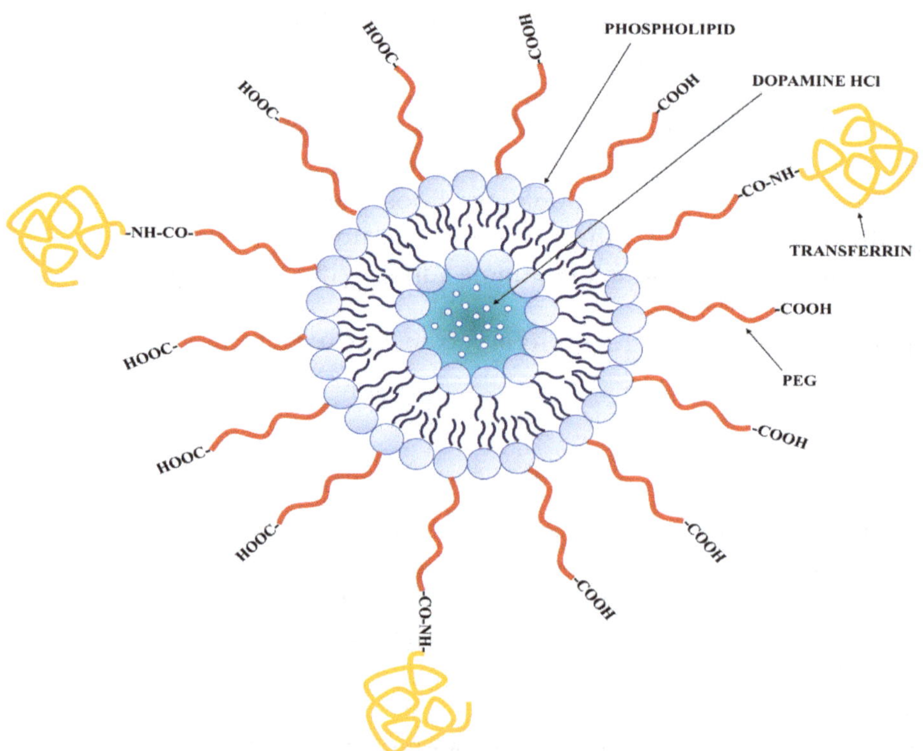

Figure 1. Schematic representation of functionalized DA·HCl-LPs. LPs are made of a phospholipid bilayer, which encloses an aqueous center. The aqueous space incorporates the hydrophilic DA·HCl. Hydrophilic polymer polyethylene glycol (PEG) coats the ligand-targeted LPs.

2. Materials and Methods

2.1. Materials

Dopamine hydrochloride (DA·HCl, MW = 189.64 g/mol), cholesterol (Chol), Triton X-100, *N*-(3-dimethylamino-propyl)-*N*′-ethylcarbodiimide hydrochloride (EDC), *N*-hydroxysulfosuccinimide (S-NHS) and Tranferrin (Tf) were bought from Sigma-Aldrich (Milan, Italy).

Hydrogenated soy phosphatidylcoline (Phospholipon 90H, PC) was a gift of Natterman Phospholipids GmbH (Koeln, Germany). 1,2-stearoyl-*sn*-glycero-3-phosphoethanolamine-*N*-[carboxy(poly(ethylene glycol)-2000)] (DSPE-PEG_{2000}-COOH) was purchased from Avanti Polar Lipids (Alabaster, AL, USA).

For cellular transport studies luciferin yellow was bought from Sigma-Aldrich (Milan, Italy); Transwell® permeable supports were from Corning (Corning, NY, USA). All the media and supplements for cell culture were bought from Life Technologies, Thermo Fisher Scientific (Waltham, MA, USA). Other materials used in this study were of analytical grade.

2.2. Quantification of DA·HCl

High-performance liquid chromatography (HPLC) analysis was used to detect and quantify DA·HCl. The HPLC station and the column were the same previously described by Lopedota et al. [24] making a change to the mobile phase which in this case was constituted by 90/10 v/v 0.020 M potassium phosphate buffer (pH 2.8)/acetonitrile mixture. The flow rate was kept at 1.0 mL/min, the eluent was continuously monitored at a wavelength of 280 nm and in these conditions DA·HCl retention time was about 6.5 min. Calibration curves were obtained solubilizing DA·HCl in the same mobile phase and were linear over the tested concentration range (from 0.85 mg/mL (4.48×10^{-3} M) to 0.0085 mg/mL (4.48×10^{-5} M)).

2.3. Preparation of Unfunctionalized LPs

Unfunctionalized LPs were made using the dehydration-rehydration method with a slight modification [25]. Briefly, PC/Chol in 7/3 molar ratio were solubilized in a chloroform/methanol (2/1 v/v) mixture and the solvents were removed by a rotary evaporator at 55 °C until a lipid film was obtained. The film was stored under vacuum for 3 h to guarantee whole elimination of the organic solvents and then rehydrated in the dark with a DA·HCl solution in phosphate buffer pH = 4.5. To avoid oxidation of DA·HCl all subsequent manipulations of the liposomal suspension were carried out in the absence of light. The resulting LPs were sized by sonication (Branson Sonifier 150, Danbury, CT, USA) alternating three cycles of 60 s each with three cooling cycles of 60 s in an ice bath. The liposomal suspension was freeze-dried for 24 h and then subjected to a controlled rehydration process with demineralized water. The un-loaded drug was removed by ultracentrifugation at 45,000 rpm for 50 min at 4 °C (Beckman L7-55, Life Science, Boston, MA, USA) and the obtained pellet was suspended in phosphate buffer pH = 4.5. Finally, dimension, zeta potential and encapsulation efficiency of the obtained vesicles were determined.

2.4. Preparation of Tf Functionalized LPs

The preparation of Tf functionalized LPs was conducted using the procedure described by Paszko et al. [26]. In detail, the initial composition of PC/Chol 7/3 molar ratio was integrated with the 2.5 mol % of DSPE-PEG_{2000}-COOH and LPs were prepared following the procedure described in the previous paragraph.

Then, LPs suspension was incubated for 10 min at room temperature with S-NHS and EDC, both dissolved in PBS pH = 4.5. Finally, 120 mg of Tf per mmol of lipid were added and incubated for 12 h at 4 °C to allow the formation of an amide bond between the carboxyl and amine groups of PEGylated lipids and Tf, respectively. The unbound Tf was separated from functionalized vesicles by ultracentrifugation at 50,000 rpm for 2 h, at 4 °C (Beckman L7-55, Life Science, Boston, MA, USA).

The recovered pellet containing LPs was suspended in PBS pH = 4.5 and stored in the dark until further manipulations.

In order to investigate the density of Tf on the LPs surface a BCA assay kit was used, evaluating the percentage of Tf exposed on external LPs surface compared to the total amount of Tf used for the conjugation. The absorbance at 595 nm was recorded (PerkinElmer 2030 multilabel reader Victor TM X3, Waltham, MA, USA) and the protein concentration was determined by comparison to a standard curve (0.5 to 30 μg/mL).

2.5. *Physicochemical Characterization of LPs*

For the determination of vesicles dimension and polydispersity index (P.I.) a Zetasizer Nano ZS (Malvern Instrument Ltd., Worcestershire, UK) was used and suspensions were appropriately diluted with demineralized water. The zeta potentials were investigated by laser Doppler velocimetry using the same instrument and diluting all samples with a 1 mM KCl solution to keep the ionic strength constant [27].

Experiments were performed in triplicate and the results were reported with the corresponding standard deviation.

2.6. *Quantification of DA·HCl into LPs*

The quantity of DA·HCl encapsulated in liposomal vesicles was expressed as the difference between the total quantity solubilized in the LPs medium and the quantity of non-encapsulated DA·HCl recovered in the aqueous suspending medium after centrifugation at 45,000 rpm for 50 min at 4 °C (Beckman L7-55, Life Science, Boston, MA, USA). DA·HCl content was determined by HPLC using the calibration curve obtained as explained in Section 2.2. Results are expressed as encapsulation efficiency (EE) determined as actual drug loading/theoretical drug loading × 100 [28]. Experiments were performed in triplicate.

2.7. *Freeze-Fracture Electron Microscopy*

A sample of DA·HCl-LPs was examined by transmission electron microscopy after freeze-fracture in the presence of 20% of glycerol as cryoprotectant. In detail, a drop of liposome dispersion, deposited in a small gold pan, was quickly frozen in liquid nitrogen. A freeze-replica apparatus at −100 °C (FR-7000A, Hitachi Science Co., Tokyo, Japan) was used to fracturing the sample and replica was realized by platinum-carbon shadowing and examined with a JEM-1200EX (Japan Electron Co., Tokyo, Japan) transmission electron microscope.

2.8. *In Vitro Release Studies*

1 mL of Tf functionalized and unfunctionalized LPs suspension containing DA·HCl was put into dialysis sacs (cut-off 3000 MW) and dialyzed against 50 mL of phosphate buffer pH = 4.5 supplemented with α-tocopherol 0.005 M to avoid DA·HCl oxidation in the release medium. The dialysis was conducted at 37 °C in a shaker bath, 100 μL of external medium were removed at predetermined times interval and analyzed by HPLC for DA·HCl content, and 100 μL of phosphate buffer were added in order to preserve the sink condition. The experiment was conducted on both functionalized and unfunctionalized LPs for at least three times.

2.9. *Stability Studies*

LPs stability was evaluated by measuring size and polydispersity index by means of light scattering for one month, after appropriate dilution with demineralized water.

2.10. Culture of hCMEC/D3 Cells and Endothelial Permeability Experiments

The *in vitro* model of the BBB, constituted by human cerebral microvascular endothelial cell line hCMEC/D3 was obtained from Dr. PO Couraud, Inserm, Paris, France. Culture of these cells was realized as reported by Lopalco et al. in a previous study. [2]. Briefly, cells at passage numbers between 25 and 30 were cultivated onto polyester Transwell® inserts and grown in supplemented media. Cell barrier integrity was verified prior to perform endothelial permeability experiments by means of trans-endothelial electrical resistance (TEER) using an EndOhm meter. Monolayers of human cerebral microvascular endothelial cells with TEER values between 65 and 89 Ohm·cm^2 were used in this study. The transport of Tf functionalized and unfunctionalized DA-LPs was examined at a concentration of 50 μg/mL of DA·HCl in LPs. The endothelial permeability of the nano-systems was performed as reported by Lopalco et al. [2]. The quantity of DA·HCl that had passed through the lipid membrane, constituted by the cell monolayer, was determined using HPLC. In order to determine the apparent permeability values across blank Transwell® inserts, experiments were performed in triplicate without seeding cells in the inserts.

Luciferin yellow transport studies were performed in the same manner explained earlier, except that the sample volumes were 200 μL. The cumulative quantity of luciferin yellow transported was measured by determining the fluorescence of the samples in phenol red-free DMEM at λ_{ex} = 480 nm and λ_{em} = 530 nm using an FLX800 microplate reader (BioTek Instruments, Inc., Winooski, VT, USA) [29]. A Gen5™ software (BioTek Instruments, Inc., Winooski, VT, USA) was used for the acquisition of the data. The relative quantity of luciferin yellow per unit of volume of solution in the basal chamber was then determined from calibration standards made by serial dilution of the luciferin yellow.

2.11. Statistical Analysis

Statistical evaluation of data has been made using GraphPad Prism version 5.0 (San Diego, CA, USA) and statistical significance ($p < 0.05$) determined using a one-way analysis of variance (ANOVA) followed by the Bonferroni post hoc tests.

3. Results and Discussion

3.1. LPs Characterization

LPs containing DA·HCl and functionalized with Tf were prepared, as described, using a modification of the Kirby and Gregoriadis procedure since this method is well known to improve entrapment of water soluble drugs [30]. Tf was conjugated to the carboxyl group of PEG on the LPs PC/Chol/DSPE-PEG-COOH surface to obtain PC/Chol/DSPE-PEG-CO-Tf according to the procedure described in the Section 2.4. Then, the fully characterization in terms of dimension, polydispersity index, zeta potential, drug loading and Tf coupling efficiency was carried out. Results are summarized in Table 1.

Table 1. Particle size ± SD, polydispersity index (PDI), zeta potential, and percent of encapsulation efficiency (EE%) of DA·HCl-LPs unfunctionalized and functionalized with Tf.

Formulation	Size (nm)	PDI	Zeta Potential (mV)	(EE%)
unfunctionalized DA·HCl-LPs	162.4 ± 3.2	0.20	+4.8 ± 0.9	41.5 ± 2.9
Tf functionalized DA·HCl-LPs	181.7 ± 7.8	0.20	+7.5 ± 1.2	35.4 ± 1.8

As can be seen, there is a difference between Tf functionalized and unfunctionalized LPs in terms of size and EE%. In particular, unfunctionalized LPs exhibit a mean diameter of 162.4 ± 3.2 nm and a EE% of 41.5 ± 2.9% while for Tf functionalized LPs we found a value of mean diameter equal to 181.7 ± 7.8 and a EE% of 35.4 ± 1.8%. This behavior is quite in agreement with data found in literature [20,31], the coupling of Tf or other ligands on the surface of liposomal vesicles leads to a slight increase in size, although the values are not different from the statistical point of view ($p > 0.05$).

In all cases the PDI was equal to 0.2 and this value indicates the existence of a very uniform liposomal population in terms of dimensional distribution.

The charge on the LPs was found to be positive and small for the two formulations (values in a range from +4.8 to +7.5 mV), with a slight increase for Tf functionalized LPs. This behavior could be ascribed to the existence of positive charged functional groups of Tf. Regarding the coupling efficiency of Tf, it was found to be equal to 48.8 ± 2.6%, compared to the total amount of Tf used for the conjugation.

In order to determine the stability of the obtained liposomal preparations, their size and PDI were evaluated one a week for 1 month, keeping them at 4 °C. Results are shown in Table 2.

Table 2. Particle size ± SD and PDI vales of DA·HCl-LPs unfunctionalized and functionalized with Transferrin.

Formulation	Week	1	Week	2	Week	3	Week	4
	Size (nm)	PDI	Size (nm)	PDI	Size (nm)	PDI	Size (nm)	PDI
unfunctionalized DA·HCl-LPs	168.4 ± 2.4	0.20	165.4 ± 1.8	0.25	159.4 ± 3.5	0.19	160.7 ± 1.2	0.21
Tf functionalized DA·HCl-LPs	186.5 ± 7.8	0.20	175.7 ± 1.3	0.18	182.4 ± 4.1	0.23	179.4 ± 0.8	0.18

It is evident that no significant variations in terms of size and PDI are highlighted, so it is possible to state that vesicles are stable and can be used for next studies.

Moreover, after one month we determined by HPLC the DA·HCl amount in LPs after vesicles disruption with 0.1% Triton X-100 and filtration with 0.22 μm cellulose acetate membrane filter (Millipore®, Milan, Italy). It was found equal to 98.2% of the initial amount with no significant loss due to drug oxidation.

Figure 2 shows the freeze fracture electron micrograph and the size distribution of unfunctionalized DA·HCl-LPs. Freeze fracture electron microscopy is a powerful technique in the characterization of nanosystems such as micelles, quantum dots, unilamellar and multilamellar liposomes, niosomes and drug crystals because it allows to distinguish between bilayer and non- bilayer structure [32]. Moreover, freeze fracture electron microscopy remains a key tool for investigation of bilayer organization, since it allows to determine the multilamellarity of liposomal systems [32]. As can be seen by micrograph, unfunctionalized DA·HCl-LPs appeared as SUV (small unilamellar vesicles), as expected having used sonication to homogenize the size distribution, with no ripples on the surface and a fairly uniform distribution in terms of size, according to what has been seen through DLS analysis.

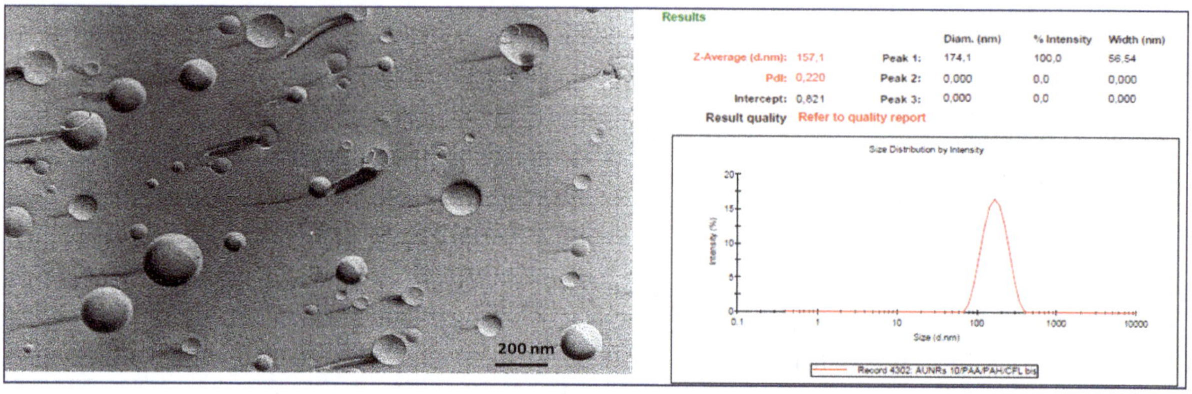

Figure 2. Freeze fracture electron micrograph and size distribution of unfunctionalized DA·HCl-LPs.

3.2. In Vitro Release Studies

In vitro release studies were carried out by dialysis and the obtained cumulative release profiles are reported in Figure 3. The percentage of DA·HCl released was found to be 59.0 ± 4.2% and 68.4 ± 2.9% for Tf functionalized and unfunctionalized LPs, respectively, after a period of 24 h, without any burst effect. The lower value found for functionalized LPs can be explained by the presence of Tf bound on the LPs surface which results in a decrease in the liposomal membrane permeability, slowing down drug release. This behavior is perfectly in line with what has been reported in the literature [20,22].

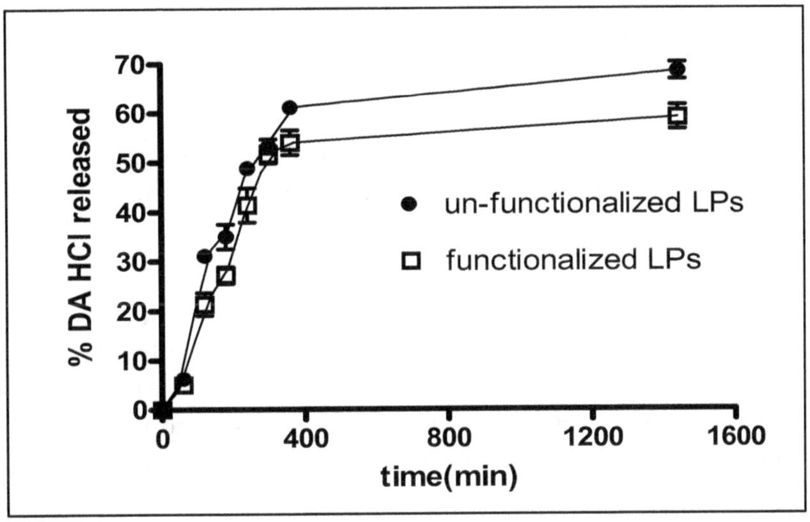

Figure 3. Release profiles of DA·HCl from LPs. Data are the mean of three determination.

3.3. In Vitro Transport Analysis

In vitro transport of formulations across the BBB was investigated using human hCMEC/D3 cell monolayers. The paracellular permeability (P_e) of luciferin yellow was evaluated to exclude alterations of the tight junction properties triggered by LPs. In the presence of both functionalized and unfunctionalized LPs the P_e value of luciferin yellow was $1.12 \pm 0.18 \times 10^{-3}$ cm/min, suggesting no adverse effect on cell monolayer integrity. The data in Table 3 show that the functionalization of LPs with Tf provide a higher permeability across the monolayer compared to unfunctionalized LPs. In detail, the permeability value registered for Tf functionalized DA·HCl-LPs turned out to be equal to $4.97 \pm 0.41 \times 10^{-3}$ cm/min versus $0.92 \pm 0.24 \times 10^{-3}$ cm/min found for unfunctionalized DA·HCl-LPs, with an increase of about 5 fold. The presence of Tf on the surface of LPs allows vesicles to exploit a mechanism of receptor-mediated endocytosis by means of the Tf receptor which is expressed on the endothelium of the cerebral capillaries (Figure 4). Five steps can describe the mechanism proposed in Figure 4. Initially, LPs decorated with transferrin bind specifically to endothelial receptor (1), resulting in their uptake or endocytosis (2). Intracellularly, LPs are transported in vesicles, that move through the endothelial cytoplasm in apical to basal direction (3), escaping degradation in lysosomes. When the opposing membrane is reached, the vesicle opens towards the basolateral compartment and releases LPs (4). The vesicle with the receptor moves through the endothelial cytoplasm in basal to apical direction (5) [33,34].

Table 3. hCMEC/D3 permeability values (P_e) of DA·HCl-LPs, functionalized DA·HCl-LPs and luciferin yellow ± standard deviation (SD).

Formulation	$P_e \pm$ SD (cm/min)
Unfunctionalized DA·HCl-LPs	$0.92 \pm 0.24 \times 10^{-3}$
Tf Functionalized DA·HCl-LPs	$4.97 \pm 0.41 \times 10^{-3}$
Luciferin yellow	$1.12 \pm 0.18 \times 10^{-3}$

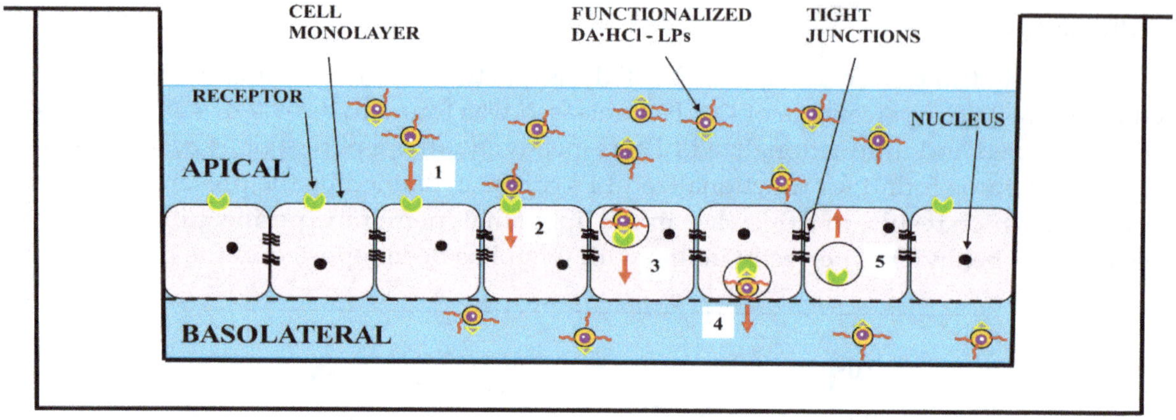

Figure 4. Representation of the endogenous Tf receptor-mediated transcytosis of DA·HCl loaded Tf functionalized LPs across an *in vitro* model of human BBB composed of hCMEC/D3 cell monolayers.

4. Conclusions

The transport of DA·HCl across the BBB represents one of the main missions for the management of Parkinson's disease. The employment of CNS targeted Tf functionalized nanoparticles such as LPs could offer a stratagem to overcome this obstacle. In this work, we have prepared both unfunctionalized and Tf functionalized LPs using a method well known to improve the capturing into the vesicles of hydrophilic drugs. Then, we evaluated their dimension, zeta potential, drug loading, Tf coupling efficiency and drug-release behavior. Finally, the permeability (P_e) through a cellular model of BBB was studied, highlighting how these vesicles are able to permeate through the cell membrane by exploiting a receptor-mediated endocytosis mechanism. The absence of cytotoxicity and the validated technique of preparation make LPs appealing candidates for brain delivery, thus improving benefits and decreasing complications to patients subjected to LD chronical treatment.

Acknowledgments: This study was funded by the Inter-University Consortium for Research (C.I.R.C.M.S.B.) and the University of Bari Aldo Moro.

Author Contributions: Annalisa Cutrignelli, Valentino Laquintana and Antonio Lopalco conceived and designed the experiments; Antonio Lopalco performed the experiments; Nunzio Denora analyzed the data; Angela Lopedota and Massimo Franco contributed reagents/materials/analysis tools; Annalisa Cutrignelli and Antonio Lopalco wrote the paper.

References

1. Spuch, C.; Navarro, C. Liposomes for targeted delivery of active agents against neurodegenerative diseases (Alzheimer's disease and Parkinson's Disease). *J. Drug Deliv.* **2011**, *2011*, 469679. [CrossRef] [PubMed]
2. Lopalco, A.; Ali, H.; Denora, N.; Rytting, E. Oxcarbazepine-loaded polymeric nanoparticles: Development and permeability studies across *in vitro* models of the blood-brain barrier and human placental trophoblast. *Int. J. Nanomed.* **2015**, *10*, 1985–1996.
3. Bjorklund, A.; Dunnett, S.B. Dopamine neuron system in the brain: An update. *Trends Neurosci.* **2007**, *30*, 194–202. [CrossRef] [PubMed]
4. Denora, N.; Cassano, T.; Laquintana, V.; Lopalco, A.; Trapani, A.; Cimmino, C.S.; Laconca, L.; Giuffrida, A.; Trapani, G. Novel codrugs with GABAergic activity for dopamine delivery in the brain. *Int. J. Pharm.* **2012**, *437*, 221–231. [CrossRef] [PubMed]
5. Cassano, T.; Lopalco, A.; de Candia, M.; Laquintana, V.; Lopedota, A.; Cutrignelli, A.; Perrone, M.; Iacobazzi, R.M.; Bedse, G.; Franco, M.; et al. Oxazepam-Dopamine Conjugates Increase Dopamine Delivery into Striatum of Intact Rats. *Mol. Pharm.* **2017**, *14*, 3178–3187. [CrossRef] [PubMed]
6. Di Stefano, A.; Sozio, P.; Iannitelli, A.; Cerasa, L.S. New drug delivery strategies for improved Parkinson's disease therapy. *Expert Opin. Drug Deliv.* **2009**, *6*, 389–404. [CrossRef] [PubMed]

7. Laquintana, V.; Denora, N.; Cutrignelli, A.; Perrone, M.; Iacobazzi, R.; Annese, C.; Lopalco, A.; Lopedota, A.; Franco, M. TSPO ligand-methotrexate prodrug conjugates: Design, synthesis, and biological evaluation. *Int. J. Mol. Sci.* **2016**, *17*, 967. [CrossRef] [PubMed]
8. Iacobazzi, R.M.; Lopalco, A.; Cutrignelli, A.; Laquintana, V.; Lopedota, A.; Franco, M.; Denora, N. Bridging Pharmaceutical Chemistry with Drug and Nanoparticle Targeting to Investigate the Role of the 18-kDa Translocator Protein TSPO. *ChemMedChem* **2017**, *12*, 1261–1274. [CrossRef] [PubMed]
9. Beesu, M.; Caruso, G.; Salyer, A.C.; Shukla, N.M.; Khetani, K.K.; Smith, L.J.; Fox, L.M.; Tanji, H.; Ohto, U.; Shimizu, T.; et al. Identification of a Human Toll-Like Receptor (TLR) 8-Specific Agonist and a Functional Pan-TLR Inhibitor in 2-Aminoimidazoles. *J. Med. Chem.* **2016**, *59*, 3311–3330. [CrossRef] [PubMed]
10. Denora, N.; Laquintana, V.; Lopalco, A.; Iacobazzi, R.M.; Lopedota, A.; Cutrignelli, A.; Iacobellis, G.; Annese, C.; Cascione, M.; Leporatti, S.; et al. *In vitro* targeting and imaging the translocator protein TSPO. *J. Control. Release* **2013**, *172*, 1111–1125. [CrossRef] [PubMed]
11. Laquintana, V.; Denora, N.; Lopalco, A.; Lopedota, A.; Cutrignelli, A.; Lasorsa, F.M.; Agostino, G.; Franco, M. Translocator protein ligand-PLGA conjugated nanoparticles for 5-fluorouracil delivery to glioma cancer cells. *Mol. Pharm.* **2014**, *11*, 859–871. [CrossRef] [PubMed]
12. Annese, C.; Abbrescia, D.I.; Catucci, L.; D'Accolti, L.; Denora, N.; Fanizza, I.; Fusco, C.; La Piana, G. Site-dependent biological activity of valinomycin analogs bearing derivatizable hydroxyl sites. *J. Pept. Sci.* **2013**, *19*, 751–757. [CrossRef] [PubMed]
13. Dawson, T.M.; Dawson, V.L. Molecular pathways of neurodegeneration in Parkinson's disease. *Science* **2003**, *302*, 819–822. [CrossRef] [PubMed]
14. Warren Olanow, C. Levodopa/dopamine replacement strategies in Parkinson's disease: Future directions. *Mov. Disord.* **2008**, *23*, S613–S622. [CrossRef] [PubMed]
15. Nutt, J.G.; Woodward, W.R. Levodopa pharmacokinetics and pharmacodynamics in fluctuating parkinsonian patients. *Neurology* **1986**, *36*, 739–744. [CrossRef] [PubMed]
16. Asanuma, M.; Miyazaki, I.; Ogawa, N. Dopamine- or L-DOPA-induced neurotoxicity: The role of dopamine quinone formation and tyrosinase in a model of Parkinson's disease. *Neurotox. Res.* **2003**, *5*, 165–176. [CrossRef] [PubMed]
17. Borah, A.; Mohanakumar, K.P. L-DOPA induced-endogenous 6-hydroxydopamine is the cause of aggravated dopaminergic neurodegeneration in Parkinson's disease patients. *Med. Hypothesis* **2012**, *79*, 271–273. [CrossRef] [PubMed]
18. Lopalco, A.; Douglas, J.; Denora, N.; Stella, V. Determination of pKa and hydration constants for a series of α-keto-carboxylic acids using nuclear magnetic resonance spectrometry. *J. Pharm. Sci.* **2016**, *105*, 664–672. [CrossRef] [PubMed]
19. Leto, I.; Coronnello, M.; Righeschi, C.; Bergonzi, M.C.; Mini, E.; Bilia, A.R. Enhanced efficacy of artemisinin loaded in transferrin-conjugated liposomes versus stealth liposomes against HCT-8 colon cancer cells. *ChemMedChem* **2016**, *11*, 1745–1751. [CrossRef] [PubMed]
20. Sonali; Singh, R.P.; Singh, N.; Sharma, G.; Vijayakumar, M.R.; Koch, B.; Singh, S.; Singh, U.; Dash, D.; Pandey, B.L.; et al. Transferrin liposomes of docetaxel for brain-targeted cancer applications: Formulation and brain theranostics. *Drug Deliv.* **2016**, *23*, 1261–1271. [CrossRef] [PubMed]
21. Nogueira-Librelotto, D.R.; Codevilla, C.F.; Farooqi, A.; Rolim, C.M.B. Transferrin-Conjugated Nanocarriers as Active-Targeted Drug Delivery Platforms for Cancer Therapy. *Curr. Pharm. Des.* **2017**, *23*, 454–466. [CrossRef] [PubMed]
22. Ulbrich, K.; Hekmatara, T.; Herbert, E.; Kreuter, J. Transferrin- and transferrin receptor-antibody-modified nanoparticles enable drug delivery across the blood–brain barrier (BBB). *Eur. J. Pharm. Biopharm.* **2009**, *71*, 251–256. [CrossRef] [PubMed]
23. Li, Y.; He, H.; Jia, X.; Lu, W.L.; Lou, J.; Wei, Y. A dual-targeting nanocarrier based on poly(amidoamine) dendrimers conjugated with transferrin and tamoxifen for treating brain gliomas. *Biomaterials* **2012**, *33*, 3899–3908. [CrossRef] [PubMed]
24. Lopedota, A.; Trapani, A.; Cutrignelli, A.; Laquintana, V.; Denora, N.; Franco, M.; Trapani, G.; Liso, G. Effect of CDs on physico-chemical and release properties of Eudragit RS 100 microparticles containing glutathione. *J. Incl. Phenom. Macrocycl. Chem.* **2007**, *57*, 425–432. [CrossRef]
25. Cutrignelli, A.; Lopedota, A.; Denora, N.; Laquintana, V.; Tongiani, S.; Franco, M. Characterization and release studies of liposomal gels containing glutathione/cyclodextrins complexes potentially useful for cutaneous administration. *J. Pharm. Sci.* **2014**, *103*, 1246–1254. [CrossRef] [PubMed]

26. Pasko, E.; Vaz Gisela, M.F.; Ehrhardt, C.; Senge, M.O. Trasferrin conjugation does not increase the efficiency of liposomal Foscan during *in vitro* photodynamic therapy of oesophageal cancer. *Eur. J. Pharm. Sci.* **2013**, *48*, 202–210. [CrossRef] [PubMed]
27. Denora, N.; Lopedota, A.; Perrone, M.; Laquintana, V.; Iacobazzi, R.M.; Milella, A.; Fanizza, E.; Depalo, N.; Cutrignelli, A.; Lopalco, A.; et al. Spray-dried mucoadhesives for intravesical drug delivery using N-acetylcysteine- and glutathione-glycol chitosan conjugates. *Acta Biomater.* **2016**, *43*, 170–184. [CrossRef] [PubMed]
28. Lopedota, A.; Cutrignelli, A.; Laquintana, V.; Denora, N.; Iacobazzi, R.M.; Perrone, M.; Fanizza, E.; Mastrodonato, M.; Mentino, D.; Lopalco, A.; et al. Spray dried chitosan microparticles for intravesical delivery of celecoxib: Preparation and characterization. *Pharm. Res.* **2016**, *33*, 2195–2208. [CrossRef] [PubMed]
29. De Campos, R.P.; Siegel, J.M.; Fresta, C.G.; Caruso, G.; Fracassi da Silva, J.A.; Lunte, S.M. Indirect detection of superoxide in RAW 264.7 macrophage cells using microchip electrophoresis coupled to laser induced fluorescence detection. *Anal. Bioanal. Chem.* **2015**, *407*, 7003–7012. [CrossRef] [PubMed]
30. Kirby, C.; Gregoriadis, G. Dehydration-Rehydration vesicles: A simple method for high yield drug entrapment in liposomes. *Nat. Biotechnol.* **1984**, *2*, 979–984. [CrossRef]
31. Anabousi, S.; Bakowsky, U.; Schneider, M.; Huwer, H.; Lehr, C.M.; Ehrhardt, C. *In vitro* assessment of transferrin-conjugated liposomes as drug delivery systems for inhalation therapy of lung cancer. *Eur. J. Pharm. Sci.* **2006**, *29*, 367–374. [CrossRef] [PubMed]
32. Bibi, S.; Kaur, R.; Henriksen-Lacey, M.; McNeil, S.E.; Wilkhu, J.; Lattmann, E.; Christensen, D.; Mohammed, A.R.; Perrie, Y. Microscopy imaging of liposomes: From coverslips to environmental SEM. *Int. J. Pharm.* **2011**, *417*, 138–150. [CrossRef] [PubMed]
33. Erazo-Oliveras, A.; Muthukrishnan, N.; Baker, R.; Wang, T.Y.; Pellois, J.P. Improving the endosomal escape of cell-penetrating peptides and their cargos: Strategies and challenges. *Pharmaceuticals* **2012**, *5*, 1177–1209. [CrossRef] [PubMed]
34. Gao, W.; Hu, C.M.J.; Fang, R.H.; Zhang, L. Liposome-like nanostructures for drug delivery. *J. Mater. Chem. B* **2013**, *1*, 6569–6589. [CrossRef] [PubMed]

8

In Vitro Anticancer Activity of Extracellular Vesicles (EVs) Secreted by Gingival Mesenchymal Stromal Cells Primed with Paclitaxel

Valentina Coccè [1,†], Silvia Franzè [2,†], Anna Teresa Brini [1,3], Aldo Bruno Giannì [1,4], Luisa Pascucci [5], Emilio Ciusani [6], Giulio Alessandri [7], Giampietro Farronato [1,8], Loredana Cavicchini [1], Valeria Sordi [9], Rita Paroni [10], Michele Dei Cas [10], Francesco Cilurzo [2,*] and Augusto Pessina [1,*]

1 CRC StaMeTec, Department of Biomedical, Surgical and Dental Sciences, University of Milan, 20133 Milan, Italy; valentina.cocce@guest.unimi.it (V.C.); anna.brini@unimi.it (A.T.B.); aldo.gianni@unimi.it (A.B.G.); giampietro.farronato@unimi.it (G.F.); loredana.cavicchini@unimi.it (L.C.)

2 Department of Pharmaceutical Science, University of Milan, 20133 Milan, Italy; silvia.franze@unimi.it

3 IRCCS Orthopedic Institute Galeazzi, 20161 Milan, Italy

4 Maxillo-Facial and Dental Unit, Fondazione Ca' Granda IRCCS Ospedale Maggiore Policlinico, 20122 Milan, Italy

5 Department of Veterinary Medicine, University of Perugia, 06123 Perugia, Italy; luisa.pascucci@unipg.it

6 Laboratory of Clinical Pathology and Medical Genetics, Fondazione IRCCS Istituto Neurologico "C. Besta", 20133 Milan, Italy; emilio.ciusani@istituto-besta.it

7 Cellular Neurobiology Laboratory, Department of Cerebrovascular Diseases, IRCCS Neurological Institute C. Besta, 20133 Milan, Italy; giulio.alessandri@istituto-besta.it

8 Unit of Orthodontics and Paediatric Dentistry, Fondazione Ca' Granda IRCCS Ospedale Maggiore Policlinico, 20122 Milan, Italy

9 Diabetes Research Institute, IRCCS San Raffaele Scientific Institute, 20132 Milan, Italy; sordi.valeria@hsr.it

10 Department of Health Sciences of the University of Milan, 20142 Milan, Italy; rita.paroni@unimi.it (R.P.); michele.deicas@unimi.it (M.D.C.)

* Correspondence: francesco.cilurzo@unimi.it (F.C.); augusto.pessina@unimi.it (A.P.);

† These authors contributed equally to this work.

Abstract: Interdental papilla are an interesting source of mesenchymal stromal cells (GinPaMSCs), which are easy to isolate and expand in vitro. In our laboratory, GinPaMSCs were isolated, expanded, and characterized by studying their secretome before and after priming with paclitaxel (PTX). The secretome of GinPaMSCs did not affect the growth of cancer cell lines tested in vitro, whereas the secretome of GinPaMSCs primed with paclitaxel (GinPaMSCs/PTX) exerted a significant anticancer effect. GinPaMSCs were able to uptake and then release paclitaxel in amounts pharmacologically effective against cancer cells, as demonstrated in vitro by the direct activity of GinPaMSCs/PTX and their secretome against both human pancreatic carcinoma and squamous carcinoma cells. PTX was associated with extracellular vesicles (EVs) secreted by cells (EVs/PTX), suggesting that PTX is incorporated into exosomes during their biogenesis. The isolation of mesenchymal stromal cells (MSCs) from gingiva is less invasive than that from other tissues (such as bone marrow and fat), and GinPaMSCs provide an optimal substrate for drug-priming to obtain EVs/PTX having anticancer activity. This research may contribute to develop new strategies of cell-mediated drug delivery by EVs that are easy to store without losing function, and could have a superior safety profile in therapy.

Keywords: gingiva mesenchymal stromal cells; paclitaxel; squamous cell carcinoma; drug delivery; exosomes

1. Introduction

A large number of sources have been considered to isolate and expand mesenchymal stromal cells (MSCs), by taking into account the accessibility and availability of stem cells as well as their biological characteristics [1,2]. Most of these studies were conducted on MSCs derived from bone marrow, adipose tissue, umbilical cord blood, and, more recently, also from oral material [3–5]. Among MSCs from the oral compartment, gingival MSCs can be easily isolated, since this tissue can be removed during dental crown lengthening and periodontal surgical procedures [4,6]. As reported, MSCs from gingival papilla (GinPaMSCs) have an interesting phenotype previously described in detail [7], a relatively low osteogenic differentiation ability [8], and have significant wound healing properties that allow tissue repair without producing significant scarring [9]. Of course, most studies on MSCs have been addressed to clinical applications for regenerative medicine. The ability of MSCs to incorporate molecules and use them as a tool for drug delivery has also been proposed and intensively studied in the last years. In fact, the drug delivery mediated by MSCs can have significant advantages in comparison to the systemic administration of free chemotherapy drugs, because MSCs may migrate towards inflammatory microenvironments and accumulate in the tumor sites [10], opening up the possibility of new therapeutic anticancer strategies based on MSCs, including engineered MSCs [11,12]. Furthermore, when used in loco-regional treatments, these systems can improve the effective drug concentration in the cancer tissue and, therefore, reduce the adverse toxic effects. Moreover, vesicles might be involved in the clearance of drugs. In fact, harmful substances such as cytotoxic drugs may be associated to the vesicles, and vesicle shedding acts as a mechanism of drug expulsion. In particular, lipophilic drugs are shuttled to the plasma membrane via vesicle-mediated traffic for the final elimination [13,14]. MSCs from different sources can uptake and release drugs without any genetic manipulation, and can incorporate a significant amount of a chemotherapeutic drug (e.g., paclitaxel) that is subsequently released in quantities sufficient to affect cancer cell proliferation both in vitro and in vivo [15,16]. This capacity has also been demonstrated for mesodermal cells isolated from gingival interdental papilla [17] and dental pulp [18], suggesting that GinPaMSCs could be an interesting potential tool for cytotherapy based on cell-mediated drug delivery. Furthermore, MSC secretomes (including extracellular vesicles (EVs)) have been recently reported to be a possible alternative to MSCs for therapeutic purposes [19], being able to release accumulated drugs not only as free molecules, but also associated to exosomes and/or microvesicles [20]. Based on these observations, the present study aimed to assess the anticancer activity of secretomes from both untreated and paclitaxel (PTX)-primed GinPaMSCs, by demonstrating that both PTX-loaded GinPaMSCs and the corresponding extracellular vesicles (EVs/PTX) were active against cancer cells. This study, performed on tongue squamous cell carcinoma cell line SCC154, provides a strong proof of concept, suggesting a possible application of the procedure to collect PTX-associated EVs from drug-primed GinPaMSC working as "natural anticancer liposomes". Among the possible different MSC sources, gingiva could be the source of choice, since MSCs obtained with minimal invasive procedures are easy to expand, with high anatomical homology to treat oral neoplasia.

2. Materials and Methods

2.1. Mesenchymal Stromal Cells

Human MSCs were isolated from gingival papilla, and after expansion were characterized as previously described [7,17]. Briefly, samples of gingival tissue obtained from reductive gingivoplasty were minced with surgical scissors, treated for 3 h with type I Collagenase (50 U/mL, Life Technologies, Monza, Italy) at 37 °C under stirring conditions, and the cells were centrifuged at 300× *g* for 10 min. The cells present in the pellets were cultured in a 25 cm^2 flask in Dulbecco's modified Eagle's medium with high glucose (DMEM HG) + 10% foetal bovine serum (FBS) and 1% L-glutamine (Euroclone, UK), at 37 °C in atmosphere of air + 5% CO_2. Primary cultures were then studied to evaluate the population doubling time (PDT), clonogenicity (CFU-F), and expression of the mesenchymal stem cell markers (CD73, CD90, and CD105). GinPaMSCs showed a mild expression of CD14, but they were CD45-negative and able to differentiate into osteogenic, adipogenic, and chondrogenic lineages.

2.2. PTX Loading in GinPaMSCs

To load GinPaMSCs with PTX, the cells were primed with a high amount of drug according to a standardized procedure previously described [7,15,17]. Briefly, cultures were obtained by seeding 2×10^4 cells/cm^2, and after 72 h, cells were exposed to 2 µg/mL PTX for 24 h. Then, after washing twice with phosphate buffered saline (PBS), the cell monolayer was trypsinized, washed in Hank's solution (HBSS)(Euroclone, Pero, Italy), and the PTX-primed cells (GinPaMSCs/PTX) were seeded in a 25 cm^2 flask in DMEM HG with 10% FBS and 2 mM L-glutamine (Euroclone, Pero, Italy) to release the drug. After 48 h of incubation into conditioned media (CM), PTX-loaded GinPaMSCs (GinPaMSCs/PTX/CM) were collected and tested in vitro for their anti-proliferative activity on different tumor cell lines (see Section 2.7). In particular, human pancreatic adenocarcinoma cell line CFPAC-1 was used as a standard laboratory assay according to the method reported below. CM from untreated MSCs were used as control.

2.3. Cell Cycle Analysis

A cell cycle study was performed by starting from GinPaMSCs after synchronization, obtained by serum starvation (48 h of culture in medium containing 0.5% FBS). Then, the cells were treated with PTX in 25 cm^2 flasks according to the above described standard conditions. DNA content for cell cycle phase detection was estimated by comparing untreated cells, 24 h PTX-primed cells, and cells trypsinized (i.e., drug uptake-phase), washed, and subcultured in the absence of PTX for 24 h (i.e., drug releasing phase). Briefly, cells were suspended in phosphate buffered saline (PBS) and fixed with 96% (*v*/*v*) ethanol for 1 h at 4 °C. After a PBS wash, cells were suspended in propidium iodide (50 µg/mL) in PBS. Cells were incubated overnight at 4 °C and analyzed by FC (FacsVantageSE, Becton-Dikinson, Franklin Lakes, NJ, USA).

2.4. Secretome Analysis and Extracellular Vesicles (EVs) Collection

To collect EVs, the medium of 72 h cultures of GinPaMSCs (6×10^4 cells/cm^2; both not primed and primed with PTX, as above described) was replaced with basal medium, namely DMEM HG + 1% L-glutamine without foetal bovine serum. Then, CM of cell cultures, the secretome, were collected at 24 and 48 h of incubation at 37 °C, 5% CO_2. To separate the PTX-loaded EVs from free PTX, aliquots of secretome were centrifuged on a 100 kDa filter device (Microsep Advance Centrifugal Devices, Life Sciences, Port Washington, NY, USA) at 5000× *g* for 15 min. The two fractions (i.e., EV: F > 100 kDa; free PTX: F < 100 kDa) were collected and characterized by the physico-chemical and biological assays reported below, using the whole secretome as control.

2.5. Extracellular Vesicles (EVs) Characterization

2.5.1. Phospholipids

The phospholipid concentrations present in the EVs were estimated as phosphate content, using the Rouser method and sodium dihydrogen phosphate as standard [21]. Test and standard samples were inserted in separate Pyrex glass tubes and heated at 100 °C until complete evaporation. An empty tube was used as control. To liberate phosphates, samples and standards were cleaved by addition of 300 µL of 70% perchloric acid and heated at 200 °C for 20 min. Then, 1 mL of purified water and 400 µL 1.25% *w*/*v* ammonium molybdate were added to each tube and mixed vigorously. Finally, 400 µL of 5% *w*/*v* ascorbic acid (Sigma-Aldrich, Darmstadt, Germany) was added and mixed before heating at 100 °C for 5 min. In the presence of phosphate, samples turned blue and the absorbance at 820 nm was measured. The phospholipid concentration in EVs were estimated to be proportional to the absorbance of a 40 nmol/µL standard. All analyses were performed at least in triplicate.

2.5.2. Particle Size and ζ-Potential

Particle size distribution and ζ-potentials of samples were determined using a Zetasizer (Nano-ZS, Malvern Instrument, Malvern, Worcestershire, UK). To perform dynamic light scattering (DLS) analyses, samples were opportunely diluted with ultrapure MilliQ® water to avoid the interference due to the culture medium coloration. Particle size measurements were carried out using a disposable cuvette and a detection angle of 173°. ζ-potentials were measured in the same sample. The results are expressed as the mean and standard deviation of three measurements.

2.5.3. EVs Concentration

The concentration of EVs was determined by a nanoparticle tracking assay (NTA, Nanosight NS300, Malvern Instrument, Malvern, Worcestershire, UK). A 25 μL sample was diluted with PBS to 1 mL and analyzed at 25 °C. The capture of the images was performed according to the following setting: Camera shutter 31.48 ms; 24.98 fps; detection threshold 7 multi. The results are expressed as the mean of five determinations.

2.5.4. Transmission Electron Microscopy (TEM)

The CM were analysed by a previously described TEM procedure [22]. Briefly, 20 μL of EV suspension was placed on Parafilm. A formvar-coated copper grid (Electron Microscopy Sciences, Hatfield, PA, USA) was gently placed on the top of the drop for about 60 min in a humidified chamber. Grids were then washed in 0.1 M cacodylate buffer (CB) at pH 7.3 and finally fixed for 10 min with 2.5% glutaraldehyde (Fluka, St. Louis, MO, USA) in CB. After washing in CB, EVs were contrasted with 2% uranyl acetate. The grids were then air dried and observed under a Philips EM208 transmission electron microscope (TEM) equipped with a digital camera (University Centre for Electron Microscopy (CUME), Perugia, Italy).

2.6. Mass Spectrometry Analysis

PTX extraction and purification from secretomes was performed by liquid–liquid extraction (LLE). Aliquots of 500 μL of secretome, or fractions, were added with 100 μL of internal standard (0.1 μg/mL PTX-d5, Cayman Chemicals, Ann Arbor, MI, USA) and with toluene in a ratio of 1:2 (v/v). After sonication for 30 min at 40 °C, samples were vigorously shaken at 50 oscillations/s for 15 min, then centrifuged at 10,000 rpm for 2 min. The organic phase was evaporated and re-dissolved with 100 μL methanol, and 10 μL was injected for LC–MS/MS analysis. The multiple reaction monitoring (MRM) analysis was run on a HPLC Dionex 3000 UltiMate (Thermo Fisher Scientific, Waltham, MA, USA) coupled to a tandem mass spectrometer AB Sciex 3200 QTRAP (AB Sciex S.r.l., Milan, Italy). Separation was attained on a reversed-phase analytical column (Luna®, 3 μm, C18(2) 50 × 2 mm, Phenomenex, CA, USA), with a linear gradient between eluent A (water + 5 mM ammonium formate + 0.1% formic acid) and eluent B (acetonitrile + 0.1% formic acid). After 2 min at 20%, eluent B was increased to 95% in 4 min, held for 0.5 min, taken back to the initial conditions in 0.5 min, and kept for 2 min at 20%. The flow rate was 0.4 mL/min, and the autosampler and the column oven were kept at 15 °C and 30 °C, respectively. The representative MRM transitions were 854.5 > 286.1 (PTX) and 859.4 > 291.5 (IS, PTX-d5).

2.7. Tumor Cell Lines

Human pancreatic adenocarcinoma cell line CFPAC-1 [23,24], glioblastoma multiforme cell line T98G [25], human meshotelioma cell line M20 [26], and human squamous cell carcinoma line SCC154 [27] were provided by Centro Substrati Cellulari (ISZLER, Brescia, Italy). Cells were maintained in the complete medium (Iscove modified Dulbecco's medium (IMDM) for CFPAC-1, T98G, and M20; DMEM HG for SCC154) supplemented with 10% FBS, by 1:5 weekly dilution. All reagents were provided by Euroclone, Pero, Italy.

2.8. *In Vitro Anticancer Assays*

The inhibitory effects of secretomes from drug-loaded GinPaMSCs, as well as the F > 100 kDa and F < 100 kDa fractions, were evaluated on the proliferation of different cancer cell lines by the MTT assay as previously described [15], taking the optical density (OD) of the cancer cell treated with EVs-unloaded GinPaMSCs as a control. The inhibitory concentration (IC_{50}) was determined according to the Reed & Muench formula [28]. To study the interaction between CFPAC-1 and GinPaMSCs, a rosette adherence assay was performed [29,30]. Briefly, 5×10^5 CFPAC-1 were mixed with GinPaMSCs or GinPaMSCs/PTX in a conical tube with 0.5 ml of IMDM + 5% foetal bovine serum (FBS; Lonza, I). The cell suspension was incubated at 37 °C in air + 5% CO_2 without stirring. After 24 h, 20 µL suspensions were collected by a micropipette from the pellet lying on the tube bottom, and then transferred on a slide in order to evaluate the rosette formation under inverted microscope (Leitz, Germany) at 100× and 200× magnifications.

2.9. *Statistical Analysis*

Data are expressed as average ± standard deviation (SD). Differences between mean values were evaluated according to Student's *t*-test performed by the GRAPHPADINSTAT program (GraphPad Software Inc., San Diego, CA, USA) or ANOVA, followed by the Tukey post-hoc analysis (OriginPro 2017, Origin US, Nothampton, MA, USA). *p* values ≤ 0.05 were considered statistically significant. The linearity of response and the correlation were studied using regression analysis, by Excel 2013 software.

3. Results

3.1. *Sensitivity of GinPaMSCs to the Cytotoxic Activity of PTX*

The sensitivity of GinPaMSCs to PTX, tested by a 24 h cytotoxic MTT assay at three logarithmic dosages of 0.1–1 and 10 µg/mL (Figure 1A), confirmed the significant resistance of MSCs to the toxic effect of PTX that did not affect significantly the cell viability. The cell cycle analysis, studied on GinPaMSCs treated with a standard dosage of 2 µg/mL for 24 h (Figure 1B), indicated a decreased number of cells in phase G0, accompanied by a significant ($p < 0.05$) increase of cells in the G2/M phase. This is compatible with the known mechanism of action of PTX, which inhibits the cell proliferation in G2/M.

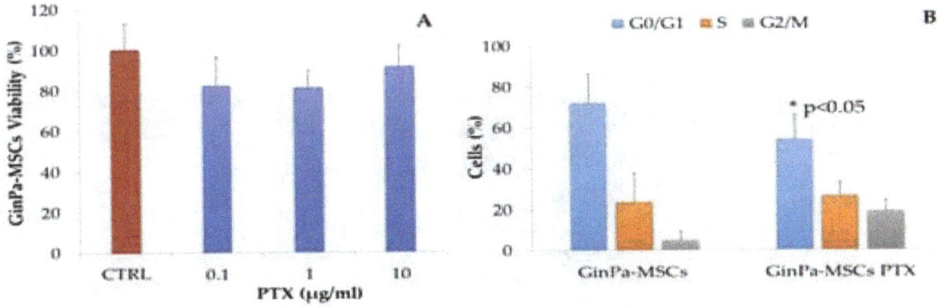

Figure 1. (**A**) Sensitivity of gingival papilla mesenchymal stem cells (GinPaMSCs) to cytotoxic activity of paclitaxel (PTX) was evaluated as cell viability at 24 h of treatment in the presence of three increasing logarithmic concentrations of the drug. The effect is expressed as percentage of the optical density measured in cultures that did not receive PTX (considered as 100%). The histogram shows the mean ± standard deviation (SD) of three independent experiments. (**B**) The histograms show the cell cycle-phase distributions of GinPaMSCs before and after treatment with 2000 ng/ml of PTX for 24 h (GinPaMSCs/PTX). Each value represents the mean ± standard deviation ($n = 3$).

3.2. *Effects Exerted on Tumor Cell Growth by Cytokines Detected in the GinPaMSCs Secretome*

The treatment of GinPaMSCs with PTX did not significantly modify the pattern of cytokine production, except for an increase of IL8 and MIF and a decrease of SCGFb. The secretome of

GinPaMSCs did not modulate the in vitro cancer cell proliferation independently of the cell line (Figure 2A). On the contrary, the secretome of cells primed with PTX (GinPaMSCs/PTX) exerted a dramatic dose–response inhibition of CFPAC-1 (pancreatic carcinoma) and SCC-154 (squamous carcinoma). Indeed, for both the cell lines, the regression analysis showed high coefficients of correlation (R^2), comparable to that of PTX (Figure 2B,C).

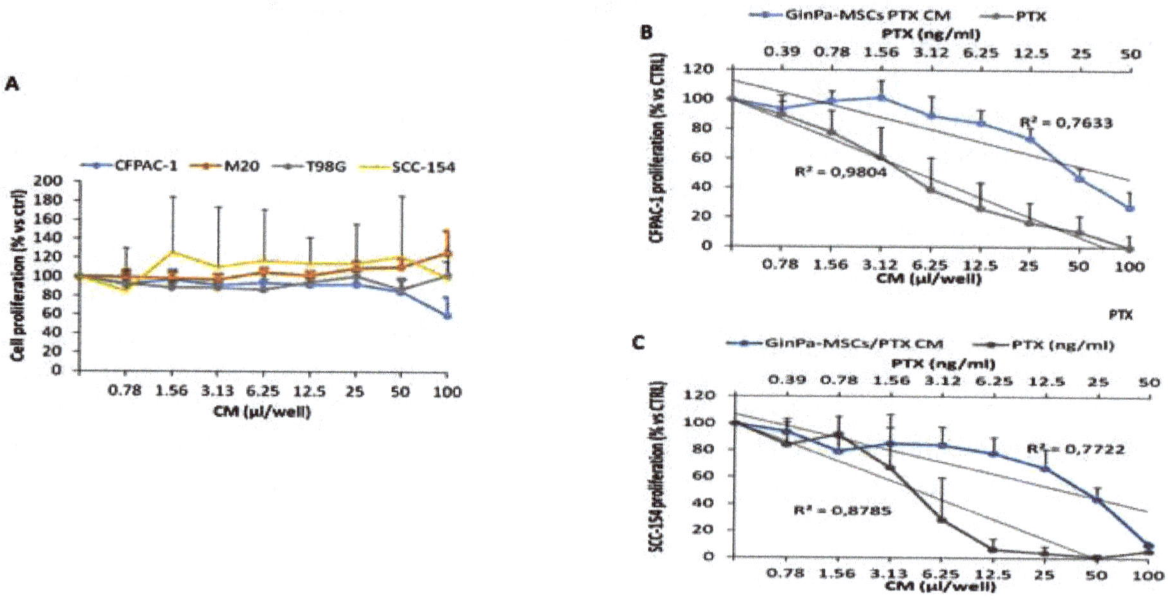

Figure 2. The activity of the GinPaMSc secretome was tested on the proliferation of four cancer cell lines (**A**). The GinPaMSCs/PTX secretome anticancer activity (blue line) and PTX solution (black line) against (**B**) pancreatic cancer cells CFPAC-1 and (**C**) squamous cell carcinoma SCC-154. The data represents the mean ± standard deviation of three independent experiments.

3.3. Direct Anticancer Activity by GinPaMSCs/PTX

The anticancer activity against CFPAC-1 and SCC-154 was confirmed by a 24 h co-culture of MSCs and cancer cells (Figure 3). Cancer cells co-cultured with GinPaMSCs did not show any sign of toxicity (Figure 3A,C), whereas many dead cancer cells were detected in the presence of GinPaMSCs/PTX, as confirmed by intracellular trypan blue uptake (Figure 3B,D).

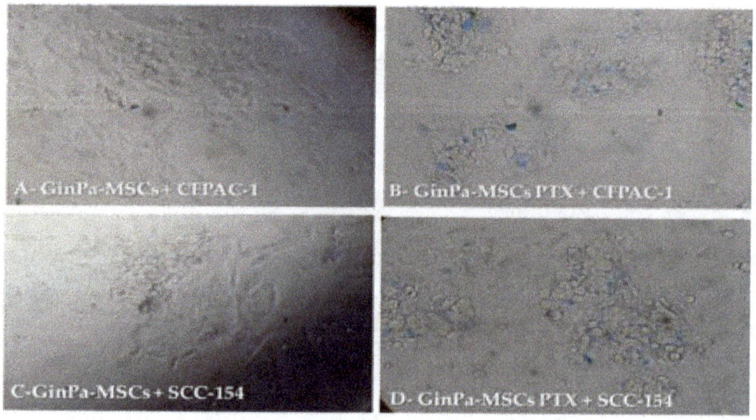

Figure 3. Direct anticancer activities of GinPaMSCs and GinPaMSCs/PTX secretomes against pancreatic cancer cells CFPAC-1 and squamous cell carcinoma SCC-154, evaluated by trypan blue in a MSCs–tumor cells co-culture system. (Panels A and C = 100× magnification, panels B and D = 200× magnification).

3.4. Characterization of EVs from GinPaMSCs and GinPaMSCs/PTX Secretome

TEM analysis of the GinPaMSCs secretome suggested the presence of EVs and exosomes with different sizes ranging from 50 to 500 nm. The treatment of GinPaMSCs with PTX did not modify the morphology of the EVs/exosome presence in either of the conditioned media (Figure 4).

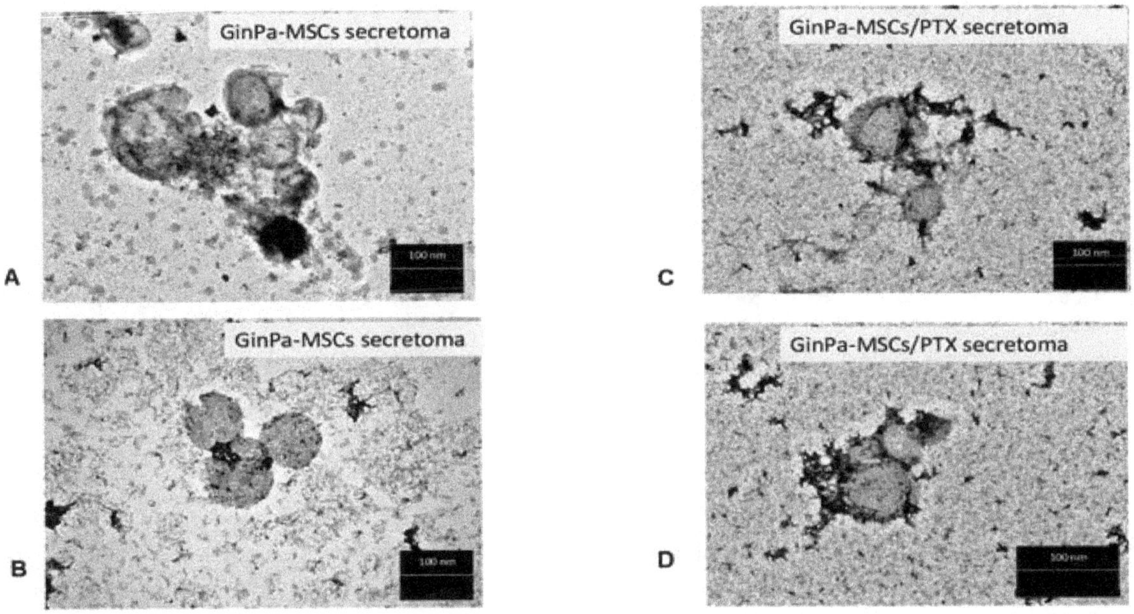

Figure 4. TEM analysis of extracellular vesicles (EVs) isolated from the secretome of cell cultures. No differences are evidenced in round-shaped morphologies of EVs from GinPaMSCs (**A**,**B**) and GinPaMSCs/PTX (**C**,**D**) with regard to size, shape, or electron density. Scale bar 100 nm.

The size distribution analysis of the isolated secretomes of GinPaMSCs was deepened both by DLS and NTA. The results of DLS analysis showed the presence of a population of microvesicles, with a particle size ranging between 200 and 300 nm, in the samples obtained from both the control and PTX-treated MSCs (Table 1). Purification by ultrafiltration led to the formation of large particles, but this increment of particle size was significant only in the case of GinPaMSCs samples (Tukey test $p = 0.0003$). This variation was not considered as a sign of particle aggregation, since the ζ-potentials showed only slight changes after purification values, maintaining the same trend (Table 1). The ζ-potential of the isolated EVs was quite negative (Table 1), and this is in line with the abundance of phosphatidylserine [31].

Table 1. Main physico-chemical features of the secretome.

Samples		D_H (nm)	ζ-potential (mV)	Phospholipids (mM)
GinPaMSCs	unfractionated	242 ± 34	−16.6 ± 0.2	0.32 ± 0.06
	Ultra-filtrated (F > 100 kDa)	430 ± 33	−20.9 ± 0.3	0.49 ± 0.07
GinPaMSCs/PTX	unfractionated	303 ± 23	−18.1 ± 2.3	0.33 ± 0.09
	Ultra-filtrated (F > 100 kDa)	385 ± 19	−22.7 ± 0.3	0.62 ± 0.15

The presence of phospholipids, which do not represent the totality of the lipid composition of extracellular vesicles, was confirmed by the Rouser assay (Table 1). No trace of vesicles was instead found in the filtrate, confirming that the purification process did not lead to the loss of some secretomes, but only allowed the removal of free PTX.

NTA analysis of the secretome evidenced the presence of different populations of vesicles and allowed us to clarify their number distribution in the samples. In particular, the whole secretome showed three different populations at about 135 nm, 200–300 nm, and 435 nm (Figure 5). The latter was not detected in the samples obtained by GinPaMSCs/PTX, which in general showed a narrowed particle size distribution, as exemplified in Figure 5. GinPaMSCs/PTX released a higher number of extracellular vesicles than untreated GinPaMSCs ($3.01 \times 10^9 \pm 1.19 \times 10^8$ versus $2.37 \times 10^9 \pm 6.80 \times 10^7$ particles/mL, respectively) but the difference was not statistically relevant.

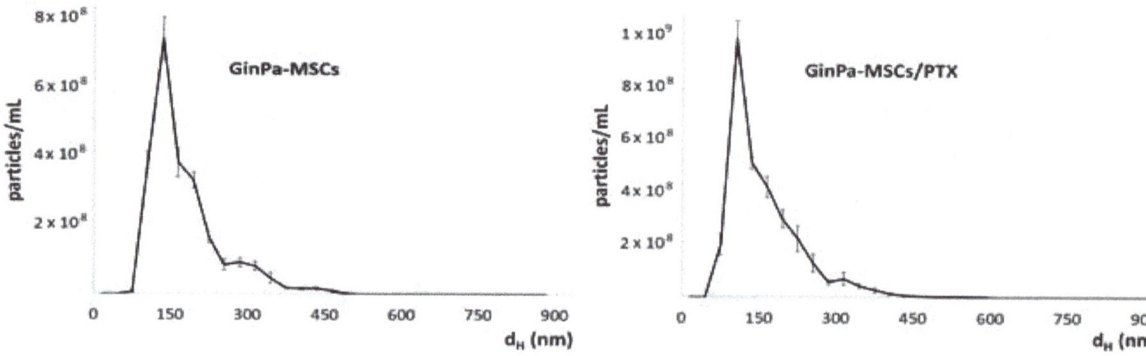

Figure 5. Size distribution analysis of the secretomes of GinPaMSCs and GinPaMSCs/PTX, analyzed by nanoparticle tracking assay (NTA). In both samples, several populations of vesicles were present at 200−300 nm.

3.5. Paclitaxel Dosage in EV Fractions of GinPaMSCs and GinPaMSCs/PTX Secretomes

The validated LC–MS/MS method was successfully applied to quantify PTX in the different samples of conditioned media from GinPaMSCs and GinPaMSCs/PTX: Unfractionated secretomes and ultra-filtered fractions (F > 100 kDa and F < 100kDa). PTX was present in both the whole secretome and the F > 100kDa fraction of PTX-treated GinPaMSCs, suggesting the incorporation or the unspecific bind of PTX to EVs (Figure 6A). No signal related to PTX was detected in the secretome of untreated GinPaMSCs used as negative controls (data not shown) or in ultra-filtered <100 GinPaMSCs/PTX samples (Figure 6C).

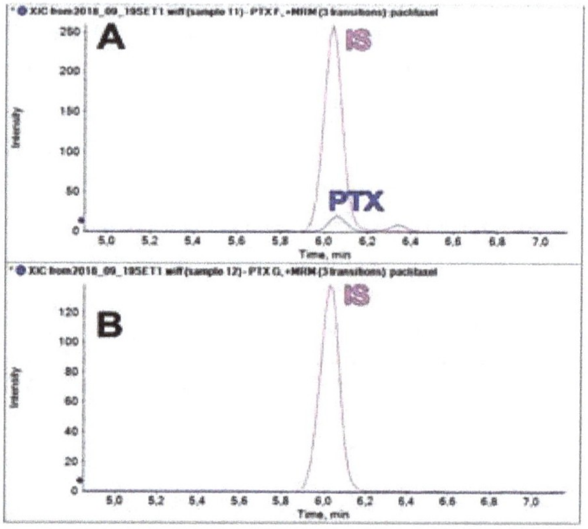

C

Sample	PTX (ng/ml)
Culture CM	< LOQ
GinPa MSCs CM	< LOQ
GinPa MSCs/PTX CM	**54.2 ± 0.3**
GinPa MSCs CM (F>100Kd)	< LOQ
GinPa MSCs CM (F<100Kd)	< LOQ
GinPa MSCs/PTX CM (F>100Kd)	**36.8 ± 3.6**
GinPa MSCs/PTX CM (F<100Kd)	< LOQ

LOQ (Limit of Quantification)= 1 ng/ml

Figure 6. PTX dosage by mass spectrometry in EV fractions. The chromatogram identification of PTX peaks by LC–MS/MS retention time: (**A**) F > 100 kDa fraction and (**B**) F < 100 kDa fraction, in which no PTX peaks were appreciable. PTX was quantified successfully in both the unfractioned secretome and the F > 100 kDa fraction of PTX-treated GinPaMSCs (**C**).

3.6. Anticancer Activity of EVs from GinPaMSCs and GinPaMSCs/PTX Secretomes

The anticancer activity of EVs secreted by GinPaMSCs/PTX was tested against squamous cancer cells (SCC154) (Figure 7). The activity is expressed as percentage of cell growth, normalized on the effect of EVs secreted by untreated GinPaMSCs used as controls. The fraction F < 100 kDa did not exert any activity against the cancer cell proliferation, with a non-significant coefficient of correlation (R^2 = 0.13). The fraction F > 100 KDa produced a significant dose-dependent inhibition of cancer cell growth, also confirmed by regression analysis (R^2 = 0.99), that is similar to the inhibition produced by the unfractioned secretome (CM) (R^2 = 0.95). These results agree with the mass spectrometry analysis that demonstrated the presence of PTX in both CM and in the F > 100 kDa (Figure 6).

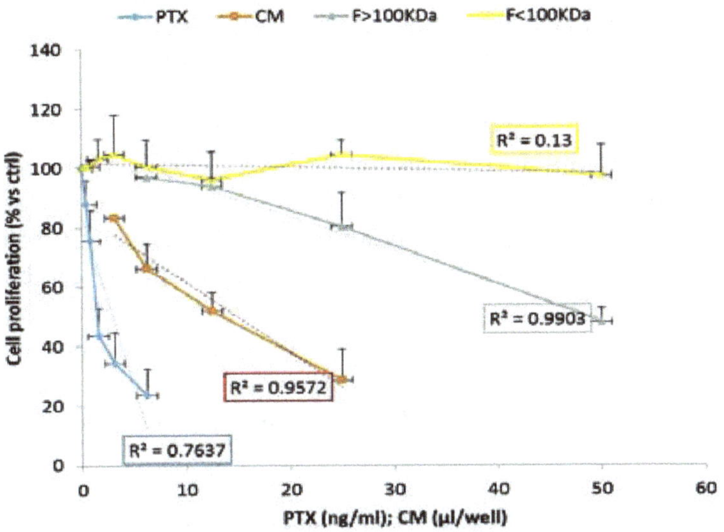

Figure 7. The anticancer activity of EVs from GinPaMSCs and GinPaMSCs/PTX tested against squamous cancer cells (SCC154). The activity is expressed as percentage of cell growth, normalized on the effect of EVs secreted by untreated GinPaMSCs used as controls (OD: 1.28 ± 0.09 was considered 100% proliferation). Data is reported as the mean ± standard deviation of three independent experiments.

4. Discussion

Our data confirm that MSCs from gingival papilla (GinPaMSCs) have a significant resistance to PTX that tested until 10,000 ng/mL, reducing the cell viability by about 20% and blocking cells in the G2/M cycle phase (Figure 1). This evidence agrees with literature data which demonstrated that the treatment of MSCs with PTX reduces their proliferation activity, migration ability, and some differentiation potentials, without significantly affecting their viability [32,33]. Of course, the analyses of secretomes of GinPaMSCs identified the presence of cytokines that did not modulate, stimulate, or inhibit the growth of four different tumor cell lines (Figure 2A). On the contrary, the secretome from the cells primed with PTX exerted a dramatic dose–response inhibition on both CFPAC-1 (pancreatic carcinoma cells) and SCC-154 (squamous carcinoma cells) (Figure 2B,C). After priming of GinPaMSCs by PTX, a little modulation of cytokine production was observed that may be considered ineffective on cancer cell growth, suggesting that the dramatic anticancer activity exerted by GinPaMSC/PTX secretomes can be mainly due to the presence of the drug secreted by PTX-primed GinPaMSCs. This result is also confirmed by the significant toxicity of GinPaMSCs/PTX only against CFPAC-1 and SCC-154, whereas cancer cells co-cultured in the presence of unprimed GinPaMSCs showed no sign of toxicity (Figure 3). Based on our previous experience with an established murine MSC line (SR4987) [20], we here investigated if primary human MSCs, particularly the gingival-derived MSCs, were able to process and then deliver PTX associated to exosomes or microvesicles. TEM analysis of GinPaMSCs secretomes demonstrated the presence of microvesicles at different sizes (Figure 4). This result was further confirmed both by dynamic light scattering (DLS) and nanoparticle tracking assay (NTA). In particular, DLS indicated the presence of a population of microvesicles ranging between 200 and 300 nm both in the secretome of GinPaMSCs and that of GinPaMSCs/PTX. Moreover, it can be assumed that isolated microvesicles shared the same origin, since the same amount of phospholipids was detected in both types of cells (Table 1). The study on size distribution by NTA evidenced three different populations in the GinPaMSCs secretome, whereas the population at about 435 nm was not detected in the Gin-PaMSCs/PTX secretome (Figure 5). This small discrepancy between NTA and DLS data depends only on the scattering intensity, because the larger the particle, the higher the contribution to the total signal. Instead, NTA allows us to provide a more reliable distribution in number. In any case, besides the slight differences in particle size distributions, it is important to highlight that the GinPaMSCs treated with PTX released a slightly higher number of EVs with respect to untreated GinPaMSCs. This difference in not statistically relevant, but this trend confirmed that PTX treatment did not affect the microvesicle biogenesis of GinPaMSCs.

The anti-proliferation activity of EVs was studied in both the unfractioned secretome (i.e., CM) and its fractions. The results confirmed that the anticancer activity was due only to the fraction containing MVs (F > 100KDa). As expected, no activity was found in the unfractioned secretomes of untreated MSCs (Figure 7), while it was a little surprising that the F < 100KDa fraction from GinPaMSCs/PTX did not contain PTX and did not present activity. This apparent discrepancy can be explained considering that a lipophilic drug, such as PTX, can be easily adsorbed and retained by filters. However, the present research was designed as a qualitative study with the main purpose to demonstrate the ability of GinPaMSCs to secrete PTX associated with EVs. A deep investigation is currently in progress to optimize the incorporation and/or release of PTX in the attempt to produce large batches of EVs by using bioreactors.

The microvesicles secreted by GinPaMSCs/PTX were active against two tumor cell lines, namely pancreatic carcinoma (CFPAC1) and tongue squamous cell carcinoma (SCC154) cell lines. As found in the preliminary screening (Figure 1), CM from GinPaMSCs/PTX was active on different tumor cell lines, and we focused the study on a human SCC model that could express an important anatomical/histological homology with the origin of MSCs generated by gingival tissue. In general, MSCs are considered as an important source of EVs and/or exosomes, and are under investigation for their role both in tumor progression and in drug delivery for tumor therapy and regenerative medicine [34–37]. As reported [20,38], upon in vitro exposure to high concentrations of PTX, MSCs can "load" the drug and deliver it by means of EVs so that the PTX-loaded EVs acquire strong anti-tumor effects on human cancers both in vitro and in vivo. Even if cancer cell-derived exosomes were proposed as effective carriers of PTX to their parental cells [39], our results demonstrated for the first time that human gingival MSCs produce a significant amount of EVs and can be considered an ideal candidate for the large production of EVs and/or exosomes. If primed with PTX, these cells can also release the drug associated to EVs and/or exosomes acting as "natural anticancer liposomes". Among the different MSC sources, our study suggests that gingival MSCs, which present an important homology with tumors originated from oral tissues (such as SCC), could be obtained with a minimally invasive procedure and easily expanded.

Currently, of paramount importance are preclinical studies, which can further corroborate the advantages of EVs. As a matter of fact, EVs could be easily manufactured in large batches by reducing the cost due to the need to personalize the cellular products, and have a superior safety profile in therapy (e.g., reduced risk related to ectopic tissue formation, microvasculature infusion toxicity, rejection) with respect to MSCs. Furthermore, the use of EVs in therapy gives the possibility to manage high drug concentrations in a minimal volume, improving the storage, the transport, and the infusion procedures [40,41].

Author Contributions: Conceptualization, A.P., G.A. and F.C.; Methodology, S.F., V.C., L.P., E.C. and V.S.; Formal Analysis, V.C., S.F.; Investigation, S.F., V.C., L.P., M.C.D. and L.C.; Data Curation, A.P., F.C. and V.C.; Vriting—Original Draft Preparation, A.P., F.C.; Writing—Review & Editing, A.P., F.C.; Supervision, R.P., A.T.B., A.B.G. and G.F.; Funding Acquisition, A.T.B., A.B.G. and G.F.

References

1. Bortolotti, F.; Ukovich, L.; Razban, V.; Martinelli, V.; Ruozi, G.; Pelos, B.; Dore, F.; Giacca, M.; Zacchigna, S. In vivo therapeutic potential of mesenchymal stromal cells depends on the source and the isolation procedure. *Stem Cell Rep.* **2015**, *4*, 332–339. [CrossRef]
2. Liu, Q.; Zhang, X.; Jiao, Y.; Liu, X.; Wang, Y.; Li, S.L.; Zhang, W.; Chen, F.M.; Ding, Y.; Jiang, C.; et al. In vitro cell behaviors of bone mesenchymal stem cells derived from normal and postmenopausal osteoporotic rats. *Int. J. Mol. Med.* **2018**, *41*, 669–678. [CrossRef]
3. Xiao, L.; Nasu, M. From regenerative dentistry to regenerative medicine: Progress, challenges, and potential applications of oral stem cells. *Stem Cells Cloning* **2014**, *7*, 89–99. [CrossRef] [PubMed]
4. Egusa, H.; Sonoyama, W.; Nishimura, M.; Atsuta, I.; Akiyama, K. Stem cells in dentistry–part I: Stem cell sources. *J. Prosthodont. Res.* **2012**, *56*, 151–165. [CrossRef]
5. Bakopoulou, A.; Apatzidou, D.; Aggelidou, E.; Gousopoulou, E.; Leyhausen, G.; Volk, J.; Kritis, A.; Koidis, P.; Geurtsen, W. Isolation and prolonged expansion of oral mesenchymal stem cells under clinical-grade, GMP-compliant conditions differentially affects stemness properties. *Stem Cell Res. Ther.* **2017**, *8*, 247. [CrossRef]
6. Fawzy El-Sayed, K.M.; Mekhemar, M.K.; Beck-Broichsitter, B.E.; Bähr, T.; Hegab, M.; Receveur, J.; Heneweer, C.; Becker, S.T.; Wiltfang, J.; Dörfer, C.E. Periodontal regeneration employing gingival margin-derived stem/progenitor cells in conjunction with IL-1ra-hydrogel synthetic extracellular matrix. *J. Clin. Periodontol.* **2015**, *42*, 448–457. [CrossRef] [PubMed]
7. Brini, A.T.; Coccè, V.; Ferreira, L.M.; Giannasi, C.; Cossellu, G.; Giannì, A.B.; Angiero, F.; Bonomi, A.; Pascucci, L.; Falchetti, M.L.; et al. Cell-mediated drug delivery by gingival interdental papilla mesenchymal stromal cells (GinPaMSCs) loaded with paclitaxel. *Expert Opin. Drug Deliv.* **2016**, *13*, 789–798.
8. Moshaverinia, A.; Chen, C.; Xu, X.; Akiyama, K.; Ansari, S.; Zadeh, H.H.; Shi, S. Bone regeneration potential of stem cells derived from periodontal ligament or gingival tissue sources encapsulated in RGD-modified alginate scaffold. *Tissue Eng. Part A* **2014**, *20*, 611–621. [CrossRef] [PubMed]
9. Larjava, H.; Wiebe, C.; Gallant-Behm, C.; Hart, D.A.; Heino, J.; Häkkinen, L. Exploring scarless healing of oral soft tissues. *J. Can. Dent. Assoc.* **2011**, *77*, b18. [PubMed]
10. Reagan, M.R.; Kaplan, D.L. Concise review: Mesenchymal stem cell tumor-homing: Detection methods in disease model systems. *Stem Cells* **2011**, *29*, 920–927. [CrossRef] [PubMed]
11. Sasportas, L.S.; Kasmieh, R.; Wakimoto, H.; Hingtgen, S.; van de Water, J.A.; Mohapatra, G.; Figueiredo, J.L.; Martuza, R.L.; Weissleder, R.; Shah, K. Assessment of therapeutic efficacy and fate of engineered human mesenchymal stem cells for cancer therapy. *Proc. Natl. Acad. Sci. USA* **2009**, *106*, 4822–48277. [CrossRef] [PubMed]
12. Stuckey, D.W.; Shah, K. TRAIL on trial: Preclinical advances in cancer therapy. *Trends Mol. Med.* **2013**, *19*, 685–694. [CrossRef] [PubMed]
13. Shedden, K.; Xie, X.T.; Chandaroy, P.; Chang, Y.T.; Rosalia, G.R. Expulsion of small molecules in vesicles shed by cancer cells: Association with gene expression and chemosensitivity profiles. *Cancer Res.* **2003**, *63*, 4331–4337. [PubMed]
14. Chen, V.Y.; Posada, M.M.; Blazer, L.L.; Zhao, T.; Rosania, G.R. The role of the VPS4A-exosome pathway in the intrinsic egress route of a DNA-binding anticancer drug. *Pharm. Res.* **2006**, *23*, 1687–1695. [CrossRef] [PubMed]
15. Pessina, A.; Bonomi, A.; Coccè, V.; Invernici, G.; Navone, S.; Cavicchini, L.; Sisto, F.; Ferrari, M.; Viganò, L.; Locatelli, A.; et al. Mesenchymal stromal cells primed with paclitaxel provide a new approach for cancer therapy. *PLoS ONE* **2011**, *6*, e28321. [CrossRef]
16. Pessina, A.; Leonetti, C.; Artuso, S.; Benetti, A.; Dessy, E.; Pascucci, L.; Passeri, D.; Orlandi, A.; Berenzi, A.; Bonomi, A.; et al. Drug-releasing mesenchymal cells strongly suppress B16 lung metastasis in a syngeneic murine model. *J. Exp. Clin. Cancer Res.* **2015**, *34*, 82. [CrossRef] [PubMed]
17. Coccè, V.; Farronato, D.; Brini, A.T.; Masia, C.; Giannì, A.B.; Piovani, G.; Sisto, F.; Alessandri, G.; Angiero, F.; Pessina, A. Drug Loaded Gingival Mesenchymal Stromal Cells (GinPaMSCs) Inhibit In Vitro Proliferation of Oral Squamous Cell Carcinoma. *Sci. Rep.* **2017**, *7*, 9376. [CrossRef] [PubMed]
18. Salehi, H.; Al-Arag, S.; Middendorp, E.; Gergely, C.; Cuisinier, F.; Orti, V. Dental pulp stem cells used to deliver the anticancer drug paclitaxel. *Stem Cell Res. Ther.* **2018**, *9*, 103. [CrossRef] [PubMed]

19. Crivelli, B.; Chlapanidas, T.; Perteghella, S.; Lucarelli, E.; Pascucci, L.; Brini, A.T.; Ferrero, I.; Marazzi, M.; Pessina, A.; Torre, M.L. Italian Mesenchymal Stem Cell Group (GISM). Mesenchymal stem/stromal cell extracellular vesicles: From active principle to next generation drug delivery system. *J. Control. Release* **2017**, *262*, 104–117. [CrossRef]
20. Pascucci, L.; Coccè, V.; Bonomi, A.; Ami, D.; Ceccarelli, P.; Ciusani, E.; Viganò, L.; Locatelli, A.; Sisto, F.; Doglia, S.M.; et al. Paclitaxel is incorporated by mesenchymal stromal cells and released in exosomes that inhibit in vitro tumor growth: A new approach for drug delivery. *J. Control. Release* **2014**, *192*, 262–270. [CrossRef]
21. Franzé, S.; Marengo, A.; Stella, B.; Minghetti, P.; Arpicco, S.; Cilurzo, F. Hyaluronan-decorated liposomes as drug delivery systems for cutaneous administration. *Int. J. Pharm.* **2018**, *535*, 333–339. [CrossRef] [PubMed]
22. Hayat, M.F. *Principles and Techniques of Electron Microscopy: Biological Applications*, 4th ed.; Cambridge University Press: Cambridge, UK, 2000.
23. McIntosh, J.C.; Schoumacher, R.A.; Tiller, R.E. Pancreatic adenocarcinoma in a patient with cystic fibrosis. *Am. J. Med.* **1988**, *85*, 592. [CrossRef]
24. Schoumacher, R.A.; Ram, J.; Iannuzzi, M.C.; Bradbury, N.A.; Wallace, R.W.; Hon, C.T.; Kelly, D.R.; Schmid, S.M.; Gelder, F.B.; Rado, T.A. A cystic fibrosis pancreatic adenocarcinoma cell line. *Proc. Natl. Acad. Sci. USA* **1990**, *87*, 4012–4016. [CrossRef] [PubMed]
25. Stein, G.H.T. 98G: An anchorage-independent human tumor cell line that exhibits stationary phase G1 arrest in vitro. *J. Cell. Physiol.* **1979**, *99*, 43–54. [CrossRef] [PubMed]
26. Treves, A.J.; Halperin, M.; Barak, V.; Bar-Tana, R.; Halimi, M.; Fibach, E.; Gamliel, H.; Leizerowitz, R.; Polliack, A. A new myelomonoblastic cell line (M20): Analysis of properties, differentiation, and comparison with other established lines of similar origin. *Exp. Hematol.* **1985**, *13*, 281–288. [PubMed]
27. Martin, C.L.; Reshmi, S.C.; Ried, T.; Gottberg, W.; Wilson, J.W.; Reddy, J.K.; Gollin, S.M. Chromosomal imbalances in oral squamous cell carcinoma. Examination of 31 cell lines and review of the literature. *Oral Oncol.* **2008**, *44*, 369–382. [CrossRef] [PubMed]
28. Reed, L.J.; Muench, H. A simple method of estimating fifty percent endpoints. *Am. J. Hyg.* **1938**, *27*, 493–497.
29. Aizawa, S.; Hojo, H.; Tsuda, A.; Sai, M.; Toyama, K. Rosette formation between stromal and hemopoietic cells: A simple assay for the supportive activity of stromal cells. *Leukemia* **1991**, *5*, 273–276. [PubMed]
30. Pessina, A.; Coccè, V.; Pascucci, L.; Bonomi, A.; Cavicchini, L.; Sisto, F.; Ferrari, M.; Ciusani, E.; Crovace, A.; Falchetti, M.L.; et al. Mesenchymal stromal cells primed with Paclitaxel attract and kill leukaemia cells, inhibit angiogenesis and improve survival of leukaemia-bearing mice. *Br. J. Haematol.* **2013**, *160*, 766–778. [CrossRef] [PubMed]
31. Van Dommelen, S.M.; Vader, P.; Lakhal, S.; Kooijmans, S.A.; van Solinge, W.W.; Wood, M.J.; Schiffelers, R.M. Microvesicles and exosomes: Opportunities for cell-derived membrane vesicles in drug delivery. *J. Control. Release* **2012**, *161*, 635–644. [CrossRef] [PubMed]
32. Bosco, D.B.; Kenworthy, R.; Zorio, D.A.R.; Sang, Q.-X.A. Human Mesenchymal Stem Cells Are Resistant to Paclitaxel by Adopting a Non-Proliferative Fibroblastic State. *PLoS ONE* **2015**, *10*, e0128511. [CrossRef] [PubMed]
33. Münz, F.; Perez, R.L.; Trinh, T.; Sisombath, S.; Weber, K.-J.; Wuchter, P.; Debus, J.; Saffrich, R.; Huber, P.E.; Nicolay, N.H. Human mesenchymal stem cellslose their functional properties after paclitaxel treatment. *Sci. Rep.* **2018**, *8*, 312.
34. Bruno, A.; Pagani, A.; Pulze, L.; Albini, A.; Dallaglio, K.; Noonan, D.M.; Mortara, L. Orchestration of angiogenesis by immune cells. *Front. Oncol.* **2014**, *4*, 131. [CrossRef]
35. Fatima, F.; Navaz, M. Stem cell-derived exosomes: Roles in stromal remodeling, tumor progression, and cancer immunotherapy. *Chin. J. Cancer* **2015**, *34*, 541–553. [CrossRef] [PubMed]
36. Lai, R.C.; Yeo, R.W.; Tan, K.H.; Lim, S.K. Exosomes for drug delivery—A novel application for the mesenchymal stem cell. *Biotechnol. Adv.* **2013**, *31*, 543–551. [CrossRef] [PubMed]
37. Li, Q.; Wijesekera, O.; Salas, S.J.; Wang, J.Y.; Zhu, M.; Aprhys, C.; Chaichana, K.L.; Chesler, D.A.; Zhang, H.; Smith, C.L.; et al. Mesenchymal stem cells from human fat engineered to secrete BMP4 are nononcogenic, suppress brain cancer, and prolong survival. *Clin. Cancer Res.* **2014**, *20*, 2375–2387. [CrossRef] [PubMed]
38. Kalimuthu, S.; Gangadaran, P.; Rajendran, R.L.; Zhu, L.; Oh, J.M.; Lee, H.W.; Gopal, A.; Baek, S.H.; Jeong, S.Y.; Lee, S.W.; et al. A New Approach for Loading Anticancer Drugs Into Mesenchymal Stem Cell-Derived Exosome Mimetics for Cancer Therapy. *Front. Pharmacol.* **2018**, *9*, 1116. [CrossRef]

39. Saari, H.; Lázaro-Ibáñez, E.; Viitala, T.; Vuorimaa-Laukkanen, E.; Siljander, P.; Yliperttula, M. Microvesicle- and exosome-mediated drug delivery enhances the cytotoxicity of Paclitaxel in autologous prostate cancer cells. *J. Control. Release* **2015**, *220*, 727–737. [CrossRef] [PubMed]
40. Akyurekli, C.; Le, Y.; Richardson, R.B.; Fergusson, D.; Tay, J.; Allan, D.S. A systematic review of preclinical studies on the therapeutic potential of mesenchymal stromal cell-derived microvesicles. *Stem Cell Rev* **2015**, *11*, 150–160. [CrossRef] [PubMed]
41. Rani, S.; Ryan, A.E.; Griffin, M.D.; Ritter, T. Mesenchymal Stem Cell-derived Extracellular Vesicles: Toward Cell-free Therapeutic Applications. *Mol. Ther.* **2015**, *23*, 812–823. [CrossRef] [PubMed]

9

Nanocarrier Lipid Composition Modulates the Impact of Pulmonary Surfactant Protein B (SP-B) on Cellular Delivery of siRNA

Roberta Guagliardo [1], Pieterjan Merckx [1], Agata Zamborlin [1], Lynn De Backer [1], Mercedes Echaide [2], Jesus Pérez-Gil [2], Stefaan C. De Smedt [1,*] and Koen Raemdonck [1,*]

1 Ghent Research Group on Nanomedicines, Laboratory of General Biochemistry and Physical Pharmacy, Department of Pharmaceutics, Ghent University, Ottergemsesteenweg 460, 9000 Ghent, Belgium

2 Departamento de Bioquímica y Biología Molecular, Facultad de Biologia, and Research Institute Hospital 12 de Octubre, Universidad Complutense, José Antonio Novais 12, 28040 Madrid, Spain

* Correspondence: stefaan.desmedt@ugent.be (S.C.D.S.); koen.raemdonck@ugent.be (K.R.);

Abstract: Two decades since the discovery of the RNA interference (RNAi) pathway, we are now witnessing the approval of the first RNAi-based treatments with small interfering RNA (siRNA) drugs. Nevertheless, the widespread use of siRNA is limited by various extra- and intracellular barriers, requiring its encapsulation in a suitable (nanosized) delivery system. On the intracellular level, the endosomal membrane is a major barrier following endocytosis of siRNA-loaded nanoparticles in target cells and innovative materials to promote cytosolic siRNA delivery are highly sought after. We previously identified the endogenous lung surfactant protein B (SP-B) as siRNA delivery enhancer when reconstituted in (proteo) lipid-coated nanogels. It is known that the surface-active function of SP-B in the lung is influenced by the lipid composition of the lung surfactant. Here, we investigated the role of the lipid component on the siRNA delivery-promoting activity of SP-B proteolipid-coated nanogels in more detail. Our results clearly indicate that SP-B prefers fluid membranes with cholesterol not exceeding physiological levels. In addition, SP-B retains its activity in the presence of different classes of anionic lipids. In contrast, comparable fractions of SP-B did not promote the siRNA delivery potential of DOTAP:DOPE cationic liposomes. Finally, we demonstrate that the beneficial effect of lung surfactant on siRNA delivery is not limited to lung-related cell types, providing broader therapeutic opportunities in other tissues as well.

Keywords: siRNA delivery; nanoparticles; pulmonary surfactant

---

1. Introduction

Over the last two decades, research in the field of RNAi therapeutics has gained attention as it allows to address diseases at the transcriptome level [1]. Once they reached the cytosol, small interfering RNAs (siRNAs) activate the RNAi machinery, leading to post-transcriptional gene silencing through sequence-specific degradation of mRNA [2,3]. High target specificity and versatility of this emerging class of therapeutics represent some of the main advantages compared to conventional small molecule drugs and monoclonal antibodies, providing a wide range of biomedical uses [1,3]. However, their application in the clinic is limited by many extra- and intracellular delivery barriers. Most importantly, negatively charged hydrophilic macromolecules like siRNAs cannot cross biological membranes, making cellular delivery challenging [1,4].

Viral vectors are often applied carriers to guide cellular delivery of nucleic acids. However, labor-intensive large-scale production and safety issues remain important drawbacks, hence encouraging research for non-viral alternatives [4–6]. Encapsulation of siRNA into synthetic nanoparticles (NPs)

allows its internalization by cells through endocytosis followed by release of the encapsulated RNA into the cytosol (i.e., endosomal escape). Among the vast number of NPs under investigation, cationic lipid nanoparticles (LNPs) currently are the preferred material for RNA delivery [7]. To date, many cationic lipid materials have been synthetized for LNP production [8–13]. However, the endosomal escape efficiency often remains poor [4,14–16]. Moreover, concerns remain regarding their safety and immunogenicity [12,17]. As such, to expedite clinical translation of this highly promising class of therapeutics, lipid-based siRNA formulations are needed to merge efficient cellular delivery with acceptable toxicity.

As synthetic polymer-and lipid-based NPs often fail to combine biocompatibility and efficacy, there is a growing interest in using bio-inspired materials [18]. We recently reported on a bio-inspired nanocomposite, composed of a siRNA-loaded polymeric matrix core surrounded by a shell of clinical pulmonary surfactant, i.e., poractant α (Curosurf®) (Figure 1) [19].

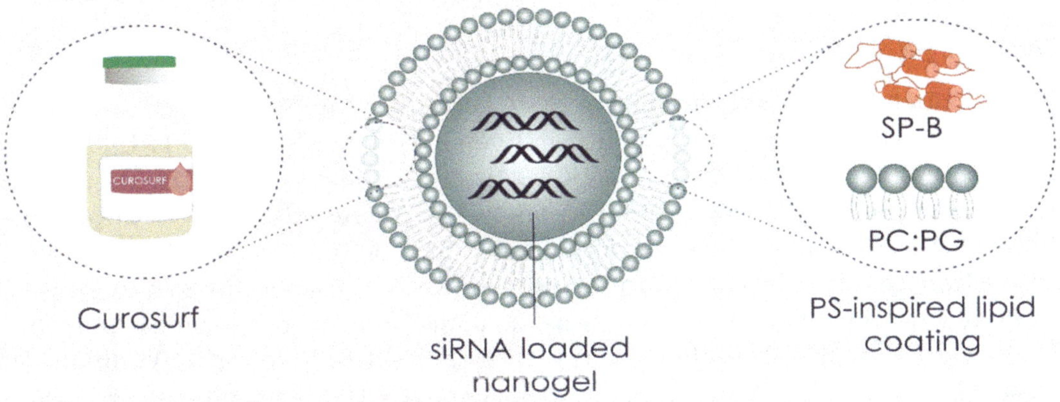

Figure 1. Visual representation of the core-shell surfactant-coated nanogel structure. SiRNA-loaded dextran nanogels (siNGs) were coated with Curosurf® (poractant α; porcine derived clinical pulmonary surfactant (PS)) or with a PS-inspired lipid coating containing the surfactant protein B (SP-B) and an anionic lipid mixture. PC = phosphatidylcholine, PG = phosphatidylglycerol.

Pulmonary surfactant (PS) is a surface-active material that is produced and secreted into the alveolar space by specialized alveolar type II epithelial cells. PS covers the entire alveolar surface and its main physiological role is to maintain low surface tension upon expiration to prevent alveolar collapse [20]. Natural human PS has a complex composition of lipids (~90 wt%) and proteins (~10 wt%). The lipid fraction mainly contains zwitterionic phosphatidylcholine (PC) (~60–70 wt%) as well as anionic phosphatidylglycerol (PG) (~10 wt%) species and neutral lipids, of which cholesterol is the most abundant (~8–10 wt%). The protein fraction consists of two major classes of specialized surfactant proteins (SPs), i.e., the larger and hydrophilic SP-A and SP-D, as well as the smaller hydrophobic SP-B and SP-C [21,22]. PS has been extensively studied mainly because of its functional role in mammalian breathing [22,23]. In the context of inhalation therapy with nanomedicines, PS is primarily regarded as one of the extracellular barriers in the deep lung that needs to be overcome to gain access to underlying target cells upon inhalation therapy [21]. Its current therapeutic use is limited to the treatment of respiratory distress syndrome in premature infants, where modified PS from animal origin (e.g., Curosurf®) is approved for so-called surfactant replacement therapy [23].

Unexpectedly, we observed that the PS outer layer in the above mentioned nanocomposites significantly enhanced intracellular siRNA delivery in lung epithelial cells and (primary) alveolar macrophages [21,24]. Although it constitutes only a minor fraction in PS, surfactant protein B (SP-B) was identified as a key component for the improved RNA delivery (Figure 1) [25]. The beneficial effect of PS and the PS-associated SP-B on RNA delivery is a very recent finding and therefore remains largely unexplored in the literature. Qiu and colleagues reported on the cationic amphiphilic peptide KL4, a synthetic SP-B mimic, as siRNA carrier for lung delivery, reaching efficient delivery *in vitro* [26]. The Anderson group covalently conjugated the truncated cationic domain of SP-B to the surface of lipidoid NPs to improve siRNA delivery [27].

Hence, many questions remain on this unique function of PS and native SP-B. First, given its natural origin, proof-of-concept on SP-B promoted siRNA delivery has been limited to lung-related cell types. Here, we sought to confirm this specific activity of SP-B on other cell types as well. In addition, our earlier data suggest that the type of lipid with which the SP-B is associated, can influence its siRNA delivery efficiency. In this report, we therefore investigated the importance of the lipid composition on the siRNA delivery activity of SP-B in more detail. In particular, the impact of cholesterol, membrane fluidity and anionic lipid type in the SP-B inspired proteolipid shell of the nanocomposites is probed. Finally, we sought to reconstitute the cationic amphiphilic SP-B in DOTAP:DOPE cationic liposomes with the aim to promote their cellular siRNA delivery efficiency.

2. Materials and Methods

2.1. Small Interfering RNAs

Twenty-one nucleotide small interfering RNA (siRNA) duplexes targeting Enhanced Green Fluorescent Protein (siEGFP), non-targeting negative control duplexes (siCTRL), protein tyrosine phosphatase receptor type C (siCD45) and pGL3 firefly luciferase (siLuc) were purchased from Eurogentec (Seraing, Belgium). For cellular uptake experiments, the siCTRL duplex was labeled with a Cy5® dye at the 5′ end of the sense strand (siCy5). The fluorescent labeling was performed and verified by Eurogentec. The concentration of the siRNA stock solutions in nuclease-free water (Ambion®-Life Technologies, Ghent, Belgium) was calculated from absorption measurements at 260 nm (1 OD260 = 40 μg/mL) with a NanoDrop 2000c UV-Vis spectrophotometer (Waltham, MA, USA). For siEGFP: sense strand = 5′-CAAGCUGACCCUGAAGUUCtt-3′; antisense strand = 5′-GAACUU CAGGGUCAGCUUGtt-3′. For siCTRL: sense strand = 5′-UGCGCUACGAUCGACGAUGtt-3′; antisense strand = 5′-CAUCGUCGAUCGUAGCGCAtt-3′. For siCD45: sense strand = 5′-GAA-GAA-UGC-UCA-CAG-AUA-A-3′; antisense strand = 5′-UUA-UCU-GUG-AGC-AUU-CUU-C-3′ (capital letters represent ribonucleotides; lower case letters represent 2′-deoxyribonucleotides). The sequence of siLuc is confidential and not available to be listed.

2.2. Synthesis of Dextran Nanogels and siRNA Complexation

Dextran hydroxyethyl methacrylate (dex-HEMA) or dextran methacrylate (dex-MA) [18,28–30] was copolymerized with a cationic methacrylate monomer [2-(methacryloyloxy)ethyl]-trimethyl-ammonium chloride (TMAEMA) to produce cationic dex-HEMA-*co*-TMAEMA (degree of substitution (DS) of 5.2) and dex-MA-*co*-TMAEMA (DS of 5.9) nanogels (hereafter abbreviated as respectively dex-HEMA NGs and dex-MA NGs), using an inverse miniemulsion photopolymerization method as previously reported [24,25,31–33]. The synthetized NGs were lyophilized and stored desiccated to ensure long term stability. To make siRNA-loaded nanogels (siNGs), 2 mg/mL of NG stock solutions were prepared by dispersing a weighed amount of the lyophilized nanoparticles in ice-cooled nuclease-free water, followed by brief sonication (Branson Ultrasonics Digital Sonifier®, Danbury, CT, USA). To allow siRNA complexation, equal volumes of siRNA and NGs in (4-(2-hydroxyethyl)-1-piperazineethanesulfonic acid) (HEPES) buffer (20 mM, pH 7.4) were mixed and incubated for ≥10 min at 4 °C.

2.3. Preparation of Proteolipid-Coated Nanogels

The commercially available clinical lung surfactant derived from minced porcine lungs, Poractant α (Curosurf®) (Chiesi Pharmaceuticals, Parma, Italy), was used to form the pulmonary surfactant (PS) outer layer on siNGs. To prepare the PS-inspired proteolipid coating the following lipids were used: 1,2-dioleoyl-*sn*-glycero-3-phosphocholine (DOPC), 1,2-dipalmitoyl-*sn*-glycero-3- phosphocholine (DPPC), 1,2-distearoyl-*sn*-glycero-3-phosphocholine (DSPC), L-α-phosphatidyl- glycerol from egg yolk (egg PG), L-α-phosphatidyl-L-serine (soy PS) and L-α-phosphatidylinositol from soy (soy PI). Soy PS was purchased from Sigma-Aldrich, all other lipids were obtained from Avanti Polar Lipids (Alabaster, AL, USA). SP-B was isolated from native porcine pulmonary surfactant following a procedure described earlier by Pérez-Gil and coworkers [34]. The lipids with or without SP-B (0.4 wt%) were mixed at the required weight ratios in chloroform and a (proteo) lipid film was obtained via nitrogen flow or rotary evaporation. The resulting lipid film was hydrated using HEPES buffer (20 mM, pH 7.4) and subsequently mixed with equal volumes of the previously formed siNGs (15 mg lipid/mg nanogel) [25]. The formation of the proteolipid coat was obtained by ≥ 10 min incubation at 4 °C and three 10″ cycles of high-energy sonication (amplitude 10%), using a probe sonicator (Branson Ultrasonics Digital Sonifier®, Danbury, CT, USA). To obtain Curosurf-coated siNGs (CS-NGs), the Curosurf® dispersion (80 mg/mL) was diluted in HEPES buffer and mixed in equal volumes with the previously formed siNGs (15 mg lipid/mg nanogel), following an identical incubation and sonication protocol as detailed above. Hydrodynamic diameter, dispersity (Đ) and ζ-potential of all formulations were measured via Dynamic Light Scattering (DLS) (Zetasizer Nano, Malvern Instruments, Worcestershire, UK).

2.4. *Preparation of Cationic Liposomes*

To prepare cationic liposomes, 1,2-dipalmitoyl-3-trimethylammonium-propane (DOTAP) and 1,2-dioleoyl-*sn*-glycero-3-phosphoethanolamine (DOPE) were purchased from Avanti Polar Lipids (AL, USA). DOTAP:DOPE liposomes (50:50 molar ratio) were prepared by mixing appropriate amount of the mentioned lipids in chloroform in a round bottom flask. In the case of DOTAP:DOPE:SP-B liposomes, 1 wt% of SP-B was added to the lipid mixture in chloroform. A lipid film was obtained via rotary evaporation and subsequently hydrated with HEPES buffer (20 mM, pH 7.4). The lipid or lipid-protein dispersion was sonicated using a probe sonicator (Branson Ultrasonics Digital Sonifier®, Danbury, CT, USA) for 30″ via a pulsed program using 10% amplitude. DOTAP:DOPE liposomes were complexed with siRNA at a charge ratio (nitrogen/phosphate ratio) equal to 8, to obtain the formation of the so-called lipoplexes (LPX). Hydrodynamic diameter, dispersity (Đ) and ζ-potential of all formulations were measured via Dynamic Light Scattering (DLS) (Zetasizer Nano, Malvern Instruments, Worcestershire, UK).

2.5. *Cell Lines and Culture Conditions*

Cell culture experiments were performed using a human non-small cell lung cancer cell line stably expressing EGFP (H1299_eGFP) [25], a human ovarian cancer cell line stably expressing luciferase (SKOV3_LUC) [35], a human hepatoma cell line stably expressing eGFP (Huh-7_eGFP) [36] and a murine alveolar macrophage cell line (MH-S). The H1299_eGFP and SKOV-3_LUC were respectively obtained from the lab of Prof. Foged (Department of Pharmacy, University of Copenhagen, Copenhagen, Denmark) and the lab of Prof. Aigner (Institute of Pharmacology, Pharmacy and Toxicology, University of Leipzig, Leipzig, Germany). The Huh-7 cell line was obtained from the lab of Prof. Lahoutte, (VUB, Brussels, Belgium). Huh-7_eGFP were generated by transfecting Huh-7 cells with the pEGFP-N2 plasmid (Clontech, Palo Alto, CA, USA). The MH-S cell line was provided by VIB-UGent. H1299_eGFP cells were cultured in RPMI 1640, supplemented with 10% fetal bovine serum, 2 mM glutamine and 100 U/mL penicillin/streptomycin. Cells were treated with medium containing 1 mg/mL Geneticin® once per month. SKOV-3_LUC were cultured in McCoy's 5A medium, supplemented with 10% FBS and 100 U/mL penicillin/streptomycin. Huh-7_eGFP cells were cultured in DMEM:F12 supplemented with 10% fetal bovine serum, 2 mM glutamine and 100 U/mL penicillin/streptomycin. MH-S were cultured in RPMI 1640 supplemented with 2 mM glutamine, 10% fetal bovine serum, 100 U/mL penicillin/streptomycin, 10 mM HEPES, 1 mM sodium pyruvate and 0.05 mM 2-mercaptoethanol. All cells were cultured at 37 °C in a humidified atmosphere containing 5% CO_2 and were passed every 3 days using a 0.25% trypsin-ethylenediaminetetraacetic acid (EDTA) solution to maintain subconfluency. All cell culture materials were purchased from Gibco®-Life Technologies, except for the serum, which was delivered by Hyclone™ (Thermo Fisher Scientific, Waltham, MA, USA).

2.6. Quantification of In Vitro Cellular siRNA Uptake by Flow Cytometry

To quantify the cellular internalization of siRNA via flow cytometry, H1299_eGFP cells (2×10^4 cells/cm^2 in 24-well plates), MH-S cells (4×10^4 cells/cm^2 in 12-well plates), Huh-7_eGFP cells (4×10^4 cells/cm^2 in 24-well plates) or SKOV-3_LUC cells (1.85×10^4 cells/cm^2 in 24-well plates) were plated (Greiner Bio-One GmbH, Kremsmünster, Austria) and allowed to settle overnight. NGs were loaded with siCTRL:siCy5 (100:0.75 mol%) and coated with a proteolipid mixture using the procedure described above. The particles were diluted 5 times in Opti-MEM to a final concentration of 30 μg/mL and incubated with the cells for 4 h (37 °C, 5% CO_2). Next, the cells were washed with dextran sulfate sodium salt (0.1 mg/mL in PBS) to remove cell surface-bound fluorescence prior to flow cytometric quantification. To quantify uptake percentage, the mean fluorescence intensity (MFI) of cells treated with coated NGs were normalized to the ones of cells treated with uncoated NGs (representing 100%). For cationic liposomes, H1299_eGFP cells were seeded in 96-well plates (SPL Lifesciences Co. Ltd., Gyeonggi-do, South Korea) at a density of 2×10^4 cells/cm^2 and allowed to settle overnight. Liposomes were used for complexation of a mixture of siCTRL:siCy5 (90:10 mol%), diluted in Opti-MEM, and incubated with the cells for 4 h (37 °C, 5% CO_2), followed by flow cytometric analysis as mentioned above. Data analysis was performed using the FlowJo™ analysis software (Treestar, Costa Mesa, CA, USA).

2.7. Quantification of eGFP Gene Silencing by Flow Cytometry

To quantify gene knockdown efficiency, H1299_eGFP cells (2×10^4 cells/cm^2) or Huh-7_eGFP (4×10^4 cells/cm^2) were plated in 24-well plates (Greiner Bio-One GMBH) and allowed to settle overnight. Particles were prepared in Opti-MEM as described above and incubated with the cells (4 h at 37 °C and 5% CO_2). Next, cells were washed with PBS and incubated with 1 mL fresh cell culture medium for 48 h. At this point, cells were prepared for flow cytometry as described above and a minimum of 10^4 cells were analyzed for each sample. The eGFP expression percentage was calculated normalizing the MFI of cells treated with siEGFP to the MFI of cells treated with siCTRL. Data analysis was performed using the FlowJo™ analysis software (Version 10.5.3, Treestar, Costa Mesa, CA, USA, 1997–2018).

2.8. Luciferase Silencing in Human Ovarian Carcinoma Cells

SKOV-3_LUC were seeded in 24-well plates at a density of 1.85×10^4 cells/cm^2 and allowed to attach overnight. Particles were prepared as described above and diluted in Opti-MEM before incubation with the cells (4 h at 37 °C and 5% CO_2). Next, cells were washed with PBS and incubated with 1 mL fresh cell culture medium for 24 h. At this time point, cell culture medium was removed and the cells were washed with PBS. Subsequently, luminescence was measured using the Luciferase Reporter Assay Kit, following the optimized Promega protocols and reagents. Luciferase activity of each sample was assayed in a GloMax™ 96 Luminometer (Promega, Madison, WI, USA).

2.9. Quantification of In Vitro CD45 Silencing in MH-S by Flow Cytometry

MH-S cells were seeded in 12-well plates and allowed to settle overnight. Particles were prepared as described above and diluted in Opti-MEM (final NG concentration of 30 μg/mL; final siRNA concentration of 100 nM) before incubation with the cells (4 h at 37 °C and 5% CO_2). Afterwards, the cells were washed with PBS and 1 mL of culture medium was added. Forty-eight hours after transfection, the cells were detached with a non-enzymatic cell dissociation buffer (10 min incubation at 37 °C). After centrifugation (7 min, 300 g), the cell pellet was resuspended in staining buffer (PBS supplemented with 5% FBS). High-affinity Fc receptors were blocked by incubation with purified anti-mouse CD16/CD32 (BD Biosciences, Erembodegem, Belgium) for 15 min at 4 °C. Subsequently, the cells were incubated with PerCP-Cy® 5.5 rat anti-mouse CD45 (BD Biosciences) diluted in staining buffer and put on a rotary shaker for 45 min at room temperature for incubation. Following three washing steps with 1 mL staining buffer, the cell pellet was resuspended in 500 μL flow buffer and placed on ice until flow cytometry analysis. Subsequently cells were analyzed using a FACSCalibur™ flow cytometer (BD Biosciences, Erembodegem, Belgium). The fluorescence for the Cy® 5.5-label was measured at 488/690 nm. Data analysis was performed using the FlowJo™ analysis software (Treestar, Costa Mesa, CA, USA).

2.10. *Statistical Analysis*

All experiments were performed in technical triplicate and with ≥ 2 independent biological repeats ($\geq n = 2$), unless otherwise stated. All data are presented as mean ± standard deviation (SD). Statistical analysis was performed via one way ANOVA, unless otherwise stated, followed by a Bonferroni multiple comparison test, using GraphPad Prism software version 8.

3. Results and Discussion

3.1. *Pulmonary Surfactant (PS) Potentiates siRNA Delivery in Non-Pulmonary Cell Lines*

As mentioned above, earlier work has demonstrated improved siRNA delivery and targeted gene silencing with PS-coated nanocomposites in both non-small cell lung cancer cells (H1299) and alveolar macrophages [21,24,25]. Corroborating these results, as shown in Figure 2a, layering cationic siNGs with a negatively charged PS bilayer (i.e., Curosurf®) strongly reduces cellular uptake in the H1299 cell line. Importantly, despite the lower intracellular siRNA dose, the same level of targeted gene knockdown is obtained (Figure 2b), indicating that the CS coat enhances the fraction of the internalized siRNA dose that is delivered into the cytosol. A comparable outcome was obtained for the murine alveolar macrophage cell line MH-S, targeting the CD45 gene (Figure 2c,d). To evaluate if PS can likewise promote siRNA delivery in cell lines derived from other organs, human ovarian carcinoma cells (SKOV-3) and human hepatoma cells (Huh-7) were treated with CS-coated siNGs (Figure 2e–h). Consistent with earlier reports, the anionic CS outer layer significantly inhibited cellular internalization of siNGs in both cell types. However, despite the ≥4-fold reduction in intracellular siRNA dose, also in these cell lines a comparable knockdown of the targeted reporter genes relative to the uncoated siNGs was observed, albeit that the Huh-7 reporter cell line in general appeared to be more difficult to transfect. These data support the notion that although the lungs constitute the natural habitat of lung surfactant, its beneficial effect on intracellular siRNA delivery is not limited to lung-related cell types and that PS-inspired drug delivery should not be restricted to the lungs as main target tissue.

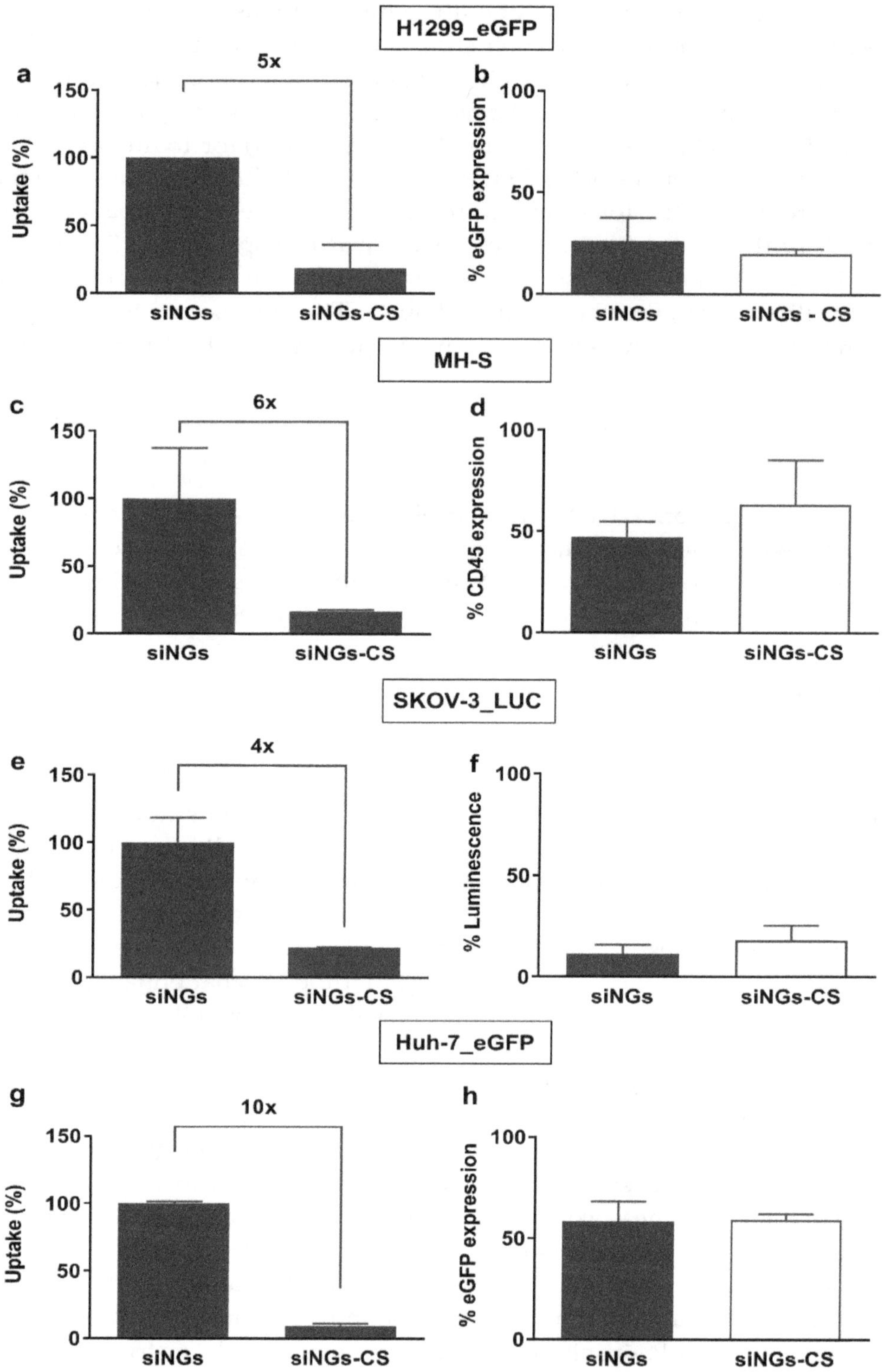

Figure 2. Biological efficacy of surfactant-coated nanogels on (non-)pulmonary cell lines. (**a,c,e,g**) Flow cytometric quantification of cellular uptake of siCy5-loaded nanogels (siNGs) with and without Curosurf® (CS) coating. (**b,d,f,h**) Gene silencing potential of siNGs and Curosurf®- coated NGs (siNGs-CS). Despite the strongly reduced cellular uptake of siNGs following Curosurf® coating, both formulations reach comparable levels of gene knockdown on the different cell lines studied. Experiments were performed with a fixed NG concentration (30 μg/mL) and siRNA concentration (50 nM), except for the MH-S cell line, for which we used a final siRNA concentration of 100 nM. Experiments on H1299_eGFP and silencing of MH-S cell lines are the result of three independent biological repeats (n = 3), other experiments are performed in technical triplicate.

3.2. *The Activity of SP-B Is Dependent on Its Lipid Microenvironment*

In recent work, Merckx et al. revealed that surfactant protein B (SP-B) is a key component in lung surfactant that dictates cellular siRNA delivery [25]. However, the activity of SP-B was proven to be strongly dependent on the type of lipids with which it is combined, with the more fluid lipid mixture DOPC:PG (85:15 wt%) clearly outperforming its more rigid counterpart DPPC:PG (85:15 wt%) in terms of *in vitro* siRNA delivery efficiency. It is postulated that less resistance against lateral movement in a less rigid proteolipid coat could promote SP-B-mediated intermembrane interactions [34,37]. To extend our understanding, siNGs were coated with DSPC:PG (85:15 wt%) of which the main lipid has a substantially higher phase transition temperature (Tc) of 55 °C, compared to DPPC (41 °C). The absence of SP-B in the lipid coat inhibited siNG-mediated gene silencing, independent of the type of lipid used. Supplementation of the DOPC:PG and DPPC:PG lipid coat with SP-B did result in reduced eGFP expression levels, albeit that the improvement in gene silencing was statistically significant solely for the more fluid DOPC-containing lipid bilayer (Figure 3a). Importantly, with DSPC as main phospholipid, no gene silencing could be observed anymore. Of note, using an identical coating protocol, the use of DSPC as main lipid component resulted in micrometer sized nanocomposites (Table 1). These data altogether suggest that the Tc of the lipid coat influences both the colloidal stability of the core-shell formulation as well as its intracellular siRNA delivery potential.

Table 1. Representative DLS data and ζ-potential of different formulations used in this study.

Sample	Hydrodynamic Diameter (nm)	Đ	ζ -Potential (mV)
NGs DOPC:PG	168 ± 2	0.24	−23 ± 1
NGs DPPC:PG	257 ± 2	0.45	−20 ± 1
NGs DSPC:PG	5480 ± 2700	1	−16 ± 0
Dex-HEMA NGs	195 ± 3	0.18	17 ± 0
Dex-HEMA NGs LIP	160 ± 1	0.24	−29 ± 1
Dex-HEMA NGs LIP SP-B	158 ± 3	0.26	−35 ± 0
Dex-MA NGs	203 ± 1	0.26	15 ± 3
Dex-MA NGs LIP	117 ± 1	0.26	−35 ± 0
Dex-MA NGs LIP SP-B	114 ± 2	0.39	−40 ± 1
DOTAP:DOPE LPX	132 ± 3	0.40	56 ± 4
DOTAP:DOPE LPX SP-B	114 ± 2	0.38	48 ± 2

Nanogels (NGs); Dextran hydroxyethyl methacrylate (dex-HEMA); dextran methacrylate (dex-MA); lipid coating DOPC:PG (LIP); Surfactant Protein B (SP-B); lipoplexes (LPX); polydispersity (Đ). Samples were measured in HEPES buffer 20 mM pH 7.4.

Natural PS contains a substantial fraction of neutral lipids, mainly cholesterol (~8 wt%), which modulate surfactant activity [38]. However, excessive cholesterol levels are known to interfere with normal surfactant function, possibly contributing to respiratory insufficiency [39,40]. As the manufacturing of Curosurf® involves depletion of neutral lipids, including cholesterol and cholesteryl esters, the data shown in Figure 2 and in earlier reports seem to indicate that the presence of cholesterol is not strictly required for the siRNA delivery-promoting effect of SP-B. However, state-of-the-art lipid formulations often contain high fractions of cholesterol (up to 40 wt%) as a stabilizing component for *in vivo* application. Therefore, we sought to probe the impact of cholesterol on SP-B mediated siRNA delivery (Figure 4). While supplementation of the DOPC:eggPG lipid mixture with physiological cholesterol levels did not negatively influence siRNA delivery efficiency, gene silencing efficiency was slightly impaired when further increasing the cholesterol fraction to ~25 wt%. Overall, we conclude that cholesterol levels exceeding the endogenous PS fractions by far, partially hamper SP-B's beneficial effect on siRNA delivery.

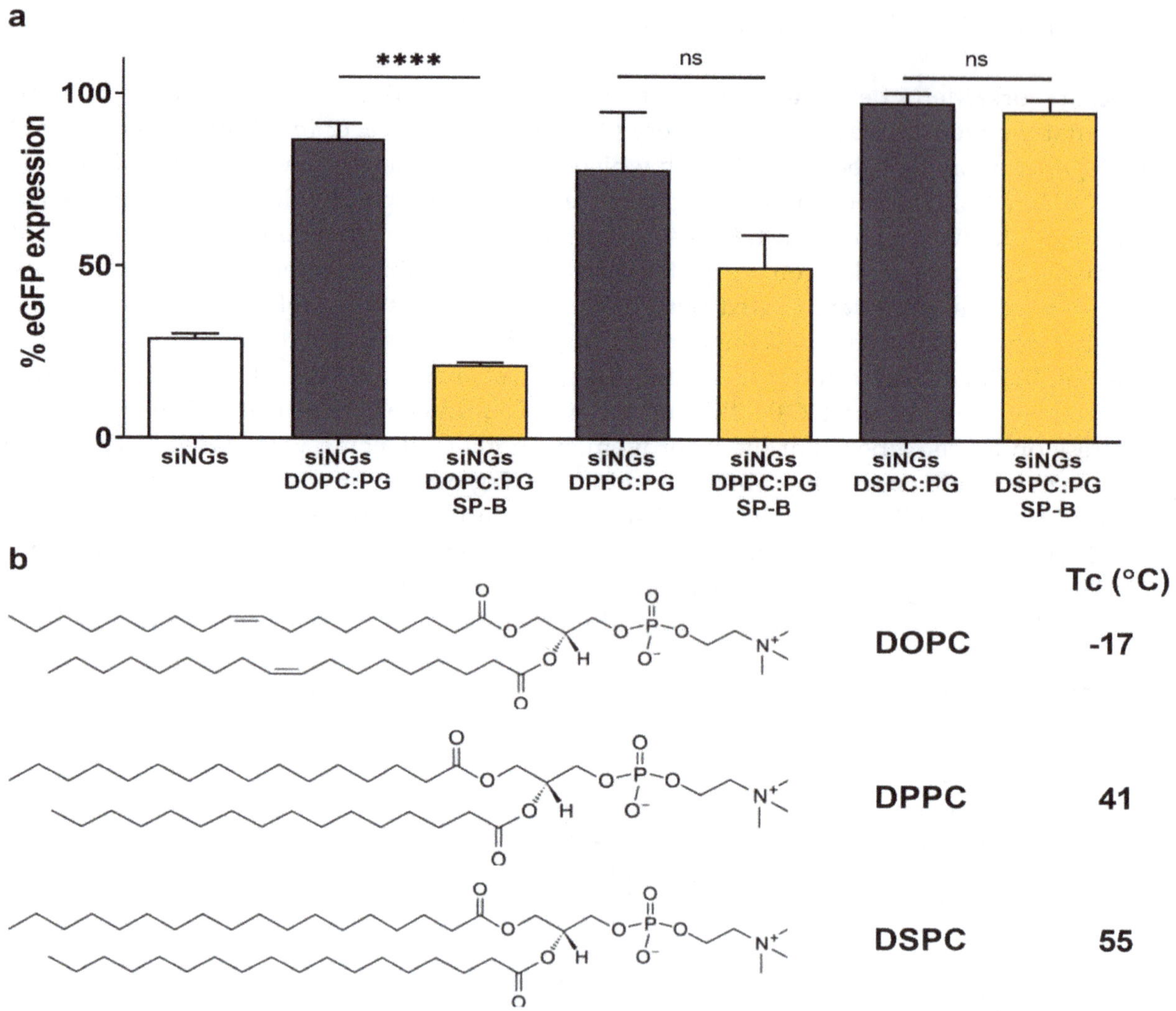

Figure 3. Impact of lipid phase transition temperature on formation and delivery efficiency of SP-B containing proteolipid-coated nanogels. (**a**) Evaluation of eGFP silencing in H1299_eGFP cells by uncoated or (proteo)lipid-coated siNGs with different lipid mixtures, supplemented with 0.4 wt% SP-B. All experiments were performed with a fixed NG concentration (30 μg/mL) and siRNA concentration (50 nM). The SP-B effect is strongly influenced by the type of lipid with which it is combined, highlighting the importance of a fluid lipid membrane in the formulation of the core-shell nanocomposites. (**b**) Chemical structures and phase transition temperatures (Tc) of the different PC lipids tested. Statistical analysis was performed via an unpaired *t*-test. Data are represented as the mean ± SD ($n = 2$) and statistical significance is indicated (**** $p < 0.0001$, ns = not significant).

While anionic phospholipids are generally present in rather low concentrations in mammalian tissues, PS represents an exception with its PG content of 7–12% by mass [41]. As mentioned above, SP-B is a cationic amphipathic protein, of which the positive charges are believed to interact with the head groups of anionic phospholipid species like PG. As previously reported, this interaction could orchestrate the distribution of SP-B in the more disordered phases of PS membranes [42,43]. It is conceivable that SP-B likewise connects electrostatically with the PG fraction in the nanocomposite proteolipid coat, mimicking the natural interaction of SP-B with lipid bilayers. However, PG does not constitute the only negative phospholipid in PS, where phosphatidylinositol (PI) and phosphatidylserine (PhS) also play a role. Of note, PI represent the main negative phospholipid in lung surfactant of other species, while in humans only fetal surfactant shows higher PI content relative to PG, which is reversed with ageing [41]. The less abundant PhS seems to be mainly involved in surfactant metabolism processes, although its exact role is still unclear [41]. Here, we aimed to evaluate the compatibility of

SP-B with other anionic lipids by replacing the PG fraction with PhS or PI in the SP-B supplemented DOPC:PG proteolipid coat of the nanocomposites (Figure 5). As expected, all coated formulations substantially reduced the cellular uptake of the siNGs (>10-fold). PI containing nanocomposites reached the highest knockdown levels, which could in part be explained by the relatively higher intracellular siRNA dose. Most importantly, independent of the type of anionic lipid, the presence of SP-B in the lipid coat significantly promotes gene silencing efficiency, indicating that the nature of the negative phospholipid is not critical for the cellular effect of SP-B (Figure 5).

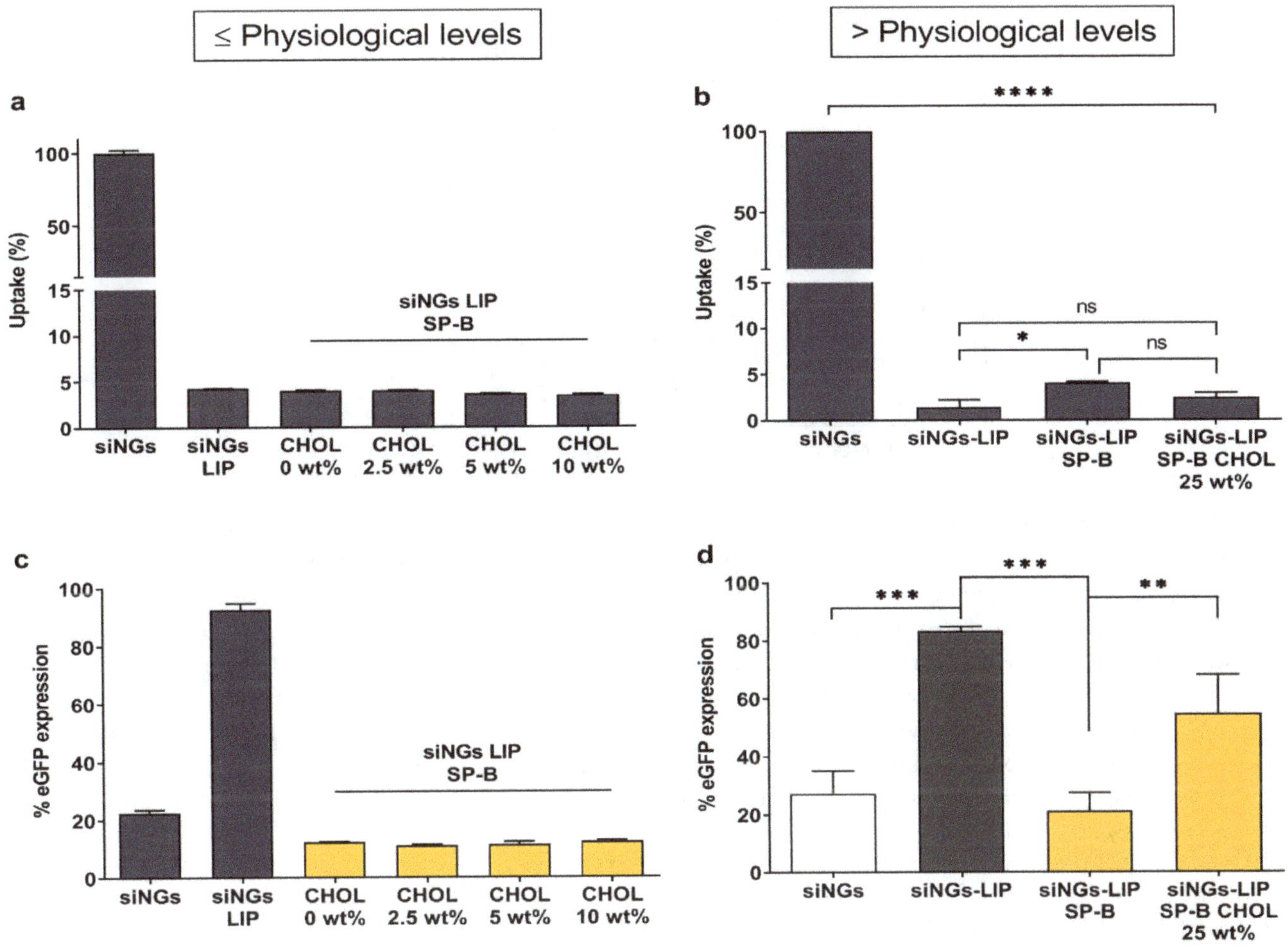

Figure 4. Impact of cholesterol on biological efficacy of proteolipid-coated nanogels. Evaluation of (**a**) cellular uptake and (**c**) gene silencing potential in H1299_eGFP cells of siRNA-loaded nanogels (siNGs) coated with lipid mixtures containing physiological cholesterol (CHOL) levels (2.5, 5 to 10 wt%). Data show one representative (technical triplicate) of two independent experiments; formulations with different siRNA concentrations showed the same trend (data not shown). Evaluation of (**b**) cellular uptake and (**d**) gene silencing potential of siNGs coated with increased cholesterol fraction in the outer layer (~25 wt%) ($n = 3$). Cholesterol exceeding physiological levels partially hinder SP-B promoted siRNA delivery. All experiments were performed with a fixed NG concentration (30 μg/mL) and siRNA concentration (50 nM). LIP = DOPC:PG (85:15); LIP SP-B = DOPC:PG (85:15) + SP-B 0.4 wt%; LIP SP-B CHOL = DOPC:CHOL:PG (60:25:15) + SP-B 0.4 wt%. Data are represented as the mean ± SD and statistical significance is indicated (* $p < 0.05$, ** $p < 0.01$, *** $p < 0.005$, **** $p < 0.0001$, ns = not significant).

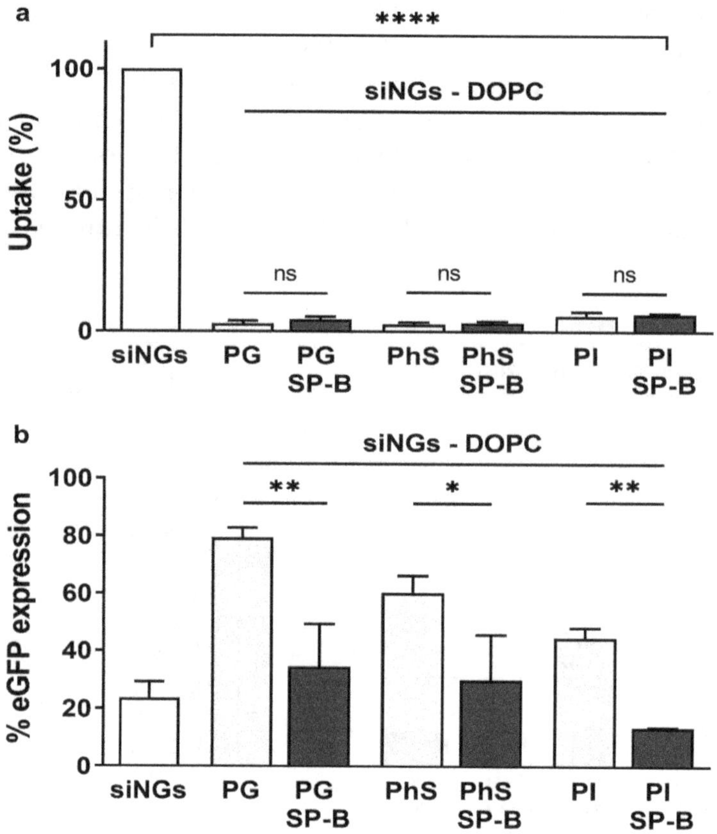

Figure 5. Role of the anionic lipid in biological efficacy of proteolipid-coated nanogels. (**a**) Cellular uptake and (**b**) gene silencing evaluated on H1299_eGFP cells via flow cytometry. SiRNA-loaded nanogels (siNGs) were coated with a mixture of DOPC:PG, DOPC:PhS or DOPC:PI (weight ratio 85:15). The presence of negatively charged lipids is required to allow the formation of the core-shell structure via electrostatic interactions. The replacement of the anionic phosphatidylglycerol (PG) with phosphatidylserine (PhS) or phosphatidylinositol (PI) does not abrogate SP-B's beneficial effect on siRNA delivery. All experiments were performed with a fixed NG concentration (30 μg/mL) and siRNA concentration (50 nM). Statistical analysis was performed via an unpaired t-test. Data are represented as the mean ± SD ($n = 3$) and statistical significance is indicated (* $p < 0.05$, ** $p < 0.01$, **** $p < 0.0001$, ns = not significant).

3.3. Degradability of the Nanogel Core Does Not Influence SP-B Activity

To date, the effect of SP-B on siRNA delivery has only been demonstrated using PS-inspired proteolipid nanocomposites with a biodegradable hydrogel core (Figure 1). To evaluate whether the degradation of the core contributes to the activity of SP-B, the hydrolysable dex-HEMA NG core was replaced by its stable dex-MA counterpart with comparable physicochemical characteristics (Figure 6) [28–30]. In line with earlier data from our group [31,44], dex-MA siNGs show a slightly reduced intrinsic siRNA delivery potential relative to dex-HEMA siNGs (due to the absence of the hydrolysable carbonate ester in the crosslinks), albeit similar uptake levels are achieved (data not shown). However, coating of the former with a SP-B proteolipid bilayer also strongly promoted siRNA delivery and target gene knockdown, indicating that degradability of the core material is not essential for SP-B's activity (Figure 6a).

In addition, intentionally degrading the dex-HEMA NG core (4 h incubation at 37 °C) after proteolipid coating but prior to transfection did not seem to affect the gene knockdown efficiency (Figure 6b). These results indicate that an intact polymeric core material in the core-shell nanocomposites is likewise not essential to the delivery-promoting effect of SP-B.

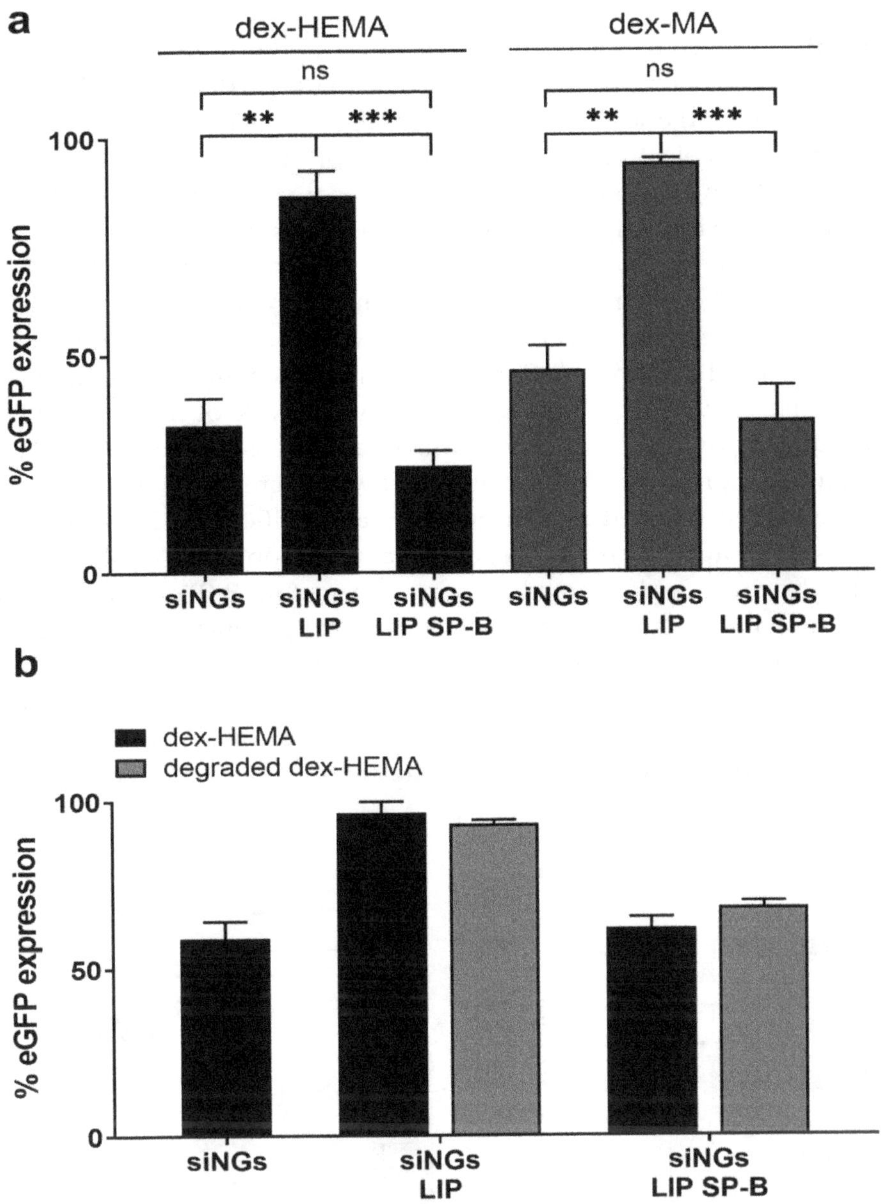

Figure 6. Impact of dextran nanogel core structure on SP-B mediated siRNA delivery. (**a**) Gene silencing potential of (proteolipid-coated) siRNA-loaded NGs (siNGs) constructed with the hydrolysable dex-HEMA or the stable dex-MA. Both formulations were coated with a mixture of DOPC:PG (85:15 wt%) here abbreviated as LIP, with or without SP-B. Although the stable dex-MA shows a less pronounced eGFP knockdown, SP-B promotes siRNA delivery equal to the degradable dex-HEMA. Data are a summary of two independent experiments. Data are represented as the mean ± SD ($n = 2$) and statistical significance is indicated (** $p < 0.01$, *** $p < 0.005$, ns = not significant). (**b**) Gene silencing of (proteo)lipid-coated dex-HEMA NGs with an intact or degraded NG core. All experiments were performed with a fixed NG concentration (30 µg/mL) and siRNA concentration (5 nM). Data show one representative graph of two independent experiments; formulations with increased SP-B fraction showed the same trend (data not shown).

3.4. Integration of SP-B into Cationic Liposomes Does Not Enhance siRNA Delivery

To form a stable core-shell nanocomposite, electrostatic interaction of a negatively charged lipid shell with the cationic NG core is required [19,24]. Here, the NG enables siRNA encapsulation in the nanocomposite and at the same time serves as a solid support for the deposition of the surfactant shell. However, as the integrity of the core material is not essential for SP-B's effect on siRNA delivery, we aimed to evaluate the impact of SP-B supplementation in cationic liposomes in which the siRNA complexation is directly achieved by the positively-charged lipids. To date, cationic lipid nanoparticles (LNPs) remain the most advanced nanoformulation for siRNA delivery [45]. LNPs are typically composed of a cationic lipid and one or more helper lipids, in which the cationic lipid is the dominant component as it enables both electrostatic complexation of the oppositely charged RNA as well as cellular delivery by facilitating cellular uptake and endosomal escape, albeit that the latter step in general lacks efficiency for the majority of siRNA nanomedicines [46]. Increasing the cytosolic delivery potential of such formulations could reduce the dose of both carrier and cargo, thus mitigating the risk of off-target effects. Here, we aimed to exploit the amphiphilic properties of SP-B to reconstitute SP-B in the bilayer of a commercially available cationic liposomal formulation (i.e., DOTAP:DOPE 50:50 mol%). To obtain the lipoplexes (LPX), the formed liposomes were incubated with siRNA solutions to obtain a charge ratio equal to 8 [47]. Adding 1 wt% of SP-B to the lipid composition seemed to slightly reduce both hydrodynamic diameter as well as surface charge (Table 1). Likewise, also the cellular internalization in the H1299 cell model was decreased when SP-B was present in the DOTAP:DOPE bilayer, albeit without reaching statistical significance. Most importantly, although higher SP-B fractions were applied here, no beneficial effect on intracellular siRNA delivery and resulting target gene silencing could be noted in the presence of SP-B (Figure 7). It is hypothesized that the high intrinsic cationic charge density of the DOTAP:DOPE liposomes might obscure the more subtle membrane destabilizing effects of the cationic amphiphilic SP-B protein. On the other hand, it cannot be excluded that electrostatic repulsion between cationic lipids and positively-charged SP-B molecules could result in a less optimal distribution of the protein to enable intracellular siRNA delivery. More detailed experiments are required to fully elucidate the contrasting effects of SP-B when reconstituted in DOTAP:DOPE cationic liposomes.

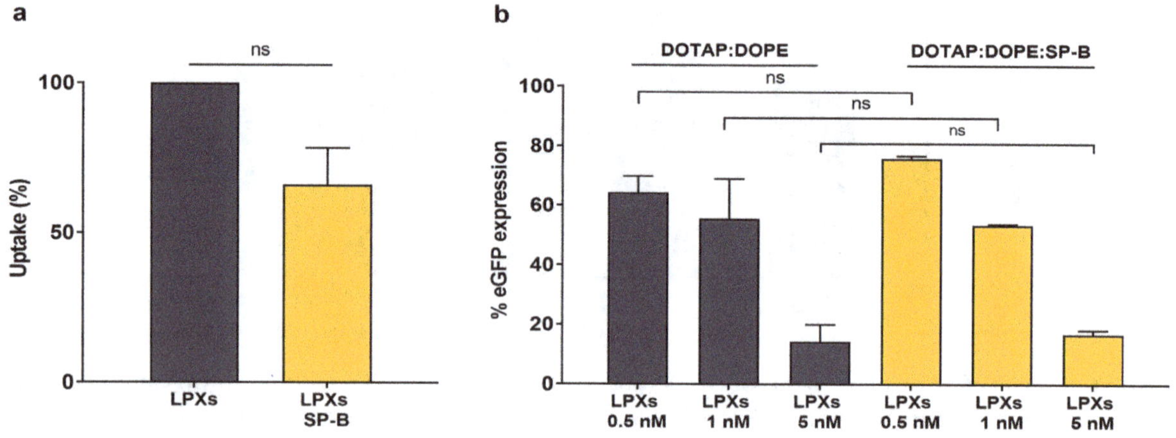

Figure 7. Evaluation of SP-B effect on DOTAP:DOPE liposomes for siRNA delivery in H1299_eGFP cells. (**a**) Cellular uptake and (**b**) gene silencing potential of DOTAP:DOPE LPXs (final concentrations siRNA are 0.5, 1 and 5 nM) with and without SP-B (1 wt%). The inclusion of SP-B in the cationic liposomal formulation does not result in any enhanced delivery effect. For uptake data, statistical analysis was performed using a one sample *t*-test. Data are represented as the mean ± SD (n = 2) and statistical significance is indicated (ns = not significant).

4. Conclusions

Previous studies have identified the endogenous surfactant protein B (SP-B) as siRNA delivery enhancer when reconstituted in lipid-coated nanogels (NGs). The mechanism of action of SP-B at the alveolar air-liquid interface has been investigated in detail, providing essential knowledge of the impact of the lipid microenvironment on SP-B's activity and, consequently, on surfactant dynamics. Contrarily, the way SP-B is able to promote intracellular delivery of siRNA and how this activity might be influenced by the lipid environment has not yet been described in detail. Here, we evaluated the influence of the main constituents of SP-B proteolipid-coated NGs, namely the lipid composition of the proteolipid coat and the degradability of the NG core, on the activity of SP-B. While the inner core degradability did not seem to be essential for SP-B promoted siRNA delivery, we showed a crucial role of the surrounding lipid membranes. Specifically, we described the importance of membrane fluidity and appropriate cholesterol levels, in analogy with the physiological interactions between SP-B and lipids occurring at the alveolar air-liquid interface. In addition, the adjuvant effect of SP-B on cellular siRNA delivery was supported by different types of anionic lipid species in the proteolipid coat. On the other hand, a formulation of commonly used DOTAP:DOPE cationic liposomes with SP-B did not result in an improved gene silencing effect. Importantly, we also showed the SP-B promoted siRNA delivery in other pulmonary cell lines, suggesting its suitability to boost siRNA delivery in extrapulmonary tissues as well. Altogether, these results provide useful insights that will support future rational design of lipid-based SP-B nanoplatforms for siRNA delivery.

Author Contributions: Conceptualization, R.G., S.C.D.S. and K.R.; Formal analysis, R.G., P.M., A.Z., L.D.B. and K.R.; Funding acquisition, S.C.D.S. and K.R.; Investigation, R.G., P.M., A.Z., L.D.B. and K.R.; Resources, M.E. and J.P.-G.; Supervision, S.C.D.S. and K.R.; Visualization, P.M., A.Z., L.D.B. and K.R.; Writing—original draft, R.G., L.D.B. and K.R.; Writing—review & editing, R.G., P.M., A.Z., J.P.-G., S.C.D.S. and K.R.

References

1. Dowdy, S.F. Overcoming cellular barriers for RNA therapeutics. *Nat. Biotechnol.* **2017**, *35*, 222–229. [CrossRef]
2. Sahin, U.; Karikó, K.; Türeci, Ö. MRNA-based therapeutics-developing a new class of drugs. *Nat. Rev. Drug Discov.* **2014**, *13*, 759–780. [PubMed]
3. Kaczmarek, J.C.; Kowalski, P.S.; Anderson, D.G. Advances in the delivery of RNA therapeutics: From concept to clinical reality. *Genome Med.* **2017**, *9*, 60.
4. Stewart, M.P.; Lorenz, A.; Dahlman, J.; Sahay, G. Challenges in carrier-mediated intracellular delivery: Moving beyond endosomal barriers. *Wiley Interdiscip. Rev. Nanomed. Nanobiotechnol.* **2016**, *8*, 465–478. [CrossRef] [PubMed]
5. Stewart, M.P.; Langer, R.; Jensen, K.F. Intracellular delivery by membrane disruption: Mechanisms, strategies, and concepts. *Chem. Rev.* **2018**, *118*, 7409–7531. [CrossRef] [PubMed]
6. Johannes, L.; Lucchino, M. Current Challenges in Delivery and Cytosolic Translocation of Therapeutic RNAs. *Nucleic Acid Ther.* **2018**, *28*, 178–193. [CrossRef]
7. Kulkarni, J.A.; Cullis, P.R.; van der Meel, R. Lipid Nanoparticles Enabling Gene Therapies: From Concepts to Clinical Utility. *Nucleic Acid Ther.* **2018**, *28*, 146–157. [CrossRef] [PubMed]
8. Akinc, A.; Zumbuehl, A.; Goldberg, M.; Leshchiner, E.S.; Busini, V.; Hossain, N.; Bacallado, S.A.; Nguyen, D.N.; Fuller, J.; Alvarez, R.; et al. A combinatorial library of lipid-like materials for delivery of RNAi therapeutics. *Nat. Biotechnol.* **2008**, *26*, 561–569. [CrossRef] [PubMed]
9. Semple, S.C.; Akinc, A.; Chen, J.; Sandhu, A.P.; Mui, B.L.; Cho, C.K.; Sah, D.W.Y.; Stebbing, D.; Crosley, E.J.; Yaworski, E.; et al. Rational design of cationic lipids for siRNA delivery. *Nat. Biotechnol.* **2010**, *28*, 172–176. [CrossRef] [PubMed]
10. Whitehead, K.A.; Dorkin, J.R.; Vegas, A.J.; Chang, P.H.; Veiseh, O.; Matthews, J.; Fenton, O.S.; Zhang, Y.; Olejnik, K.T.; Yesilyurt, V.; et al. Degradable lipid nanoparticles with predictable in vivo siRNA delivery activity. *Nat. Commun.* **2014**, *5*, 4277. [CrossRef]
11. Yin, H.; Kanasty, R.L.; Eltoukhy, A.A.; Vegas, A.J.; Dorkin, J.R.; Anderson, D.G. Non-viral vectors for gene-based therapy. *Nat. Rev. Genet.* **2014**, *15*, 541–555. [CrossRef] [PubMed]
12. Rietwyk, S.; Peer, D. Next-Generation Lipids in RNA Interference Therapeutics. *ACS Nano* **2017**, *11*, 7572–7586. [CrossRef] [PubMed]
13. Fenton, O.S.; Kauffman, K.J.; McClellan, R.L.; Kaczmarek, J.C.; Zeng, M.D.; Andresen, J.L.; Rhym, L.H.; Heartlein, M.W.; DeRosa, F.; Anderson, D.G. Customizable Lipid Nanoparticle Materials for the Delivery of siRNAs and mRNAs. *Angew. Chem. Int. Ed.* **2018**, *57*, 13582–13586. [CrossRef] [PubMed]

14. Gilleron, J.; Querbes, W.; Zeigerer, A.; Borodovsky, A.; Marsico, G.; Schubert, U.; Manygoats, K.; Seifert, S.; Andree, C.; Stöter, M.; et al. Image-based analysis of lipid nanoparticle–mediated siRNA delivery, intracellular trafficking and endosomal escape. *Nat. Biotechnol.* **2013**, *31*, 638–646. [CrossRef] [PubMed]
15. Sahay, G.; Querbes, W.; Alabi, C.; Eltoukhy, A.; Sarkar, S.; Zurenko, C.; Karagiannis, E.; Love, K.; Chen, D.; Zoncu, R.; et al. Efficiency of siRNA delivery by lipid nanoparticles is limited by endocytic recycling-supp. *Nat. Biotechnol.* **2013**, *31*, 653–658. [CrossRef] [PubMed]
16. Mizrahy, S.; Hazan-Halevy, I.; Dammes, N.; Landesman-Milo, D.; Peer, D. Current Progress in Non-viral RNAi-Based Delivery Strategies to Lymphocytes. *Mol. Ther.* **2017**, *25*, 1491–1500. [CrossRef]
17. Sabnis, S.; Kumarasinghe, E.S.; Salerno, T.; Mihai, C.; Ketova, T.; Senn, J.J.; Lynn, A.; Bulychev, A.; McFadyen, I.; Chan, J.; et al. A Novel Amino Lipid Series for mRNA Delivery: Improved Endosomal Escape and Sustained Pharmacology and Safety in Non-human Primates. *Mol. Ther.* **2018**, *26*, 1509–1519. [CrossRef]
18. Raemdonck, K.; Braeckmans, K.; Demeester, J.; De Smedt, S.C. Merging the best of both worlds: Hybrid lipid-enveloped matrix nanocomposites in drug delivery. *Chem. Soc. Rev.* **2014**, *43*, 444–472. [CrossRef]
19. De Backer, L.; Naessens, T.; De Koker, S.; Zagato, E.; Demeester, J.; Grooten, J.; De Smedt, S.C.; Raemdonck, K. Hybrid pulmonary surfactant-coated nanogels mediate efficient in vivo delivery of siRNA to murine alveolar macrophages. *J. Control. Release* **2015**, *217*, 53–63. [CrossRef]
20. Parra, E.; Pérez-Gil, J. Composition, structure and mechanical properties define performance of pulmonary surfactant membranes and films. *Chem. Phys. Lipids* **2015**, *185*, 153–175. [CrossRef]
21. De Backer, L.; Cerrada, A.; Pérez-Gil, J.; De Smedt, S.C.; Raemdonck, K. Bio-inspired materials in drug delivery: Exploring the role of pulmonary surfactant in siRNA inhalation therapy. *J. Control. Release* **2015**, *220*, 642–650. [CrossRef]
22. Guagliardo, R.; Pérez-Gil, J.; De Smedt, S.; Raemdonck, K. Pulmonary surfactant and drug delivery: Focusing on the role of surfactant proteins. *J. Control. Release* **2018**, *291*, 116–126. [CrossRef] [PubMed]
23. Johansson, J.; Curstedt, T. Synthetic surfactants with SP-B and SP-C analogues to enable worldwide treatment of neonatal respiratory distress syndrome and other lung diseases. *J. Intern. Med.* **2019**, *285*, 165–186. [PubMed]
24. De Backer, L.; Braeckmans, K.; Stuart, M.C.A.; Demeester, J.; De Smedt, S.C.; Raemdonck, K. Bio-inspired pulmonary surfactant-modified nanogels: A promising siRNA delivery system. *J. Control. Release* **2015**, *206*, 177–186. [CrossRef]
25. Merckx, P.; De Backer, L.; Van Hoecke, L.; Guagliardo, R.; Echaide, M.; Baatsen, P.; Olmeda, B.; Saelens, X.; Pérez-Gil, J.; De Smedt, S.C.; et al. Surfactant protein B (SP-B) enhances the cellular siRNA delivery of proteolipid coated nanogels for inhalation therapy. *Acta Biomater.* **2018**, *78*, 1–11. [CrossRef] [PubMed]
26. Qiu, Y.; Chow, M.Y.T.; Liang, W.; Chung, W.W.Y.; Mak, J.C.W.; Lam, J.K.W. From Pulmonary Surfactant, Synthetic KL4 Peptide as Effective siRNA Delivery Vector for Pulmonary Delivery. *Mol. Pharm.* **2017**, *14*, 4606–4617. [CrossRef] [PubMed]
27. Karagiannis, E.D.; Urbanska, A.M.; Sahay, G.; Pelet, J.M.; Jhunjhunwala, S.; Langer, R.; Anderson, D.G. Rational design of a biomimetic cell penetrating peptide library. *ACS Nano* **2013**, *7*, 8616–8626. [CrossRef]
28. Van Dijk-Wolthuis, W.N.E.; Kettenes-van Den Bosch, J.J.; Van Der Kerk-van Hoof, A.; Hennink, W.E. Reaction of dextran with glycidyl methacrylate: An unexpected transesterification. *Macromolecules* **1997**, *30*, 3411–3413. [CrossRef]
29. van Dijk-Wolthuis, W.N.E.; Franssen, O.; Talsma, H.; van Steenbergen, M.J.; Kettenes-van den Bosch, J.J.; Hennink, W.E. Synthesis, Characterization, and Polymerization of Glycidyl Methacrylate Derivatized Dextran. *Macromolecules* **1995**, *28*, 6317–6322. [CrossRef]
30. van Dijk-Wolthuls, W.N.E.; Tsang, S.K.Y.; Kettenes-van den Bosch, W.E.; Hennink, J.J. A new class of polymerizable dextrans with hydrolyzable groups: Hydroxyethyl methacrylated dextran with and without oligolactate spacer. *Polymer* **2002**, *38*, 6235–6242. [CrossRef]
31. Raemdonck, K.; Naeye, B.; Buyens, K.; Vandenbroucke, R.E.; Høgset, A.; Demeester, J.; Smedt, S.C.D. Biodegradable dextran nanogels for RNA interference: Focusing on endosomal escape and intracellular siRNA delivery. *Adv. Funct. Mater.* **2009**, *19*, 1406–1415. [CrossRef]
32. De Backer, L.; Braeckmans, K.; Demeester, J.; De Smedt, S.C.; Raemdonck, K. The influence of natural pulmonary surfactant on the efficacy of siRNA-loaded dextran nanogels. *Nanomedicine* **2013**, *8*, 1625–1638. [CrossRef] [PubMed]

33. Raemdonck, K.; Naeye, B.; Høgset, A.; Demeester, J.; De Smedt, S.C. Prolonged gene silencing by combining siRNA nanogels and photochemical internalization. *J. Control. Release* **2010**, *145*, 281–288. [CrossRef] [PubMed]
34. Olmeda, B.; García-Álvarez, B.; Gómez, M.J.; Martínez-Calle, M.; Cruz, A.; Pérez-Gil, J.; Garcia-Alvarez, B.; Gomez, M.J.; Martinez-Calle, M.; Cruz, A.; et al. A model for the structure and mechanism of action of pulmonary surfactant protein B. *FASEB J.* **2015**, *29*, 4236–4247. [CrossRef] [PubMed]
35. Dakwar, G.R.; Braeckmans, K.; Ceelen, W.; De Smedt, S.C.; Remaut, K. Exploring the HYDRAtion method for loading siRNA on liposomes: The interplay between stability and biological activity in human undiluted ascites fluid. *Drug Deliv. Transl. Res.* **2017**, *7*, 241–251. [CrossRef] [PubMed]
36. Naeye, B.; Raemdonck, K.; Remaut, K.; Sproat, B.; Demeester, J.; De Smedt, S.C. PEGylation of biodegradable dextran nanogels for siRNA delivery. *Eur. J. Pharm. Sci.* **2010**, *40*, 342–351. [CrossRef] [PubMed]
37. Schürch, D.; Ospina, O.L.; Cruz, A.; Pérez-Gil, J. Combined and independent action of proteins SP-B and SP-C in the surface behavior and mechanical stability of pulmonary surfactant films. *Biophys. J.* **2010**, *99*, 3290–3299. [CrossRef] [PubMed]
38. Gómez-Gil, L.; Pérez-Gil, J.; Goormaghtigh, E. Cholesterol modulates the exposure and orientation of pulmonary surfactant protein SP-C in model surfactant membranes. *Biochim. Biophys. Acta Biomembr.* **2009**, *1788*, 1907–1915. [CrossRef] [PubMed]
39. Al-Saiedy, M.; Pratt, R.; Lai, P.; Kerek, E.; Joyce, H.; Prenner, E.; Green, F.; Ling, C.C.; Veldhuizen, R.; Ghandorah, S.; et al. Dysfunction of pulmonary surfactant mediated by phospholipid oxidation is cholesterol-dependent. *Biochim. Biophys. Acta Gen. Subj.* **2018**, *1862*, 1040–1049. [CrossRef]
40. Zuo, Y.Y.; Veldhuizen, R.A.W.; Neumann, A.W.; Petersen, N.O.; Possmayer, F. Current perspectives in pulmonary surfactant—Inhibition, enhancement and evaluation. *Biochim. Biophys. Acta Biomembr.* **2008**, *1778*, 1947–1977. [CrossRef]
41. Alcorn, J.L. Pulmonary Surfactant Trafficking and Homeostasis. In *Lung Epithelial Biology in the Pathogenesis of Pulmonary Disease*; Elsevier: Amsterdam, The Netherlands, 2017; pp. 59–75. ISBN 9780128038819.
42. Nag, K.; Taneva, S.G.; Perez-Gil, J.; Cruz, A.; Keough, K.M.W. Combinations of fluorescently labeled pulmonary surfactant proteins SP- B and SP-C in phospholipid films. *Biophys. J.* **1997**, *72*, 2638–2650. [CrossRef]
43. Pérez-Gil, J.; Casals, C.; Marsh, D. Interactions of Hydrophobic Lung Surfactant Proteins SP-B and SP-C with Dipalmitoylphosphatidylcholine and Dipalmitoylphosphatidylglycerol Bilayers Studied by Electron Spin Resonance Spectroscopy. *Biochemistry* **1995**, *34*, 3964–3971. [CrossRef] [PubMed]
44. Raemdonck, K.; Van Thienen, T.G.; Vandenbroucke, R.E.; Sanders, N.N.; Demeester, J.; De Smedt, S.C. Dextran microgels for time-controlled delivery of siRNA. *Adv. Funct. Mater.* **2008**, *18*, 993–1001. [CrossRef]
45. Lin, Q.; Chen, J.; Zhang, Z.; Zheng, G. Lipid-based nanoparticles in the systemic delivery of siRNA. *Nanomedicine* **2014**, *9*, 105–120. [CrossRef] [PubMed]
46. Du, Z.; Munye, M.M.; Tagalakis, A.D.; Manunta, M.D.I.; Hart, S.L. The Role of the helper lipid on the DNA transfection efficiency of lipopolyplex formulations. *Sci. Rep.* **2014**, *4*, 7107. [CrossRef] [PubMed]
47. Dakwar, G.R.; Braeckmans, K.; Demeester, J.; Ceelen, W.; De Smedt, S.C.; Remaut, K. Disregarded Effect of Biological Fluids in siRNA Delivery: Human Ascites Fluid Severely Restricts Cellular Uptake of Nanoparticles. *ACS Appl. Mater. Interfaces* **2015**, *7*, 24322–24329. [CrossRef]

10

Silver Nanoparticles: Synthetic Routes, In Vitro Toxicity and Theranostic Applications for Cancer Disease

Valeria De Matteis [1,*], Mariafrancesca Cascione [2], Chiara Cristina Toma [1] and Stefano Leporatti [3,*]

1 Dipartimento di Matematica e Fisica "E. De Giorgi", Università del Salento, Via Monteroni, 73100 Lecce, Italy; chiara.toma@unisalento.it
2 Dipartimento di Scienze Biomediche e Oncologia Umana, Università degli Studi di Bari "Aldo Moro", p.zza G. Cesare, 70124 c/o Policlinico Bari, Italy; mariafrancesca.cascione@unisalento.it
3 CNR Nanotec-Istituto di Nanotecnologia, c/o Campus Ecotekne, Via Monteroni, 73100 Lecce, Italy
* Correspondence: valeria.dematteis@unisalento.it (V.D.M.); stefano.leporatti@nanotec.cnr.it (S.L.)

Abstract: The large use of nanomaterials in many fields of application and commercial products highlights their potential toxicity on living organisms and the environment, despite their physico-chemical properties. Among these, silver nanoparticles (Ag NPs) are involved in biomedical applications such as antibacterial agents, drug delivery vectors and theranostics agents. In this review, we explain the common synthesis routes of Ag NPs using physical, chemical, and biological methods, following their toxicity mechanism in cells. In particular, we analyzed the physiological cellular pathway perturbations in terms of oxidative stress induction, mitochondrial membrane potential alteration, cell death, apoptosis, DNA damage and cytokines secretion after Ag NPs exposure. In addition, their potential anti-cancer activity and theranostic applications are discussed.

Keywords: silver nanoparticles; synthetic routes; toxicity; theranostics

---

1. Introduction

The unique physico-chemical properties of silver nanoparticles (Ag NPs) have attracted increasing interest from the scientific community [1] due to their high thermal conductivity, plasmonic properties, chemical stability and antibacterial ability [2]. The use of Ag is not new; it dates to the times of Hippocrates, who used it as antibacterial to manage ulcers [3]. Nowadays, Ag NPs are used in many commercial products including soaps, plastics, food, textiles, catheters, and bandages. It is calculated that around 383 products are based on nano Ag globally, corresponding to 24% of all nano-products in use. For this reason, researchers are attempting to understand the adverse effects on living organisms: numerous in vitro and in vivo studies have demonstrated their toxicity occurring by means of cellular pathway perturbations [4]; nevertheless, their mechanism of action is still unclear. A lot of factors (size, shape, morphology, surface chemistry, charge, coating/capping agents, agglomeration, purity) influence the biological activity of Ag NPs and as consequence the adverse effects are different in different cell types [5].

Another important feature of Ag NPs is their involvement in cancer treatment. Cancer is a disease characterized by uncontrolled cellular growth and spread, during which cells become unresponsive to the usual check-points, leading to tumor growth and metastasis [6]. However, chemotherapy does not specifically target drugs to cancerous sites, therefore exposing healthy cells to undesirable effects. Moreover, a large dose is required owing to its rapid elimination and nonspecific distribution [7]. For these reasons, the goal of nanomedicine is to identify cost-effective molecules that have high specificity and sensitivity in cells **[8]**. With this in mind, Ag NPs are a promising tool as anticancer agents in diagnostics and probing [9], with strong effects against different cancer cell lines offering many advantages [10]. Their better penetration, and the possibility to track Ag NPs in the body make them a more efficient tool in cancer treatment with less risk compared to standard therapeutic procedures [11]. The unique Ag NP properties, such as easy surface functionalization, optical properties, reproducible synthetic routes and high surface: volume ratio, makes them suitable for cancer treatment [12]. The optical properties can be tuned to have an absorption at specific wavelengths that is useful for imaging and photothermal applications in tissue [13]. Ag NPs can also be functionalized with different molecules such as DNA/RNA to selectively target different cells [14] and antibodies or polymers [15]. These last agents are important to extend the half-life time for in vivo circulation that is critical in drug and gene delivery applications [16]. In addition, Ag NPs are used as an ablation tool for cancer cells due their ability to convert radiofrequencies into heat [17].

Starting from these assumptions, in this review we focused on the synthetic routes used for the synthesis of Ag NPs (physical, chemical and green methods), the mechanism of their toxicity in cells and their potential applications in theranostics for cancer.

2. Principal Routes of Ag NPs Synthesis

Engineering nanoparticles (NPs) can be synthetized by different approaches: "top-down", and "bottom-up". The first means the nanoparticle synthesis comes from a bulk system, while bottom-up means they are obtained from nanoscaled materials starting from atomic level. The top-down is exploited in synthesis based on physical methods, whereas the bottom-up approach is useful for chemical or green procedures, and it is more suitable for obtaining monodispersed nanostructures with fewer defects [18].

2.1. *Physical Synthesis*

The use of physical methods allows the synthesis of nanoparticles in the absence of solvent, permitting the uniformity of Ag NPs size distribution compared to chemical routes [19].

The main routes of synthesis are listed below:

- Evaporation-condensation

One of the common physical routes is the evaporation-condensation method, using a tube furnace at atmospheric pressure, where the source material is centered in a furnace and vaporized into a carrier gas. Many types of NPs are synthetized using this technique, including Ag NPs [20]. However, this procedure presents many limitations, among them high consumption of energy, large time to achieve the operating temperature. Together with bulky shape instrumentation, this makes this technique of little use.

- Laser ablation

Ag NPs can be produced by laser ablation method, which permits the obtaining of uncontaminated colloids, even if the control of size is difficult. This method uses a laser beam as the energy source to induce ablation on a solid target material, which vaporizes into atoms and clusters, and successively the NPs are assembled in ambient media (gas or liquid) [21]. Pyatenko et al. [22] synthetized Ag NPs by a laser ablation, irradiating a bulk Ag with a 532 nm laser beam in pure water. They obtained 2–5 nm Ag NPs after use of high laser power and small spot sizes. Tsuji et al. [23] used focused and unfocused laser beam irradiation with two intensities (12 and 900 mJ/cm^2 respectively). They demonstrated a reduction in terms of NP diameter (from 29 nm to 12 nm) with the decrease of laser wavelength. Amendola et al. [24] obtained stable solutions of Ag NPs in pure acetonitrile and *N,N*-dimethylformamide by laser ablation of the bulk metal with a size of (1.9 ± 1.5) nm and (2.2 ± 2.5) nm respectively (Figure 1a).

- Thermal decomposition

Thermal decomposition is an endothermic chemical reaction induced by heat. The substances have a specific thermal decomposition that cause chemical decomposition. Therefore, the process permits the break-up of large molecules into smaller ones due to heat in an oxygen-restricted environment [25]. Ag NPs have also been synthesized using thermal decomposition method by Lee and Kang [26], using a solution of $AgNO_3$ and sodium oleate. The synthesis of spherical Ag NPs with a size ranging from 9.5 nm to 0.7 nm was obtained by changing the temperature from room temperature to 290 °C for 1 h. Navaladian et al. achieved [27] spherical crystalline Ag NPs (10 nm) by thermal decomposition of Ag oxalate in water and in ethylene glycol, using polyvinyl-alcohol (PVA) as a capping agent, which reduces Ag oxalate. The Ag NPs became smaller when the PVA concentration increased.

- Ultrasonic spray pyrolysis

Another physical approach is ultrasonic spray pyrolysis, which allows the obtaining of NPs with a controlled size through the production of aerosol from a dilute aqueous metal salt solution. Pluym et al. [28] produced pure and monodispersed micron-sized Ag NPs by spray pyrolysis with an ultrasonic generator at 600 °C (using N_2 carrier gas), and above 900 °C (using air carrier gas). Pingali et al. [29] proposed a one-step synthesis of Ag NPs with a diameter ranging from 20 nm to 300 nm, by pyrolysis of ultrasonically atomized spray of $AgNO_3$ solution, maintaining a temperature of 650 °C with a tube furnace. Different sizes were obtained tuning the concentration of $AgNO_3$ solution and ultrasound power.

- Arc discharge method

Arc discharge method is mostly used to synthetize carbon nanotubes (CNTs): a current arc voltage is applied between two graphite electrodes that vaporize carbon in the presence of a catalyst immersed in an inert gas (helium or argon) [30]. Recently, this method is used for synthesis of metallic NPs such as Ag NPs.

Arc discharge method requires vacuum apparatus with an efficient cooling system. Tien et al. [31] used it to produce Ag NPs into ultrapure water. They adopted two Ag electrodes that, after melting at high temperature, were converted into Ag NPs with a size ranging from 5 nm to 45 nm. Another study [32] described the production of spherical Ag NPs (3–5) nm by direct metal sputtering into propane-1,2,3-triol (glycerol).

Although physical methods were consistent for obtaining good Ag NPs without the use of hazardous chemicals, their use is often unfeasible due to the limitations of large energy consumption and long times required to reach thermal stability [33].

2.2. *Chemical Approach*

- Chemical reduction

The most used chemical approach is chemical reduction, which permits synthesis of Ag NPs in solution (water or organic solvents) in presence of (i) metal precursors, (ii) reducing agents sodium citrate, ascorbate, sodium borohydride ($NaBH_4$), elemental hydrogen, polyol process, Tollens reagent, *N*,*N*-dimethylformamide (DMF), poly(ethyleneglycol)—block co polymer (PLGA-PEG-PLGA), and (iii) stabilizing/capping agents poly(vinyl alcohol) (PVA), poly(vinyl pyrrolidone) (PVP), poly(ethyleneglycol) PEG, poly(methacrylic acid) (PMAA), poly(methyl methacrylate) (PMMA) [31].

The reduction of Ag salts induces the formation of colloidal solutions: this process occurs in two steps (nucleation and growth) that strongly influence the shape and the size of Ag NPs. These two critical steps are controlled by pH, temperature, stabilizing agents and reduction agents [34,35]. Dadosh [36] developed a one-step synthesis of Ag NPs using tannic acid as reducing agent together with sodium citrate. The modification of tannic acid concentrations induced the formation of different sized (from 18 nm to 30 nm) Ag NPs. Based on this procedure, De Matteis et al. [37]

optimized the synthetic route, in terms of $AgNO_3$ concentration and temperature. Zhang et al. [38] used a hyper-branched poly(methylene bisacrylamide aminoethyl piperazine) with terminal dimethylamine groups (HPAMAM-N$(CH_3)_2$) to produce Ag NPs. Wang et al. [39] proposed the generation of Ag NPs using a solution of PVP and $AgNO_3$ with glucose as reducing agent. The solution was completed with NaOH to increase the speed of reaction. The stability of solution took placed when the mole ratio of NaOH and $AgNO_3$ varied between 1.4 and 1.6, without Ag^+. Suriati et al. [40] obtained Ag NPs (35–80 nm) using trisodium citrate and ascorbic acid as surfactants. The increase of ascorbic concentration induced the formation of polygonal NPs with a large size while the size was reduced increasing the trisodium citrate amount, and the shape was quasi-spherical. The use of gallic acid as reducing and stabilizing agent was adopted to obtain 7, 29, and 89 nm of Ag NPs from $AgNO_3$ [41]. The authors used two pH values (11 and 10) to obtain 7 and 29 nm respectively. Also, another method allowed the synthesis of Ag NPs (24 nm) by exploiting hydrazine hydrate and sodium citrate as reducing agents [42] and sodium dodecyl sulphate as stabilizing agent in presence of $AgNO_3$ 8% (*w*/*w*). In other routes, tri-sodium citrate and $NaBH_4$ acted as stabilizer and the reducing agent respectively, in presence of $AgNO_3$ [43,44]. Agnihotri et al. [45] synthetized monodispersed Ag NPs (5, 7, 10, 15, 20, 30, 50, 63, 85, and 100 nm) with a co-reduction employing sodium borohydride ($NaBH_4$) as a primary reductant and trisodium citrate (TSC), as secondary reductant and a stabilizing agent. $NaBH_4$ allowed to form instant nuclei generation, while TSC was important to control the particles size (Figure 1b).

- Microemulsion

Microemulsion method is a reproducible technique that allows the obtaining of uniform size NPs and it is based on the use of three precursors: (i) polar phase that commonly is water, (ii) non-polar phase as hydrocarbon liquid or oil, and (iii) surfactant [46]. The two phases are separated by the presence of surfactant, which forms an interfacial layer, reducing the interfacial tension between the microemulsion, and inhibiting the coalescence of the droplets. This technique (water-in-oil (w/o) or oil-in-water (o/w) depending on the surfactant) allows the obtaining of monodispersed and stable Ag NPs using two microemulsions: one with water core of $AgNO_3$ (as Ag^+ source) and the other water core with hydrazine hydrate (as reducing agent) [47,48]. The reaction starts with the addition of non-toxic dodecane (oil phase) and sodium bis (2-ethylhexyl) sulfosuccinate (AOT, surfactant). Pileni et al. [49] used w/o droplets to tune the size of Ag NPs that were extracted from reverse micelles and mixed in nonpolar solvent. They found that the diameter of NPs changed from 2 nm to 7 nm, after increasing the size of water drops. Chen et al. [50] reduced $AgNO_3$ with AOT, obtaining cubic shaped Ag NPs, with diameters less of 10 nm.

- Sonochemical method

Many NPs of different materials were synthetized by sonochemical method, which have the advantages of eliciting rapidity of reaction time and formation of small NPs. The method includes three steps: formation, growth and implosive collapse of microcavities [51]. Ultrasound waves perturb chemical reactions derived from high temperature (5000 K) and pressure (1000 atm), inducing the collapse of microscopic bubbles (cavities), which expand during the decompression step and implode in the compression phase [52,53]. Gutierrez et al. [54] used this method to produce Ag NPs from a solution of Ag^+ by sonication at 1 MHz under argon-hydrogen atmosphere. Wani and co-workers [55] synthetized Ag NPs using two reducing agents (sodium borohydride and sodium citrate) in two separate reactions irradiated with the same 20 KHz ultrasound waves. Spherical Ag NPs (10 nm) were obtained using $NaBH_4$, while smaller NPs (3 nm) were formed in the presence of sodium citrate.

- Sol-gel

The sol-gel process is a colloidal chemistry technology, which is widely applied to synthetized metal and metal oxide NPs at low temperature. In the first phase, the monomers of materials are converted into a colloidal solution (sol), which represents the precursor (metal alkoxides or chlorides) for gel formation, which in turn formed particles or polymers. To obtain colloids, the precursors are hydrolysed and polycondensed [56].

Zhai et al. [57] used a sol-gel route to synthetize Ag NPs embedding hybrid materials with organicosilica precursors (tetraethoxysilane, mercaptopropyltrimethoxysilane and polymethyl hydrosiloxane) in alcoholic conditions. The three precursors act as framework constructor, a complexing agent toward metal ions and an in situ reducing agent for Ag^+. Lkhagvajav et al. [58] prepared Ag NPs using $AgNO_3$ and glucose as a reducing agent, which were first mixed in distilled water. The formation of NPs was showed when the solution become transparent.

- Electrochemical synthetic method

Electrochemical synthetic method is used to synthetize Ag NPs with a controllable size. In fact, the size can vary by electrolysis parameters modifications, while the monodispersion grade depends on the electrolytic compositions [31]. The detailed protocol of this method was described by Reetz and Helbig [59]. The authors reported Ag NPs synthesis in which a metal sheet was anodically dissolved, thus the formed metal was reduced at the cathode, giving rise to metallic particles stabilized by tetra alkylammonium salts. Ma et al. [60] obtained spherical Ag NPs (10–20 nm) in aqueous solution, choosing PVP to stabilize the Ag clusters and to reduce agglomerations. The application of rotating platinum cathode permitted the obtaining of a high monodispersity route, while the sodium dodecyl benzene sulfonate enhanced particle size distribution. This method was also adopted for the synthesis of the Ag NPs in acetonitrile containing tetrabutylammonium salts [61].

The possibility of obtaining monodisperse NPs with a tunable size is an advantage in the use of chemical methods, together with low cost and rapidity of steps [33]. However, the disadvantages of these methods are the hazardous and toxic elements employed in the synthetic routes and difficulty in purification. Although chemical and physical methods are considered suitable methods to synthetize well-defined nanoparticles, the scientific community is moving towards green synthesis of NPs.

2.3. Green Synthesis

The use of natural products as a source of reagents for NP synthesis is defined as green synthesis [62]. The natural source useful for synthetized Ag NPs can be divided in three categories:

(a) microorganisms (fungi, yeasts, bacteria, and actinomycetes),
(b) plants and plant extract,
(c) membranes, viruses' DNA, and diatoms.

Microorganisms are able to produce metallic NPs by enzymes that contribute to physiological cellular activities. Depending on the NPs localization, the synthesis can take place intracellularly or extracellularly [62]. The intracellular synthesis of Ag NPs are due to the transfer of metal ions into the microorganism, while the extracellular route includes the localization of metal ions onto the cell surface. The enzymes, functional groups, proteins and enzymes are designated to reduce ions [63].

- *Bacteria*

Bacillus licheniformis was used to synthetized 50 nm Ag NPs by Kalimuthu et al. [64] in the presence of an aqueous solution of $AgNO_3$, with enzyme nitrate as a stabilizer. Culture supernatants of *Staphylococcus aureus* as well as supernatants derived from *Enterobacteriaceae* were exploited to synthetize Ag NPs [65]. Many lactic acid bacteria (*Lactobacillus* spp., *Pediococcus pentosaceus* and *Enterococcus faecium*) have the ability to produce glucose, galactose, mannose and fructose, thus they are involved in redox reactions to obtain Ag NPs [66]. Ag NPs with different physico-chemical properties were also synthetized from *Escherichia coli* [67], *Klebsiella pneumonia* [68], *Pseudomonas stutzeri* [69], *Brevibacterium casei* [70], *Bacillus megaterium* [71], *Proteus mirsabilis* [72], *Plectonema boryanum* [73], and *Enterobacter cloacae* [74].

- *Fungi*

Fungi are considered useful tools for Ag NPs synthesis, due to their ability to quickly collect and uptake metals as well as the easy set-up equipment in the laboratory compared to bacteria. The large number of enzymes produced by fungi allow the reduction of $AgNO_3$ solution on their surface [75]. Bhangale et al. [76] used biomass derived from *Aspergillus flavus* for the synthesis of spherical Ag NPs with a size of 7.13 nm. Vigneshwaran and co-workers [77] reported a similar synthesis of NPs with a size of (8.92 ± 1.61) nm. *Penicillium fellutanum* produces the enzyme nitrate reductase in culture filtrate, which was involved in reduction of Ag^+ [78]. At the same time, the fungus *Aspergillus niger* was used to produce Ag NPs extracellularly [79]. In this case, the combination of reductase enzyme and quinine induced a transfer of electrons extracellularly [80]. In some cases, Ag NPs are not obtained in the solution, but on the surface of fungus where Ag+ are confined. This phenomenon is probably induced by the presence of wall proteins with carboxylate groups that have negative charge. In addition, the proteins contributed to the Ag nuclei formation that increase flowing the Ag^+ reduction [81]. Ag NPs are also derived from fungi as *Aspergillus terreus* [82], *Bryophilous rhizoctoni* [83], *Pleurotus ostreatus* [84], *Aspergillus flavus* [77].

- *Plants*

The non-toxic and eco-friendly method of synthetizing NPs is biosynthesis, which includes the reduction of Ag^+ by biomolecules (saponins, proteins, tannins, amino polysaccharides, enzymes, alkaloids, vitamins, etc.) from plant extracts [85]. In general, adding plant extracts to $AgNO_3$ solution induces the reduction of Ag^+, and this phenomenon can be visualized with Ultra-violet Visible (UV-VIS) spectroscopy in time points. Many portions of flora are employed to obtain Ag NPs. Extracts of *Alternanthera dentate* have permitted the rapid obtaining of spherical Ag NPs with a size ranging from 50 nm to 100 nm, with antibacterial activity [86]. Dried roasted *Coffea arabica* seed extract in the presence of $AgNO_3$ induced a reduction of Ag^+ showing a color changing from yellow to dark brown. By this approach, the nano Ag exhibited spherical (20 nm) and ellipsoidal (30 nm) shape [87]. Tribulus terrestris was used to obtain spherical Ag NPs (16–28 nm) due to the mix of extracts and $AgNO_3$. Also, in this case, the NPs have strong antibacterial properties against *Escherichia coli*, *Staphylococcus aureus*, *Pseudomonas aeruginosa* and *Bacillus subtilis* [88]. Krishnaraj et al. synthetized spherical Ag NPs (15–50 nm) from the leaf extract of *Acalypha indica* [89]. Some researchers exploited orange peel (*Citrussinensis*) to obtain nanomaterials derived from food waste. They obtained spherical NPs with an average size of 6 nm [90]. Khalil et al. [91] used olive leaf to reduce $AgNO_3$ in order to obtain Ag NPs. The authors observed a significant synthetic route with the increase of pH and temperature that contributed to spherical Ag NPs with a size of (20–25) nm. A concentration of (0.03–0.07) mg/mL of NPs induced several toxic effects against *Staphylococcus aureus*, *Pseudomonas aeruginosa*, and *Escherichia coli*. In a recent work, Rashid et al. [92] employed *Ferula latisecta* leaf extract and 1 mM-aqueous $AgNO_3$ to obtain Ag NPs with a diameter of about 20 nm (Figure 1c). Green synthesis is a promising route for synthesis of biocompatible and stable nanoparticles that minimizes the waste and energy costs and reduces the toxicity in comparison with physical and chemical methods [93]. Indeed, this method is environmentally friendly, easily scaled up for large-scale syntheses of nanoparticles, and is low cost. In addition, in the synthetic routes do not involve high temperatures, pressures, energy or toxic chemicals [94]. However, some disadvantages should be considered: for example, in the case of plants, they produce low yield of secreted proteins, which decreases the synthetic rate [95], while the manipulation of bacteria presupposes the use of specific set-up that, in many cases, is expensive. Representative Transmission electron microscopy (TEM) images of Ag NPs obtained with different methods were showed in Figure 2a–d.

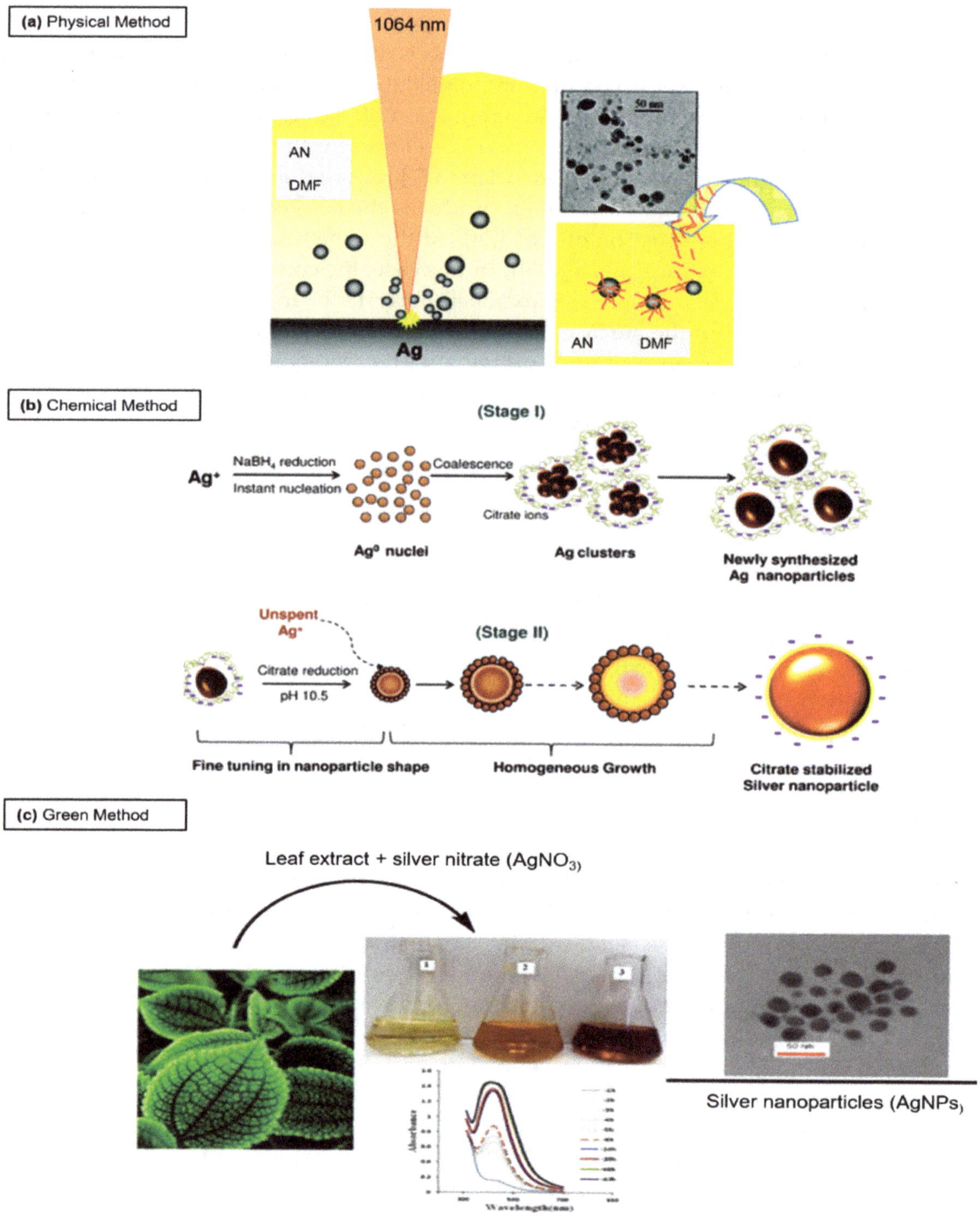

Figure 1. Schematic representation of common routes to synthetize Ag NPs with different approaches: (**a**) physical approach (laser ablation) adapted from [24] with permission from American Chemical Society, Copyright 2007: a laser pulses of 1064 nm focused with a 10 cm focus lens on Ag plate in pure acetonitrile (AN) and *N,N*-dimethylformamide (DMF) was used in order to obtain Ag NPs with a size of 5 nm, (**b**) chemical approach (chemical reduction), adapted from [45] with permission from The Royal Society of Chemistry, 2014: Ag NPs were obtained from a solution of $AgNO_3$ using $NaBH_4$ as a primary reductant and trisodium citrate, both as secondary reductant as well as stabilizing agent, and (**c**) green approach (plant extract) adapted from [92] with permission from The Royal Society of Chemistry, 2016: Ag NPs (20–30 nm) were synthetized by adding *Ferula latisecta* leaves extract to 1 mM aqueous $AgNO_3$ solution. The solution turned from yellow to dark brown.

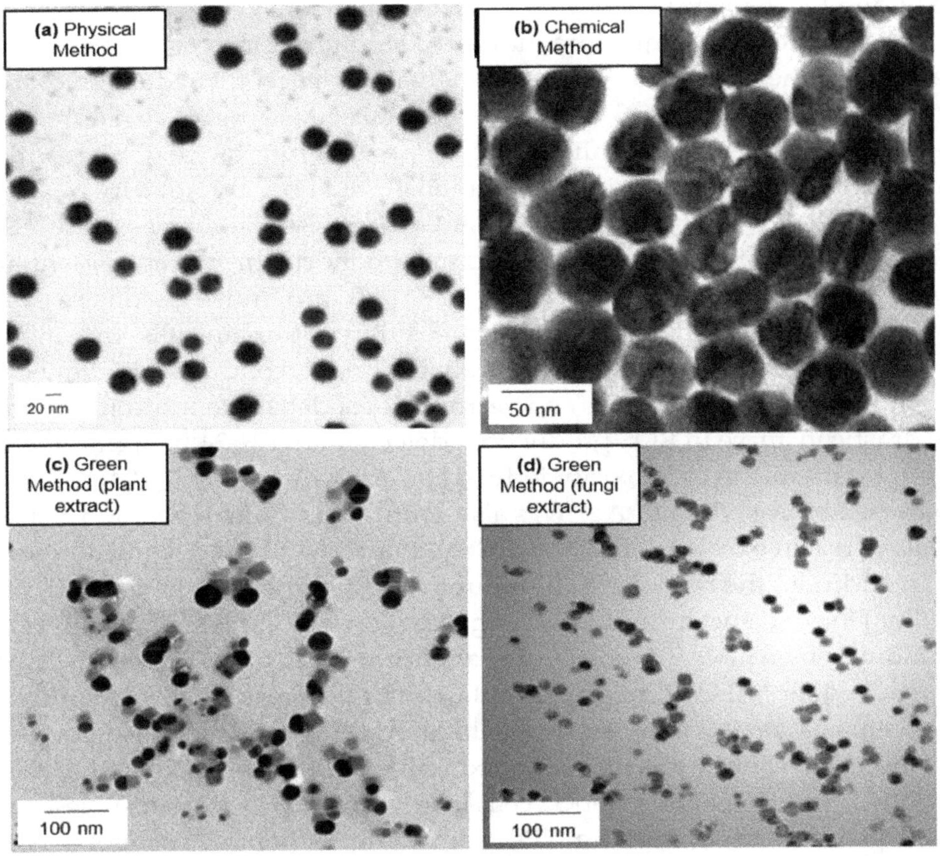

Figure 2. Representative TEM images of Ag NPs synthetized by different synthetic routes: (**a**) Ag NPs (9.4 ± 5.9) nm obtained by 532 nm laser ablation of a Ag rod using 60 mJ/pulse at 1.0×10^{-3} M of CTAB. Adapted/reprinted from [96], Copyright (2002), with permission from Elsevier; (**b**) Ag NPs (130 nm) produced by chemical method with ascorbic acid reduction at pH 10. Adapted/reprinted from [97], Copyright (2010), with permission from Elsevier; (**c**) Ag NPs (from 3 nm to 44 nm) synthesized from fresh *Codium capitatum* extract. Adapted from [98], Creative Commons Attribution License (CC BY) (**d**) Ag NPs (5–25) nm obtained from *Penicillium fellutanum Biourge*. Adapted from [78] with permission of Elsevier, 2009.

3. In Vitro Cytotoxicity Mechanism Induced by Ag NPs

The level of cytotoxicity relating to the rate of internalized NPs was influenced by their size; this evidence was confirmed in the Ag NPs case [99–101]. In particular, Liu and co-workers demonstrated the size-dependent cytotoxicity of Ag NPs (approximately 5, 20 and 50 nm) in terms of cell morphology, cell viability, cellular membrane integrity, oxidative stress and cell cycle progression, in four human cell lines (A549, SGC-7901, HepG2 and MCF-7). The obtained results, with quantified EC50 values, ensured a greater cytotoxic response to the nano Ag size [99]. Furthermore, as obtained by Hsin et al. [100], the decreased viability in NIH_3T_3 mouse fibroblast, A10 rat vascular smooth muscle and HCT116 human colon cancer cells was induced only from Ag particles having a size smaller than a 100 nm. Several studies reported in the literature suggest how the Ag NP toxicity occurs in sequential steps. When the Ag NPs were endocitated, they undergo a degradation process that induce a release of Ag^+ causing Reactive Oxygen Species (ROS) generation and glutathione (SGH) level reduction. The augmentation of cellular superoxide radicals triggers the alterations in the transmembrane potential of mitochondria and influences the signal transduction pathways, which play an important role in apoptosis program activation and cell death [102] (Figure 3a). Carlson et al. evaluated alterations, in terms of mitochondrial and cell membrane viability, in alveolar macrophages cells after 24 h of exposure to Ag NPs (NPs, Ag-15 nm, Ag-30 nm, and Ag-55 nm), quantifying ROS production [103].

In this work, MTT and LDH analysis indicated the size-dependent cytotoxic effects following Ag NPs exposure demonstrating how only Ag-15nm induced a significant increase of ROS level. The authors suggested different hypothesis to justify the experimental evidence: the reduction of the macrophages abilities to protect themselves from ROS caused by the total cell –SH reactive nature, the stronger ROS generation due to the possible unquenching of Ag-15 nm by glutathione (GSH), or the activation of apoptosis pathways. Previously, Hussain et al. demonstrated how cytotoxicity of Ag (15, 100 nm) in BRL 3A rat liver cells is likely to be mediated through oxidative stress: increase in ROS levels is related to a significant depletion of GSH level and reduced mitochondrial membrane potential [101]. In vitro effects provoked by exposure to PVP-coated Ag NPs (~70 nm) and Ag^+ ions released by solution of $AgNO_3$ were evaluated by Foldbjerg et al. on two different human cells line: monocytic cell line (THP-1) and alveolar cell line (A549) [104,105]. Study on THP-1, conducted by flow cytometric assay, showed how the induction of cell apoptosis and necrosis depended on concentration and exposure time. In addition, the drastic increase in ROS production, detected after 6–24 h, highlighted that oxidative stress plays an important role in cytotoxicity induced by Ag NPs and Ag^+ [104]. The dose-dependent cellular toxicity caused by Ag NPs and Ag^+ was also confirmed in A549 cells, and a strictly correlation between the levels of reactive oxygen species (ROS) and mitochondrial dysfunctions or apoptosis was demonstrated. In addition, the role of Ag compounds as ROS-induced genotoxicity was suggested by increased bulky DNA adduct amount after Ag exposure [105]. Hsin et al. [100] showed that the apoptotic effect induced by nano Ag exposure was a mitochondria-dependent mechanism. Specifically, this effect was reported for NIH3T3 mouse fibroblast, A10 rat vascular smooth muscle and HCT116 human colon cancer cells treated with Ag NPs (<100 nm) for 72 h at increasing concentration (from 0.5 ng/mL to 0.5 mg/mL). The key role played by oxidative stress in cytoxicity induced by nano Ag was also demonstrated in human hepatoma HepG2 cells [106]. Kim and co-workers investigated the toxicity events due to 24 h' exposure to Ag^+ and Ag NPs (from ~5 nm to 10 nm). The most cytotoxic effect was shown for free Ag^+ ions in comparison with Ag NPs, as suggested by metal-responsive metallothionein 1b (MT1b) mRNA expression. Nevertheless, intracellular oxidative stress level was increased also following Ag NPs treatment. However, the use of the antioxidant *N*-acetyl-L-cysteine (NAC) prevented Ag toxicity and DNA-damage in HepG2 cells. The authors concluded that the oxidative stress was the first phenomena involved in Ag NPs cytotoxicity and it was independent of Ag+ ions adverse effects. Avalos et al. [107] investigated cytotoxicity induced to Ag NPs, having two different size: 4.7 nm and 42 nm, on normal human dermal fibroblasts. Smaller particles were more toxic than larger ones, as confirmed by MTT and lactate dehydrogenase (LDH) assays. In both case, the preventive addition of NAC strongly reduced the adverse effects of nano Ag exposure. Foldbjerg et al. [108] performed a systematic study by microarray technique on altered A549 cell transcriptome upon 12.1 μg/mL Ag NPs and 1.3 μg/mL Ag+ stimulation at two different time points (24 h and 48 h). They found that Ag NP altered the regulation of more than 1000 genes, whereas Ag+ only 133: different gene members of the metallothionein, heat shock protein, and histone families were upregulated. In addition, Ag+ and Ag NP treatment influenced cell cycle progression and ROS production. The authors concluded by suggesting that the cellular response to Ag^+ was faster but less stable than Ag NP treatment. At the same time, Piao et al. [109] demonstrated that the Ag-induced toxicity in human Chang liver cells was higher after free Ag^+ compared with NPs, having size of ranging from 5 nm to 10 nm. After 24 h of Ag exposure, ROS level increased and concurrently the GSH decreased. This elicited damage against various cellular components, such as DNA breaks, lipid membrane peroxidation, and protein carbonylation. In addition, alteration of mitochondrial membrane potential was detected by cytochrome c release from the mitochondria, resulting in the activation of caspases 9 and 3. Finally, the apoptotic effect was exerted via the activation of c-Jun $NH_{(2)}$-terminal kinase (JNK) causing the formation of apoptotic bodies and DNA fragmentation. The DNA damage, cell cycle arrest and apoptosis events were observed in human Jurkat T cells by Eom et al. [110]. These effects were induced by activation of p38 mitogen-activated protein kinase through nuclear factor-E2-related factor-2 and nuclear factor-κB signaling pathways. Nishanth et al. [111] examined the inflammatory responses of RAW 264.7 mouse macrophages due to exposure at different time points of many kinds of NPs, such as Ag at concentrations of 5 μg/mL, having different size (~15 nm, ~40 nm). This study reveals the high propensity of Ag NPs in inflammation induction, suggested by a significant increase in IL-6, reactive oxygen species (ROS) generation, nuclear translocation of nuclear factor-κB (NF-κB), and tumor necrosis factor-alpha (TNF-α) expression. AshaRani and colleagues [112] explored the potential molecular mechanisms involved in Ag NPs toxicity in normal human lung cells (IMR-90) and human brain cancer cells (U251). In their work, it was demonstrated that nano Ag interacts with cytosolic proteins, which were adsorbed on nanoparticle surfaces, influencing the gene and protein expression profiles. In particular, in the two cell lines, Ag NP exposure provoked downregulation of both cyclin B and cyclin E, which were involved in cell cycle progression, and many DNA damage response/repair factors (XRCC1 and 3, FEN1, RAD51C, RPA1). Moreover, apoptosis pathway was activated by down regulation of p53 and caspase 3 cleavage. Finally, the Ag NPs triggered an inflammatory response through IL-8 and IL-6 cytokines secretions, and macrophages stimulations. Many studies suggest that surface modifications of Ag NPs influenced their interactions with cellular components. Ahamed et al. [113] reported that polysaccharide-coated and -uncoated Ag NPs induced genotoxic effects in two mammalian cell lines: mouse embryonic stem (mES) cells and mouse embryonic fibroblasts (MEF). The different chemical surface functionalization induced a different effect in terms of toxicity: a major damage of DNA was obtained in coated nanoparticles. Even so, the annexin V protein expression and MTT assay showed a decrease of cell viability in both NPs types. Chichova and co-workers [114] analyzed the effects on rat liver mitochondrial oxidative phosphorylation due to exposure to Ag NPs coated with polysaccharide starch (Ag NPs/Starch, Dav = 15.4 $\pm$ 3.9 nm) and trisaccharide raffinose (Ag NPs/Raff, Dav = 24.8 $\pm$ 6.8 nm). Both types of Ag NPs showed decoupling effects on intact mitochondria through the alteration of ATP synthase and ATPase activities, suggesting their ability to cross the inner mitochondrial membrane. De Matteis et al. [37] investigated the mechanism of toxicity induced by citrate-capped Ag NPs with a hydrodynamic diameter of around 20 nm in HeLa and A549 cells at concentrations of 0.06, 0.3 and 0.6 nM after 48 and 96 h. The authors firstly confirmed the negative effects on cell viability, ROS production, apoptotic pathway stimulation and DNA damage and after, they investigated the in situ degradation of Ag NPs using a fluorescent probe. They found an intracellular "heavy metal type" mechanism due to ionization of NPs in Ag^+ in lysosomes and the consecutive release in the cytosol, which explains the stronger toxicity behavior of Ag NPs. In addition, the activation of metallothioneins upon Ag NPs demonstrated a link between ions and cell death (Figure 3b,c).

a.

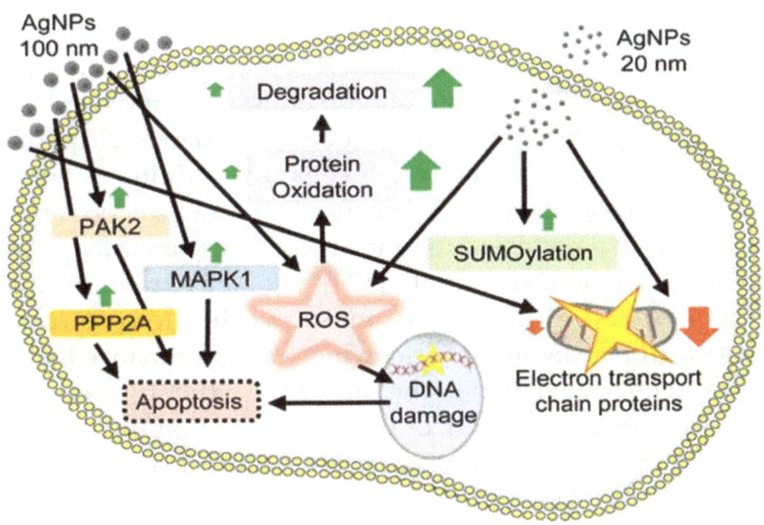

Figure 3. *Cont.*

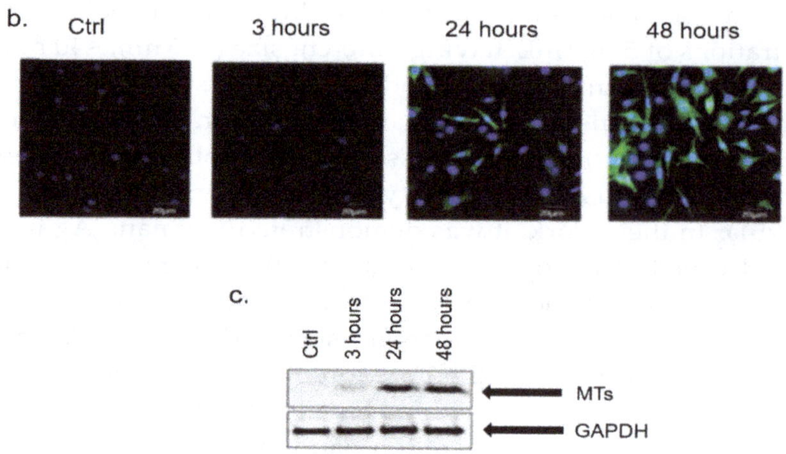

Figure 3. (**a**) Schematic representation mechanism of toxicity induced by AgNPs in cell. Reprinted/adapted with permission from [102], Copyright (2014) American Chemical Society (**b**) Representative images of Hela cell lines exposed to AgNPs at different time points and immunostained to detect metallothionein expression. Nuclei are stained by DAPI staining and metallothioneins with a primary anti-metallothioneins antibody coupled with a FITC-labeled secondary antibody. The expression of metallothioneins in cells is dependent on time. (**c**) Western blot analysis of metallothionein expression in HeLa cells treated with AgNPs. Adapted from [37] with permission from Elsevier, 2015.

4. AgNPs and Theranostics

While the early efforts in nanomedicine were focused on improving the properties of already available therapeutic and diagnostic modalities, more novel strategies have emerged through the supramolecular assembly of simpler components, by means of nanoscale engineering [115,116]. Theranostics is a new technological field which develops molecular diagnostics integrated with targeted therapeutics. It comprises nanosize structures, combining targeting properties, i.e., control of the spatial and temporal release of therapeutic agents, and monitoring modalities for the response to the treatment, and assessing the effectiveness of these agents [116]. Because of its properties, theranostics increases drug efficacy and safety, and therefore it is of great interest in cancer research, becoming one of the key topics in this field [117–120]. Nowadays, much research effort has been made in order to synthetize anticancer drugs and design proper vehicles, guiding them more precisely to tumor cells and away from sites of toxicity, optimizing drug concentration and limiting size-adverse effects [117]. Moreover, an imaging function is often added to delivery vehicles by attaching contrast agents for use in non-invasive methods of imaging, including X-ray-based computer-assisted tomography (CT), positron emission tomography (PET), single photon emission tomography and magnetic resonance imaging (MRI) [121]. With respect to conventional modalities, nanoscale particles and nanovehicles are increasingly being tested for their effects on cancer cells [122]. Multifunctional nanomaterials are used as drug-delivery agents and diagnostic tools, because they offer the possibility to deliver and release drugs, targeting cancer cells in a regulated manner and at the same time allow the detection of cancer cells with enormous specificity and sensitivity [123]. Ag NPs exhibit unique physical and chemical features that make them suitable for cancer theranostic applications. As other metallic NPs, Ag NPs have a larger surface area and area:volume ratio, which in turn enhance their catalytic activity. Owing to their nanosize, they can be vehiculated to the tumor site either by passive targeting (exploiting the enhanced permeability and retention effect), or by active targeting (by means of proper ligand surface functionalization) [124]. Ag NPs are reported to have anticancer property; furthermore, Ag NPs elicit various damaging effects on structures and functions of cells, which finally induce cytotoxicity, genotoxicity, immunological responses, and even cell death. Gonipanath et al. [125] demonstrated the cytotoxic effect of Ag NPs exerted on living cells; in fact, they found that Ag NPs induced apoptosis on cancerous HT29 as well as non-cancerous BHK21 cells. Interestingly, they observed a synergistic effect on apoptosis using uracil phosphoribosyltransferase (UPRT)-expressing cells and non-UPRT expressing cells in the presence of the drug fluorouracil (5-FU), suggesting that Ag NPs, combined with traditional cancer treatment modalities, enhanced their performance. By means of biotechnology and nanotechnology, nanomaterials could be properly bioconjugated, exhibiting new features in tumor treatment [126,127]. Proper functionalized nanomaterials could affect cell growth and viability based on the size, capping or coating materials, color, surface chemistry, and dose [128]. Starting from these observations, Ag NPs were often used in combination with polymers for the delivery to cancer cells. Sanpui et al. reported the synthesis of a chitosan (CS) nanocarrier (NC)-based delivery of Ag NPs able to induce apoptosis at very low concentrations of the NPs in human colon cancer cells (HT 29) [129]. They demonstrated that Ag CS NCs induced the production of intracellular ROS also at low concentration, compared to the use of free Ag NPs.

Other experimental research has proved the synergistic effect of Ag NPs and polymers concerning cancer treatment. For example, PVP-coated Ag NPs inhibited the growth of acute myeloid leukemia (AML), inducing a cytotoxic effect due to the production of reactive oxygen species (ROS), losses of mitochondrial membrane potential and DNA damage [130]. The same molecular mechanisms were reported for starch-coated Ag NPs, which were studied in normal human lung fibroblast cells (IMR-90), and human glioblastoma cells (U251) showing anticancer properties [131]. In a recent study, Liang et al., investigated the effect of Ag NPs on human glioma U251 cells and its role in the combinational use with Temozolomide (TMZ), an imidazotetrazine derivative of the alkylating agent dacarbazine, against glioma cells. They found that Ag NPs could have a potential application in enhancing chemotherapy for glioma. In fact, Ag NPs showed dose-dependent cytotoxicity on U251 cells owing to their ability to enhance the drug-sensitivity of TMZ on U251 cells [132]. Protein-conjugated Ag sulfide nano-particles, nano-rods and nano-wires were reported to inhibit the C6 glioma cells and human hepatocellular carcinoma Bel-7402 cells significantly; moreover, the effect of nano-crystals on tumor cells was crystal size-dependent [128]. Among the modalities used for reached tumor sites, targeted therapy has recently become the most attractive strategy for cancer treatment. Locatelli et al. synthetized multifunctional nanocomposites consisting of polymeric nanoparticles (PNPs) containing two cytotoxic agents (the drug alisertib and Ag NPs), conjugated with a chlorotoxin, an active targeting 36-amino acid-long peptide that specifically binds to MMP-2, a receptor overexpressed by brain cancer cells. They demonstrated the strong toxicity ability of these composite nanostructures in a human glioblastoma-astrocytoma epithelial-like cell line (U87MG) [133]. Not only chemistry synthetized Ag NPs elicited cytotoxic effects on cancer cells, but also biologically derived Ag NPs showed anticancer properties [134]. In fact, the anticancer property of bacterial (B-Ag NPs) and fungal extract-produced Ag NPs (F-Ag NPs) was demonstrated in human breast cancer MDA-MB-231 and MCF-7 cells [135–137]. Plant extract-mediated synthesis of Ag NPs exhibited more pronounced toxic effects in human lung carcinoma cells (A549) compared to non-cancer cells such as human lung cells, indicating that Ag NPs could target cell-specific toxicity. This mechanism could be due to the typical acidic pH value in cancer cells [138]. The interesting ability of Ag NPs to selectively affect cell viability was also confirmed by other experimental evidenc. Zureberek et al. [139] investigated the role of respiration in Ag NP-induced oxidative stress. Considering that cancer cells rely on glucose as the main source of energy supply, the authors demonstrated that glucose availability was strictly related to NP toxicity. They found that Ag NPs induced dose-dependent generation of H_2O_2. In addition, Ag NP toxicity for the cells maintained in the low-glucose medium was significantly lower compared to cells growing in the high-glucose concentration. This result indicated that scarceness of glucose supply resulted in upregulation of the endogenous antioxidant defense mechanisms, which in turn affected ROS generation and toxicity induced by Ag NPs. Moreover, because hydrogen peroxide is continuously formed at micromolar levels and participates in redox homeostasis [140], He and co-workers [141] studied the interaction between H_2O_2 and Ag NPs, examining the effects of Ag NPs upon generation of ROS and oxygen over a physiologically relevant pH range. Their results demonstrated the alteration of the balance between hydroxyl radicals, oxygen and hydrogen peroxide influenced the effects of Ag NPs. In addition, Ag NPs [142] are known to strongly interact with electromagnetic radiation (i.e., photons) [143,144] resulting in a localized surface plasmonic resonance (LSPR) [145,146] (Figure 4a). The local electric fields generated on the NP surfaces are the product of enhanced light-matter interaction, occurring only at specific resonant frequencies [147,148]. The elevated fields raise a high number of electron–hole pairs, which in turn can induce photochemical transformations [149]. However, the plasmonic resonance of conventionally spherical Ag NPs is restricted only in the visible range of the spectrum (400–550 nm) [150], and its employment in biological tissues is thus rather limited because of the high tissue-mediated visible light absorption [151]. Ag exhibits the highest efficiency of plasmonic excitation among the three metals displaying plasmonic resonance (Ag, Au, and Cu) [152]. In addition, the plasmonic peak can be tuned, varying the shape and sizes of Ag-based nanomaterials (Figure 4b).

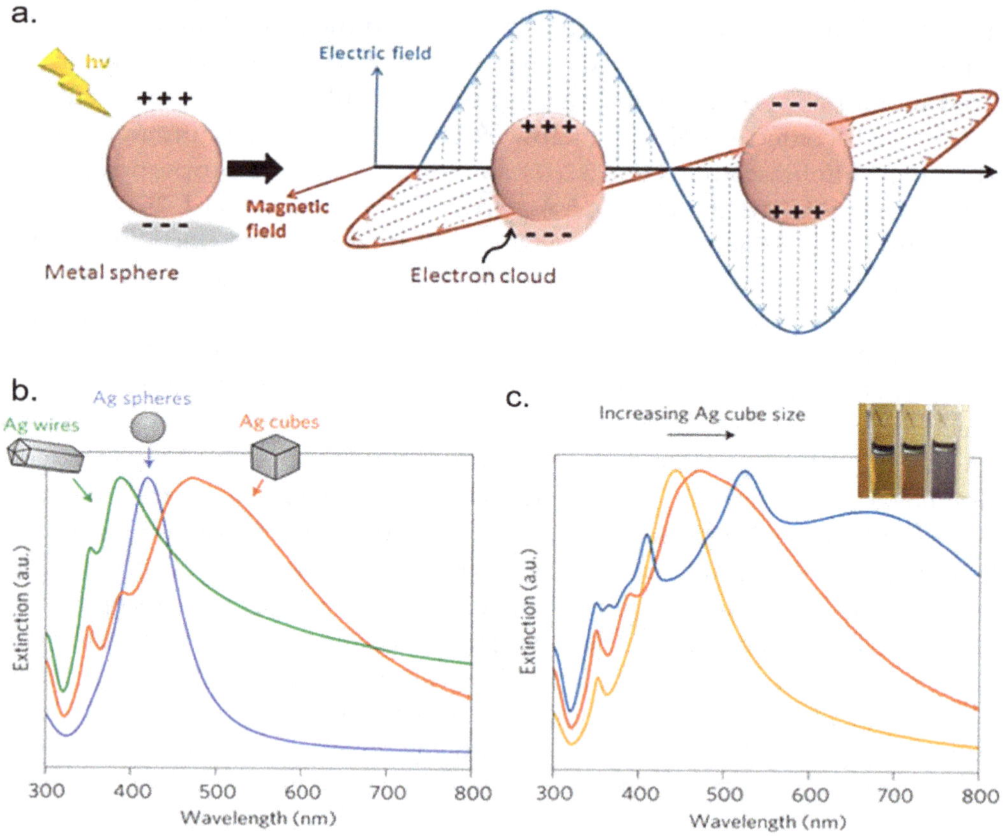

Figure 4. (**a**) Schematic representation of a localized surface plasmon resonance (LSPR), reproduced from [153] with permission of The Royal Society of Chemistry. (**b**,**c**) The change of shape and size exhibited different extinction properties. Adapted from [154] with permission from Macmillan Publishers (Nature Materials), 2015.

Mukherjee et al. developed green synthesized Ag NPs with multifunctional activities, using *Olaz scandens* leaf extracts. Ag NPs exhibited anticancer activity against different cancer cells (A549: human lung cancer cell lines, B16: mouse melanoma cell line and MCF7: human breast cancer cells). In addition to that, they were biocompatible to rat cardiomyoblast normal cell line (H9C2), human umbilical vein endothelial cells (HUVEC) and Chinese hamster ovary cells (CHO). At the same time, Ag NPs showed bright red fluorescence, which could be used to detect the localization of drug molecules inside cancer cells. For these reasons, Ag NPs could act not only as anticancer drugs but also as drug delivery vehicle and imaging facilitator [155]. Farrag et al. [156] functionalized Ag NPs with PVP and antitumoral drug Doxorubicin (DOX) to quickly track by ^{125}I isotope their localization in the tumor site. They showed the double use of this Ag vector, which is both diagnostic and therapeutic (Figure 5a). In another study, Boca-Farcau et al. [157] developed newly synthesized chitosan-coated Ag nanotriangles (Chit-Ag NTs) with strong resonances in near infrared (NIR), investigating their ability to operate as photothermal agents against a line of human non-small lung cancer cells (NCI-H460). By the hyperthermia experiments, they found that the rate of cell mortality in the presence of Chit-AgNTs was higher than in the presence of thiolated poly(ethylene) glycol capped gold nanorods (PEG-AuNRs) (a common hyperthermia agent used as reference). No destructive effects were detected on the control sample (cells without nanoparticles) under identical irradiation conditions. Kovács et al. [158] synthetized Ag NPs (5 and 35 nm) to test their ability to kill tumor suppressor-deficient osteosarcoma cancer cells. They found that NPs induced apoptosis in wild-type p53-containing U2Os and p53-deficient Saos-2 cells demonstrating the potential novel chemotherapeutic approaches based on Ag NPs (Figure 5b). Schrand et al. examined the chemical and biological properties of Ag NPs of similar sizes, differing in their surface chemistry (hydrocarbon versus polysaccharide), for their potential use as biological labels in neuroblastoma cells. We observed strong optical labelling of the cells in high-illumination light microscopy. Ag NPs were able to bind to plasma membrane and be uptaken and localized into intracellular vacuoles, suggesting that they could be involved in a cell labelling procedure. The major drawbacks of this approach relied on the induction of ROS, the degradation of mitochondrial membrane integrity, and the disruption of the actin cytoskeleton system after 24 h of Ag NPs exposure [159]. The large use of Ag NPs for cancer diagnosis and treatment raises concerns over their potential short- and long-term toxicity, above all in view of the application into clinical practice. Nevertheless, information about the mechanism of cytotoxicity derived mainly from in vitro studies and the impact of Ag NPs on animal models is still unclear. As reviewed elsewhere, Ag NPs elicited many toxicological responses (including effects on circulatory, respiratory, central nervous and hepatic systems) in laboratory rodents exposed to Ag NPs [160]. Results showed that the cytotoxic and genotoxic effect of Ag NPs was strictly linked to their concentration, size, surface-coating, exposure time and environmental factors [161]. Adult male C57BL/6N mice exposed to Ag NPs exhibited oxidative stress-induced neurotoxicity in brain regions [162] and other experimental evidence reported that liver and bile ducts are accumulation sites for Ag NPs [163]. Another study in zebrafish embryos suggested that the toxicity of Ag NPs was associated with bioavailable Ag^+ [164]. More recently, Munger et al. orally administered Ag NPs in healthy volunteers and they evaluated human biodistribution, bioprocessing and possible toxicity of Ag NPs. They demonstrated that in vivo oral exposure to Ag NPs solutions did not produce clinically severe changes in human metabolic, hematologic, urine, physical findings or imaging morphology [165]. This work opened a new scenario for the use of Ag NPs in cancer theranostics in the near future.

a.

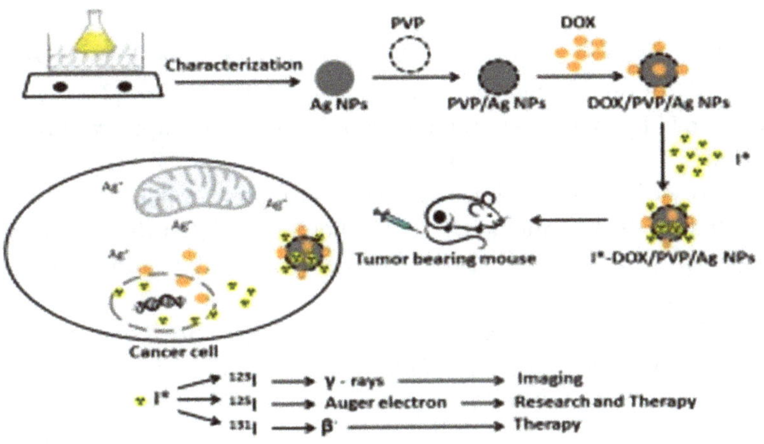

Figure 5. *Cont.*

b.

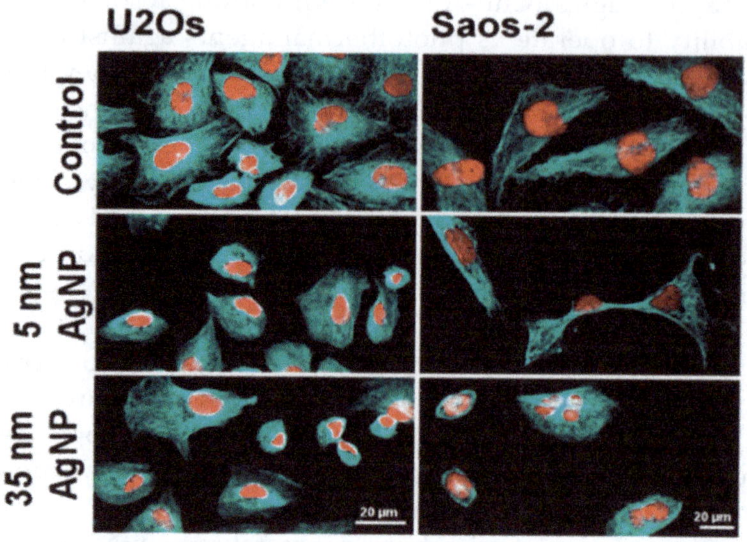

Figure 5. (**a**) AgNPs with PVP coating and Doxorubicin (DOX) loaded polymeric NPs (DOX/PVP/Ag NPs) AND iodine-125 isotope to tracking in vivo the NPs after intravenously injection in normal and solid tumor bearing mice. NPs specifically targeted tumor site for a long period of time making Ag-based NPs as tumor-specific agents for both diagnostic and therapeutic applications. Reprinted from Publication [156] with permission from Elsevier, 2017. (**b**) Confocal images showed the effect of AgNPs on tubulin by apoptotic events induction in U2Os and Saos-2 cells. Adapted from [158] with permission of Springer Nature, 2016.

5. Conclusions

In this work, we have first studied the main methods (physical, chemical and green) to synthetize Ag NPs by using bottom-up and top-down approaches. These methods are aimed at obtaining Ag NPs in a reproducible manner and with specific physico-chemical properties, suitable for various applications. We also analyzed the most recent literature concerning the toxicity mechanisms at the cellular level of Ag NPs, which makes it useful as an anti-cancer tool, combining a good intracellular and intra-tissue tracking with a therapeutic effect. Future challenges are finalized to develop Ag-based anti-tumor nanomaterials for personalized medicine treatment.

References

1. Beyene, H.D.; Werkneh, A.A.; Bezabh, H.K.; Ambaye, T.G. Synthesis paradigm and applications of silver nanoparticles (Ag NPs), a review. *Sustain. Mater. Technol.* **2017**, *13*, 18–23.
2. Chen, X.; Schluesener, H.J. Nanosilver: A nanoproduct in medical application. *Toxicol. Lett.* **2008**, *176*, 1–12. [CrossRef] [PubMed]
3. Alexander, J.W. History of the medical use of silver. *Surg. Infect.* **2009**, *10*, 289–292. [CrossRef] [PubMed]
4. Bhattacharya, S.; Zhang, Q.; Carmichael, P.L.; Boekelheide, K.; Andersen, M.E. Toxicity testing in the 21 century: Defining new risk assessment approaches based on perturbation of intracellular toxicity pathways. *PLoS ONE* **2011**, *6*, e20887. [CrossRef] [PubMed]
5. Jo, D.H.; Kim, J.H.; Lee, T.G.; Kim, J.H. Size, surface charge, and shape determine therapeutic effects of nanoparticles on brain and retinal diseases. *Nanomed. Nanotechnol. Biol. Med.* **2015**, *11*, 1603–1611. [CrossRef] [PubMed]
6. Rai, M.; Kon, K.; Ingle, A.; Duran, N.; Galdiero, S.; Galdiero, M. Broad-spectrum bioactivities of silver nanoparticles: The emerging trends and future prospects. *Appl. Microbiol. Biotechnol.* **2014**, *98*, 1951–1961. [CrossRef] [PubMed]

7. Jurj, A.; Braicu, C.; Pop, L.A.; Tomuleasa, C.; Gherman, C.D.; Berindan-Neagoe, I. The new *era* of nanotechnology, an alternative to change cancer treatment. *Drug Des. Dev. Ther.* **2017**, *11*, 2871–2890. [CrossRef] [PubMed]
8. Riehemann, K.; Schneider, S.W.; Luger, T.A.; Godin, B.; Ferrari, M.; Fuchs, H. Nanomedicine–challenge and perspectives. *Angew. Chem.* **2009**, *48*, 872–897. [CrossRef] [PubMed]
9. Huang, Y.; Fan, C.Q.; Dong, H.; Wang, S.M.; Yang, X.C.; Yang, S.M. Current applications and future prospects of nanomaterials in tumor therapy. *Int. J. Nanomed.* **2017**, *12*, 1815–1825. [CrossRef] [PubMed]
10. Conde, J.; Doria, G.; Baptista, P. Noble metal nanoparticles applications in cancer. *J. Drug Deliv.* **2012**, *2012*, 751075. [CrossRef] [PubMed]
11. Bhattacharyya, S.; Kudgus, R.A.; Bhattacharya, R.; Mukherjee, P. Inorganic nanoparticles in cancer therapy. *Pharm. Res.* **2011**, *28*, 237–259. [CrossRef] [PubMed]
12. Sau, T.K.; Rogach, A.L.; Jackel, F.; Klar, T.A.; Feldmann, J. Properties and applications of colloidal nonspherical noble metal nanoparticles. *Adv. Mater.* **2010**, *22*, 1805–1825. [CrossRef] [PubMed]
13. Lee, K.S.; El-Sayed, M.A. Gold and silver nanoparticles in sensing and imaging: Sensitivity of plasmon response to size, shape, and metal composition. *J. Phys. Chem. B* **2006**, *110*, 19220–19225. [CrossRef] [PubMed]
14. Sperling, R.A.; Parak, W.J. Surface modification, functionalization and bioconjugation of colloidal inorganic nanoparticles. *Philos. Trans. Ser. A Math. Phys. Eng. Sci.* **2010**, *368*, 1333–1383. [CrossRef] [PubMed]
15. Pelaz, B.; del Pino, P.; Maffre, P.; Hartmann, R.; Gallego, M.; Rivera-Fernandez, S.; de la Fuente, J.M.; Nienhaus, G.U.; Parak, W.J. Surface functionalization of nanoparticles with polyethylene glycol: Effects on protein adsorption and cellular uptake. *ACS Nano* **2015**, *9*, 6996–7008. [CrossRef] [PubMed]
16. Nishiyama, N. Nanomedicine: Nanocarriers shape up for long life. *Nat. Nanotechnol.* **2007**, *2*, 203–204. [CrossRef] [PubMed]
17. Day, E.S.; Morton, J.G.; West, J.L. Nanoparticles for thermal cancer therapy. *J. Biomech. Eng.* **2009**, *131*, 074001. [CrossRef] [PubMed]
18. De Matteis, V.; Rinaldi, R. Toxicity assessment in the nanoparticle *era*. *Adv. Exp. Med. Biol.* **2018**, *1048*, 1–19. [PubMed]
19. Iravani, S.; Korbekandi, H.; Mirmohammadi, S.V.; Zolfaghari, B. Synthesis of silver nanoparticles: Chemical, physical and biological methods. *Res. Pharm. Sci.* **2014**, *9*, 385–406. [PubMed]
20. Gurav, A.S.; Kodas, T.T.; Wang, L.-M.; Kauppinen, E.I.; Joutsensaari, J. Generation of nanometer-size fullerene particles via vapor condensation. *Chem. Phys. Lett.* **1994**, *218*, 304–308. [CrossRef]
21. Kim, M.; Osone, S.; Kim, T.; Higashi, H.; Seto, T. Synthesis of nanoparticles by laser ablation: A review. *KONA Powder Part. J* **2017**, 80–90. [CrossRef]
22. Pyatenko, A.; Shimokawa, K.; Yamaguchi, M.; Nishimura, O.; Suzuki, M. Synthesis of silver nanoparticles by laser ablation in pure water. *Appl. Phys. A* **2004**, *79*, 803–806. [CrossRef]
23. Tsuji, T.; Iryo, K.; Watanabe, N.; Tsuji, M. Preparation of silver nanoparticles by laser ablation in solution: Influence of laser wavelength on particle size. *Appl. Surf. Sci.* **2002**, *202*, 80–85. [CrossRef]
24. Amendola, V.; Polizzi, S.; Meneghetti, M. Free silver nanoparticles synthesized by laser ablation in organic solvents and their easy functionalization. *Langmuir ACS J. Surf. Colloids* **2007**, *23*, 6766–6770. [CrossRef] [PubMed]
25. Balboul, B.A. Thermal decomposition study of erbium oxalate hexahydrate. *Thermochim. Acta* **2000**, *351*, 55–60. [CrossRef]
26. Lee, D.K.; Kang, Y.S. Preparation and characterization of magnetic nanoparticles by γ-irradiation. *Mater. Sci. Eng. C* **2004**, *24*, 107–111. [CrossRef]
27. Navaladian, S.; Viswanathan, B.; Viswanath, R.; Varadarajan, T. Thermal decomposition as route for silver nanoparticles. *Nanoscale Res. Lett.* **2006**, *2*, 44–48. [CrossRef] [PubMed]
28. Pluym, T.; Powell, Q.; Gurav, A.; Ward, T.; Kodas, T.; Wang, L.; Glicksman, H. Solid silver particle production by spray pyrolysis. *J. Aerosol Sci.* **1993**, *24*, 383–392. [CrossRef]
29. Pingali, K.C.; Rockstraw, D.A.; Deng, S. Silver nanoparticles from ultrasonic spray pyrolysis of aqueous silver nitrate. *Aerosol Sci. Technol.* **2005**, *39*, 1010–1014. [CrossRef]
30. Sharma, R.; Sharma, A.K.; Sharma, V. Synthesis of carbon nanotubes by Arc discharge and chemical vapor deposition method with analysis of its morphology, dispersion and functionalization characteristics. *Cogent Eng.* **2015**, *2*, 1094017. [CrossRef]

31. Tien, D.-C.; Tseng, K.-H.; Liao, C.-Y.; Huang, J.-C.; Tsung, T.-T. Discovery of ionic silver in silver nanoparticle suspension fabricated by Arc discharge method. *J. Alloys Compd.* **2008**, *463*, 408–411. [CrossRef]
32. Siegel, J.; Kvítek, O.; Ulbrich, P.; Kolská, Z.; Slepička, P.; Švorčík, V. Progressive approach for metal nanoparticle synthesis. *Mater. Lett.* **2012**, *89*, 47–50. [CrossRef]
33. Zhang, X.-F.; Liu, Z.-G.; Shen, W.; Gurunathan, S. Silver nanoparticles: Synthesis, characterization, properties, applications, and therapeutic approaches. *Int. J. Mol. Sci.* **2016**, *17*, 1534. [CrossRef] [PubMed]
34. Chen, S.-F.; Zhang, H. Aggregation kinetics of nanosilver in different water conditions. *Adv. Nat. Sci. Nanosci. Nanotechnol.* **2012**, *3*, 035006. [CrossRef]
35. Dang, T.M.D.; Le, T.T.T.; Fribourg-Blanc, E.; Dang, M.C. Influence of surfactant on the preparation of silver nanoparticles by polyol method. *Adv. Nat. Sci. Nanosci. Nanotechnol.* **2012**, *3*, 035004. [CrossRef]
36. Dadosh, T.; Sperling, J.; Bryant, G.W.; Breslow, R.; Shegai, T.; Dyshel, M.; Haran, G.; Bar-Joseph, I. Plasmonic control of the shape of the raman spectrum of a single molecule in a silver nanoparticle dimer. *ACS Nano* **2009**, *3*, 1988–1994. [CrossRef] [PubMed]
37. De Matteis, V.; Malvindi, M.A.; Galeone, A.; Brunetti, V.; De Luca, E.; Kote, S.; Kshirsagar, P.; Sabella, S.; Bardi, G.; Pompa, P.P. Negligible particle-specific toxicity mechanism of silver nanoparticles: The role of Ag^+ ion release in the cytosol. *Nanomedicine Nanotechnol. Biol. Med.* **2015**, *11*, 731–739. [CrossRef] [PubMed]
38. Zhang, Y.; Peng, H.; Huang, W.; Zhou, Y.; Yan, D. Facile preparation and characterization of highly antimicrobial colloid Ag or Au nanoparticles. *J. Colloid Interface Sci.* **2008**, *325*, 371–376. [CrossRef] [PubMed]
39. Wang, H.; Qiao, X.; Chen, J.; Ding, S. Preparation of silver nanoparticles by chemical reduction method. *Colloids Surf. A Physicochem. Eng. Asp.* **2005**, *256*, 111–115. [CrossRef]
40. Suriati, G.; Mariatti, M.; Azizan, A. Synthesis of silver nanoparticles by chemical reduction method: Effect of reducing agent and surfactant concentration. *Int. J. Autom. Mech. Eng.* **2014**, *10*, 1920. [CrossRef]
41. Martinez-Castanon, G.; Nino-Martinez, N.; Martinez-Gutierrez, F.; Martinez-Mendoza, J.; Ruiz, F. Synthesis and antibacterial activity of silver nanoparticles with different sizes. *J. Nanopart. Res.* **2008**, *10*, 1343–1348. [CrossRef]
42. Guzmán, M.G.; Dille, J.; Godet, S. Synthesis of silver nanoparticles by chemical reduction method and their antibacterial activity. *Int. J. Chem. Biomol. Eng.* **2009**, *2*, 104–111.
43. Pinto, V.V.; Ferreira, M.J.; Silva, R.; Santos, H.A.; Silva, F.; Pereira, C.M. Long time effect on the stability of silver nanoparticles in aqueous medium: Effect of the synthesis and storage conditions. *Colloids Surf. A Physicochem. Eng. Asp.* **2010**, *364*, 19–25. [CrossRef]
44. Jana, N.R.; Gearheart, L.; Murphy, C.J. Wet chemical synthesis of high aspect ratio cylindrical gold nanorods. *J. Phys. Chem. B* **2001**, *105*, 4065–4067. [CrossRef]
45. Agnihotri, S.; Mukherji, S.; Mukherji, S. Size-controlled silver nanoparticles synthesized over the range 5–100 nm using the same protocol and their antibacterial efficacy. *RSC Adv.* **2014**, *4*, 3974–3983. [CrossRef]
46. Dhand, C.; Dwivedi, N.; Loh, X.J.; Ying, A.N.J.; Verma, N.K.; Beuerman, R.W.; Lakshminarayanan, R.; Ramakrishna, S. Methods and strategies for the synthesis of diverse nanoparticles and their applications: A comprehensive overview. *RSC Adv.* **2015**, *5*, 105003–105037. [CrossRef]
47. Solanki, J.N.; Murthy, Z.V.P. Controlled size silver nanoparticles synthesis with water-in-oil microemulsion method: A topical review. *Ind. Eng. Chem. Res.* **2011**, *50*, 12311–12323. [CrossRef]
48. Zhang, W.; Qiao, X.; Chen, J. Synthesis of nanosilver colloidal particles in water/oil microemulsion. *Colloids Surf. A Physicochem. Eng. Asp.* **2007**, *299*, 22–28. [CrossRef]
49. Pileni, M.; Taleb, A.; Petit, C. Silver metal nanosized particles: Control of particle size, self assemblies in 2d and 3d superlattices and optical properties. *J. Dispers. Sci. Technol.* **1998**, *19*, 185–206. [CrossRef]
50. Chen, D.-H.; Wu, S.-H. Synthesis of nickel nanoparticles in water-in-oil microemulsions. *Chem. Mater.* **2000**, *12*, 1354–1360. [CrossRef]
51. Zhanjiang, Z.; Jinpei, L. Synthesis and characterization of silver nanoparticles by a sonochemical method. *Rare Met. Mater. Eng.* **2012**, *41*, 1700–1705. [CrossRef]
52. Okitsu, K.; Yue, A.; Tanabe, S.; Matsumoto, H.; Yobiko, Y. Formation of colloidal gold nanoparticles in an ultrasonic field: Control of rate of gold (iii) reduction and size of formed gold particles. *Langmuir ACS J. Surf. Colloids* **2001**, *17*, 7717–7720. [CrossRef]
53. Zhu, J.; Palchik, O.; Chen, S.; Gedanken, A. Microwave assisted preparation of CdSe, PbSe, and $Cu_{2-x}Se$ nanoparticles. *J. Phys. Chem. B* **2000**, *104*, 7344–7347. [CrossRef]

54. Gutierrez, M.; Henglein, A.; Dohrmann, J.K. Hydrogen atom reactions in the sonolysis of aqueous solutions. *J. Phys. Chem.* **1987**, *91*, 6687–6690. [CrossRef]

55. Wani, I.A.; Ganguly, A.; Ahmed, J.; Ahmad, T. Silver nanoparticles: Ultrasonic wave assisted synthesis, optical characterization and surface area studies. *Mater. Lett.* **2011**, *65*, 520–522. [CrossRef]

56. Brinker, C.J.; Scherer, G.W. *Sol-Gel Science: The Physics and Chemistry of Sol-Gel Processing*; Academic Press: New York, NY, USA, 2013.

57. Zhai, S.-R.; Shao, X.; Zhou, D.; Zhai, B.; An, Q.-D. Sol-gel synthesis of nanosilver embedded hybrid materials using combined organosilica precursors. *J. Sol-Gel Sci. Technol.* **2012**, *62*, 281–286. [CrossRef]

58. Lkhagvajav, N.; Yasa, I.; Celik, E.; Koizhaiganova, M.; Sari, O. Antimicrobial activity of colloidal silver nanoparticles prepared by sol-gel method. *Dig. J. Nanomater. Biostruct.* **2011**, *6*, 149–154.

59. Reetz, M.T.; Helbig, W. Size-selective synthesis of nanostructured transition metal clusters. *J. Am. Chem. Soc.* **1994**, *116*, 7401–7402. [CrossRef]

60. Ma, H.; Yin, B.; Wang, S.; Jiao, Y.; Pan, W.; Huang, S.; Chen, S.; Meng, F. Synthesis of silver and gold nanoparticles by a novel electrochemical method. *ChemPhysChem* **2004**, *5*, 68–75. [CrossRef] [PubMed]

61. Rodriguez-Sanchez, L.; Blanco, M.; Lopez-Quintela, M. Electrochemical synthesis of silver nanoparticles. *J. Phys. Chem. B* **2000**, *104*, 9683–9688. [CrossRef]

62. Rafique, M.; Sadaf, I.; Rafique, M.S.; Tahir, M.B. A review on green synthesis of silver nanoparticles and their applications. *Artif. Cells Nanomed. Biotechnol.* **2017**, *45*, 1272–1291. [CrossRef] [PubMed]

63. Zhang, X.; Yan, S.; Tyagi, R.; Surampalli, R. Synthesis of nanoparticles by microorganisms and their application in enhancing microbiological reaction rates. *Chemosphere* **2011**, *82*, 489–494. [CrossRef] [PubMed]

64. Kalimuthu, K.; Babu, R.S.; Venkataraman, D.; Bilal, M.; Gurunathan, S. Biosynthesis of silver nanocrystals by bacillus licheniformis. *Colloids Surf. B Biointerfaces* **2008**, *65*, 150–153. [CrossRef] [PubMed]

65. Nanda, A.; Saravanan, M. Biosynthesis of silver nanoparticles from staphylococcus aureus and its antimicrobial activity against mrsa and mrse. *Nanomed. Nanotechnol. Biol. Med.* **2009**, *5*, 452–456. [CrossRef] [PubMed]

66. Saravanan, C.; Rajesh, R.; Kaviarasan, T.; Muthukumar, K.; Kavitake, D.; Shetty, P.H. Synthesis of silver nanoparticles using bacterial exopolysaccharide and its application for degradation of azo-dyes. *Biotechnol. Rep.* **2017**, *15*, 33–40. [CrossRef] [PubMed]

67. El-Shanshoury, A.E.-R.R.; ElSilk, S.E.; Ebeid, M.E. Extracellular biosynthesis of silver nanoparticles using escherichia coli ATCC 8739, bacillus subtilis atcc 6633, and streptococcus thermophilus esh1 and their antimicrobial activities. *ISRN Nanotechnol.* **2011**, *2011*, 385480. [CrossRef]

68. Mokhtari, N.; Daneshpajouh, S.; Seyedbagheri, S.; Atashdehghan, R.; Abdi, K.; Sarkar, S.; Minaian, S.; Shahverdi, H.R.; Shahverdi, A.R. Biological synthesis of very small silver nanoparticles by culture supernatant of klebsiella pneumonia: The effects of visible-light irradiation and the liquid mixing process. *Mater. Res. Bull.* **2009**, *44*, 1415–1421. [CrossRef]

69. Klaus, T.; Joerger, R.; Olsson, E.; Granqvist, C.-G. Silver-based crystalline nanoparticles, microbially fabricated. *Proc. Natl. Acad. Sci. USA* **1999**, *96*, 13611–13614. [CrossRef] [PubMed]

70. Kalishwaralal, K.; Deepak, V.; Pandian, S.R.K.; Kottaisamy, M.; BarathManiKanth, S.; Kartikeyan, B.; Gurunathan, S. Biosynthesis of silver and gold nanoparticles using brevibacterium casei. *Colloids Surf. B Biointerfaces* **2010**, *77*, 257–262. [CrossRef] [PubMed]

71. Fu, J.-K.; Zhang, W.; Liu, Y.-Y.; Lin, Z.-Y.; Yao, B.-X.; Weng, S.-Z.; Zeng, J.-L. Characterization of adsorption and reduction of noble metal ions by bacteria. *Chem. J. Chin. Univ.* **1999**, *20*, 1452–1454.

72. Samadi, N.; Golkaran, D.; Eslamifar, A.; Jamalifar, H.; Fazeli, M.R.; Mohseni, F.A. Intra/extracellular biosynthesis of silver nanoparticles by an autochthonous strain of proteus mirabilis isolated fromphotographic waste. *J. Biomed. Nanotechnol.* **2009**, *5*, 247–253. [CrossRef] [PubMed]

73. Lengke, M.F.; Fleet, M.E.; Southam, G. Biosynthesis of silver nanoparticles by filamentous cyanobacteria from a silver (i) nitrate complex. *Langmuir ACS J. Surf. Colloids* **2007**, *23*, 2694–2699. [CrossRef] [PubMed]

74. Minaeian, S.; Shahverdi, A.; Nouhi, A.A.; Shahverdi, H.R. Extracellular biosynthesis of silver nanoparticles by somebacteria. *J. Sci. I. U. A. (JSIAU)* **2008**, *17*, 66.

75. Kowshik, M.; Ashtaputre, S.; Kharrazi, S.; Vogel, W.; Urban, J.; Kulkarni, S.K.; Paknikar, K. Extracellular synthesis of silver nanoparticles by a silver-tolerant yeast strain mky3. *Nanotechnology* **2002**, *14*, 95. [CrossRef]

76. Bhangale, H.; Sarode, K.; Patil, A.; Patil, D. *Microbial Synthesis of Silver Nanoparticles Using Aspergillus Flavus and Their Characterization*; Techno-Societal 2016, International Conference on Advanced Technologies for Societal Applications; Springer: Berlin, Germany, 2016; pp. 463–470.
77. Vigneshwaran, N.; Ashtaputre, N.; Varadarajan, P.; Nachane, R.; Paralikar, K.; Balasubramanya, R. Biological synthesis of silver nanoparticles using the fungus *Aspergillus Flavus*. *Mater. Lett.* **2007**, *61*, 1413–1418. [CrossRef]
78. Kathiresan, K.; Manivannan, S.; Nabeel, M.; Dhivya, B. Studies on silver nanoparticles synthesized by a marine fungus, penicillium fellutanum isolated from coastal mangrove sediment. *Colloids Surf. B Biointerfaces* **2009**, *71*, 133–137. [CrossRef] [PubMed]
79. Kathiresan, K.; Alikunhi, N.M.; Pathmanaban, S.; Nabikhan, A.; Kandasamy, S. Analysis of antimicrobial silver nanoparticles synthesized by coastal strains of *Escherichia Coli* and aspergillus niger. *Can. J. Microbiol.* **2010**, *56*, 1050–1059. [CrossRef] [PubMed]
80. Gade, A.; Bonde, P.; Ingle, A.; Marcato, P.; Duran, N.; Rai, M. Exploitation of *Aspergillus Niger* for synthesis of silver nanoparticles. *J. Biobased Mater. Bioenergy* **2008**, *2*, 243–247. [CrossRef]
81. De Souza, A.O.; Rodrigues, A.G. Biosynthesis of silver nanoparticles by fungi. *Fungal Biomol. Sources Appl. Recent Dev.* **2015**, 115–135. [CrossRef]
82. Li, G.; He, D.; Qian, Y.; Guan, B.; Gao, S.; Cui, Y.; Yokoyama, K.; Wang, L. Fungus-mediated green synthesis of silver nanoparticles using Aspergillus terreus. *Int. J. Mol. Sci.* **2011**, *13*, 466–476. [CrossRef] [PubMed]
83. Raudabaugh, D.B.; Tzolov, M.B.; Calabrese, J.P.; Overton, B.E. Synthesis of silver nanoparticles by a bryophilous rhizoctonia species. *Nanomater. Nanotechnol.* **2013**, *3*, 2. [CrossRef]
84. Devika, R.; Elumalai, S.; Manikandan, E.; Eswaramoorthy, D. Biosynthesis of silver nanoparticles using the fungus *Pleurotus Ostreatus* and their antibacterial activity. *Open Access Sci. Rep.* **2012**, *1*, 557.
85. Kulkarni, N.; Muddapur, U. Biosynthesis of metal nanoparticles: A review. *J. Nanotechnol.* **2014**, *2014*, 510246. [CrossRef]
86. Kumar, D.A.; Palanichamy, V.; Roopan, S.M. Green synthesis of silver nanoparticles using alternanthera dentata leaf extract at room temperature and their antimicrobial activity. *Spectrochim. Acta Part A Mol. Biomol. Spectrosc.* **2014**, *127*, 168–171. [CrossRef] [PubMed]
87. Dhand, V.; Soumya, L.; Bharadwaj, S.; Chakra, S.; Bhatt, D.; Sreedhar, B. Green synthesis of silver nanoparticles using coffea arabica seed extract and its antibacterial activity. *Mater. Sci. Eng. C* **2016**, *58*, 36–43. [CrossRef] [PubMed]
88. Gopinath, V.; MubarakAli, D.; Priyadarshini, S.; Priyadharsshini, N.M.; Thajuddin, N.; Velusamy, P. Biosynthesis of silver nanoparticles from tribulus terrestris and its antimicrobial activity: A novel biological approach. *Colloids Surf. B Biointerfaces* **2012**, *96*, 69–74. [CrossRef] [PubMed]
89. Krishnaraj, C.; Jagan, E.; Rajasekar, S.; Selvakumar, P.; Kalaichelvan, P.; Mohan, N. Synthesis of silver nanoparticles using acalypha indica leaf extracts and its antibacterial activity against water borne pathogens. *Colloids Surf. B Biointerfaces* **2010**, *76*, 50–56. [CrossRef] [PubMed]
90. Veeraputhiran, V. Bio-catalytic synthesis of silver nanoparticles. *Int. J. ChemTech Res.* **2013**, *5*, 255–2562.
91. Khalil, M.M.; Ismail, E.H.; El-Baghdady, K.Z.; Mohamed, D. Green synthesis of silver nanoparticles using olive leaf extract and its antibacterial activity. *Arab. J. Chem.* **2014**, *7*, 1131–1139. [CrossRef]
92. Rashid, Z.; Moadi, T.; Ghahremanzadeh, R. Green synthesis and characterization of silver nanoparticles using ferula latisecta leaf extract and their application as a catalyst for the safe and simple one-pot preparation of spirooxindoles in water. *New J. Chem.* **2016**, *40*, 3343–3349. [CrossRef]
93. Roy, N.; Gaur, A.; Jain, A.; Bhattacharya, S.; Rani, V. Green synthesis of silver nanoparticles: An approach to overcome toxicity. *Environ. Toxicol. Pharmacol.* **2013**, *36*, 807–812. [CrossRef] [PubMed]
94. Ahmed, S.; Ahmad, M.; Swami, B.L.; Ikram, S. A review on plants extract mediated synthesis of silver nanoparticles for antimicrobial applications: A green expertise. *J. Adv. Res.* **2016**, *7*, 17–28. [CrossRef] [PubMed]
95. Makarov, V.V.; Love, A.J.; Sinitsyna, O.V.; Makarova, S.S.; Yaminsky, I.V.; Taliansky, M.E.; Kalinina, N.O. "Green" nanotechnologies: Synthesis of metal nanoparticles using plants. *Acta Nat.* **2014**, *6*, 35–44.
96. Chen, Y.-H.; Yeh, C.-S. Laser ablation method: Use of surfactants to form the dispersed ag nanoparticles. *Colloids Surf. A Physicochem. Eng. Asp.* **2002**, *197*, 133–139. [CrossRef]
97. Qin, Y.; Ji, X.; Jing, J.; Liu, H.; Wu, H.; Yang, W. Size control over spherical silver nanoparticles by ascorbic acid reduction. *Colloids Surf. A Physicochem. Eng. Asp.* **2010**, *372*, 172–176. [CrossRef]

98. Kannan, R.; Stirk, W.; Van Staden, J. Synthesis of silver nanoparticles using the seaweed *Codium Capitatum P.C. Silva (Chlorophyceae). S. Afr. J. Bot.* **2013**, *86*, 1–4. [CrossRef]
99. Liu, W.; Wu, Y.; Wang, C.; Li, H.C.; Wang, T.; Liao, C.Y.; Cui, L.; Zhou, Q.F.; Yan, B.; Jiang, G.B. Impact of silver nanoparticles on human cells: Effect of particle size. *Nanotoxicology* **2010**, *4*, 319–330. [CrossRef] [PubMed]
100. Hsin, Y.H.; Chen, C.F.; Huang, S.; Shih, T.S.; Lai, P.S.; Chueh, P.J. The apoptotic effect of nanosilver is mediated by a ROS- and JNK-dependent mechanism involving the mitochondrial pathway in NIH3T3 cells. *Toxicol. Lett.* **2008**, *179*, 130–139. [CrossRef] [PubMed]
101. Hussain, S.M.; Hess, K.L.; Gearhart, J.M.; Geiss, K.T.; Schlager, J.J. In Vitro toxicity of nanoparticles in BRL 3a rat liver cells. *Toxicology In Vitro* **2005**, *19*, 975–983. [CrossRef] [PubMed]
102. Verano-Braga, T.; Miethling-Graff, R.; Wojdyla, K.; Rogowska-Wrzesinska, A.; Brewer, J.R.; Erdmann, H.; Kjeldsen, F. Insights into the cellular response triggered by silver nanoparticles using quantitative proteomics. *ACS Nano* **2014**, *8*, 2161–2175. [CrossRef] [PubMed]
103. Carlson, C.; Hussain, S.M.; Schrand, A.M.; Braydich-Stolle, L.K.; Hess, K.L.; Jones, R.L.; Schlager, J.J. Unique cellular interaction of silver nanoparticles: Size-dependent generation of reactive oxygen species. *J. Phys. Chem. B* **2008**, *112*, 13608–13619. [CrossRef] [PubMed]
104. Foldbjerg, R.; Olesen, P.; Hougaard, M.; Dang, D.A.; Hoffmann, H.J.; Autrup, H. PVP-coated silver nanoparticles and silver ions induce reactive oxygen species, apoptosis and necrosis in THP-1 monocytes. *Toxicol. Lett.* **2009**, *190*, 156–162. [CrossRef] [PubMed]
105. Foldbjerg, R.; Dang, D.A.; Autrup, H. Cytotoxicity and genotoxicity of silver nanoparticles in the human lung cancer cell line, a549. *Arch. Toxicol.* **2011**, *85*, 743–750. [CrossRef] [PubMed]
106. Kim, S.; Choi, J.E.; Choi, J.; Chung, K.H.; Park, K.; Yi, J.; Ryu, D.Y. Oxidative stress-dependent toxicity of silver nanoparticles in human hepatoma cells. *Toxicology In Vitro* **2009**, *23*, 1076–1084. [CrossRef] [PubMed]
107. Avalos, A.; Haza, A.I.; Mateo, D.; Morales, P. Interactions of manufactured silver nanoparticles of different sizes with normal human dermal fibroblasts. *Int. Wound J.* **2016**, *13*, 101–109. [CrossRef] [PubMed]
108. Foldbjerg, R.; Irving, E.S.; Hayashi, Y.; Sutherland, D.S.; Thorsen, K.; Autrup, H.; Beer, C. Global gene expression profiling of human lung epithelial cells after exposure to nanosilver. *Toxicol. Sci.* **2012**, *130*, 145–157. [CrossRef] [PubMed]
109. Piao, M.J.; Kang, K.A.; Lee, I.K.; Kim, H.S.; Kim, S.; Choi, J.Y.; Choi, J.; Hyun, J.W. Silver nanoparticles induce oxidative cell damage in human liver cells through inhibition of reduced glutathione and induction of mitochondria-involved apoptosis. *Toxicol. Lett.* **2011**, *201*, 92–100. [CrossRef] [PubMed]
110. Eom, H.J.; Choi, J. P38 mapk activation, DNA damage, cell cycle arrest and apoptosis as mechanisms of toxicity of silver nanoparticles in jurkat t cells. *Environ. Sci. Technol.* **2010**, *44*, 8337–8342. [CrossRef] [PubMed]
111. Nishanth, R.P.; Jyotsna, R.G.; Schlager, J.J.; Hussain, S.M.; Reddanna, P. Inflammatory responses of raw 264.7 macrophages upon exposure to nanoparticles: Role of ROS-NFkB signaling pathway. *Nanotoxicology* **2011**, *5*, 502–516. [CrossRef] [PubMed]
112. Asharani, P.; Sethu, S.; Lim, H.K.; Balaji, G.; Valiyaveettil, S.; Hande, M.P. Differential regulation of intracellular factors mediating cell cycle, DNA repair and inflammation following exposure to silver nanoparticles in human cells. *Genome Integr.* **2012**, *3*, 2. [CrossRef] [PubMed]
113. Ahamed, M.; Karns, M.; Goodson, M.; Rowe, J.; Hussain, S.M.; Schlager, J.J.; Hong, Y. DNA damage response to different surface chemistry of silver nanoparticles in mammalian cells. *Toxicol. Appl. Pharmacol.* **2008**, *233*, 404–410. [CrossRef] [PubMed]
114. Chichova, M.; Shkodrova, M.; Vasileva, P.; Kirilova, K.; Doncheva-Stoimenova, D. Influence of silver nanoparticles on the activity of rat liver mitochondrial atpase. *J. Nanopart. Res.* **2014**, *16*, 1–14. [CrossRef]
115. Lee, D.Y.; Li, K.C. Molecular theranostics: A primer for the imaging professional. *AJR Am. J. Roentgenol.* **2011**, *197*, 318–324. [CrossRef] [PubMed]
116. Svenson, S. Theranostics: Are we there yet? *Mol. Pharm.* **2013**, *10*, 848–856. [CrossRef] [PubMed]
117. Lim, E.K.; Kim, T.; Paik, S.; Haam, S.; Huh, Y.M.; Lee, K. Nanomaterials for theranostics: Recent advances and future challenges. *Chem. Rev.* **2015**, *115*, 327–394. [CrossRef] [PubMed]
118. Bardhan, R.; Lal, S.; Joshi, A.; Halas, N.J. Theranostic nanoshells: From probe design to imaging and treatment of cancer. *Acc. Chem. Res.* **2011**, *44*, 936–946. [CrossRef] [PubMed]

119. Cole, A.J.; Yang, V.C.; David, A.E. Cancer theranostics: The rise of targeted magnetic nanoparticles. *Trends Biotechnol.* **2011**, *29*, 323–332. [CrossRef] [PubMed]
120. Davis, M.E.; Chen, Z.G.; Shin, D.M. Nanoparticle therapeutics: An emerging treatment modality for cancer. *Nat. Rev. Drug Discov.* **2008**, *7*, 771–782. [CrossRef] [PubMed]
121. Ferrari, M. Cancer nanotechnology: Opportunities and challenges. *Nat. Rev. Cancer* **2005**, *5*, 161–171. [CrossRef] [PubMed]
122. Verma, S.K.; Mani, P.; Sharma, N.R.; Krishnan, A.; Kumar, V.V.; Reddy, B.S.; Chaudhuri, A.; Roy, R.P.; Sarkar, D.P. Histidylated lipid-modified sendai viral envelopes mediate enhanced membrane fusion and potentiate targeted gene delivery. *J. Biol. Chem.* **2005**, *280*, 35399–35409. [CrossRef] [PubMed]
123. Acharya, S.; Sahoo, S.K. PLGA nanoparticles containing various anticancer agents and tumour delivery by EPR effect. *Adv. Drug Deliv. Rev.* **2011**, *63*, 170–183. [CrossRef] [PubMed]
124. Sharma, H.; Mishra, P.K.; Talegaonkar, S.; Vaidya, B. Metal nanoparticles: A theranostic nanotool against cancer. *Drug Discov. Today* **2015**, *20*, 1143–1151. [CrossRef] [PubMed]
125. Gopinath, P.; Gogoi, S.K.; Chattopadhyay, A.; Ghosh, S.S. Implications of silver nanoparticle induced cell apoptosis for in vitro gene therapy. *Nanotechnology* **2008**, *19*, 075104. [CrossRef] [PubMed]
126. Kerr, S.L.; Sharp, B. Nano-particle labelling of nucleic acids for enhanced detection by inductively-coupled plasma mass spectrometry (ICP-MS). *Chem. Commun.* **2007**, 4537–4539. [CrossRef] [PubMed]
127. Whaley, S.R.; English, D.S.; Hu, E.L.; Barbara, P.F.; Belcher, A.M. Selection of peptides with semiconductor binding specificity for directed nanocrystal assembly. *Nature* **2000**, *405*, 665–668. [CrossRef] [PubMed]
128. Wang, H.J.; Yang, L.; Yang, H.Y.; Wang, K.; Yao, W.G.; Jiang, K.; Huang, X.L.; Zheng, Z. Antineoplastic activities of protein-conjugated silver sulfide nano-crystals with different shapes. *J. Inorg. Biochem.* **2010**, *104*, 87–91. [CrossRef] [PubMed]
129. Sanpui, P.; Chattopadhyay, A.; Ghosh, S.S. Induction of apoptosis in cancer cells at low silver nanoparticle concentrations using chitosan nanocarrier. *ACS Appl. Mater. Interfaces* **2011**, *3*, 218–228. [CrossRef] [PubMed]
130. Guo, D.; Zhu, L.; Huang, Z.; Zhou, H.; Ge, Y.; Ma, W.; Wu, J.; Zhang, X.; Zhou, X.; Zhang, Y. Anti-leukemia activity of PVP-coated silver nanoparticles via generation of reactive oxygen species and release of silver ions. *Biomaterials* **2013**, *34*, 7884–7894. [CrossRef] [PubMed]
131. AshaRani, P.V.; Low Kah Mun, G.; Hande, M.P.; Valiyaveettil, S. Cytotoxicity and genotoxicity of silver nanoparticles in human cells. *ACS Nano* **2009**, *3*, 279–290. [CrossRef] [PubMed]
132. Liang, P.; Shi, H.; Zhu, W.; Gui, Q.; Xu, Y.; Meng, J.; Guo, X.; Gong, Z.; Chen, H. Silver nanoparticles enhance the sensitivity of temozolomide on human glioma cells. *Oncotarget* **2017**, *8*, 7533–7539. [CrossRef] [PubMed]
133. Locatelli, E.; Naddaka, M.; Uboldi, C.; Loudos, G.; Fragogeorgi, E.; Molinari, V.; Pucci, A.; Tsotakos, T.; Psimadas, D.; Ponti, J.; et al. Targeted delivery of silver nanoparticles and alisertib: In vitro and in vivo synergistic effect against glioblastoma. *Nanomedicine* **2014**, *9*, 839–849. [CrossRef] [PubMed]
134. Ortega, F.G.; Fernandez-Baldo, M.A.; Fernandez, J.G.; Serrano, M.J.; Sanz, M.I.; Diaz-Mochon, J.J.; Lorente, J.A.; Raba, J. Study of antitumor activity in breast cell lines using silver nanoparticles produced by yeast. *Int. J. Nanomed.* **2015**, *10*, 2021–2031.
135. Gurunathan, S.; Han, J.W.; Eppakayala, V.; Jeyaraj, M.; Kim, J.H. Cytotoxicity of biologically synthesized silver nanoparticles in MDA-MB-231 human breast cancer cells. *BioMed Res. Int.* **2013**, *2013*, 535796. [CrossRef] [PubMed]
136. Gurunathan, S.; Park, J.H.; Han, J.W.; Kim, J.H. Comparative assessment of the apoptotic potential of silver nanoparticles synthesized by *bacillus tequilensis* and *calocybe indica* in MDA-MB-231 human breast cancer cells: Targeting p53 for anticancer therapy. *Int. J. Nanomed.* **2015**, *10*, 4203–4222. [CrossRef] [PubMed]
137. Gurunathan, S.; Han, J.W.; Dayem, A.A.; Eppakayala, V.; Park, J.H.; Cho, S.-G.; Lee, K.J.; Kim, J.-H. Green synthesis of anisotropic silver nanoparticles and its potential cytotoxicity in human breast cancer cells (MCF-7). *J. Ind. Eng. Chem.* **2013**, *19*, 1600–1605. [CrossRef]
138. Gurunathan, S.; Jeong, J.K.; Han, J.W.; Zhang, X.F.; Park, J.H.; Kim, J.H. Multidimensional effects of biologically synthesized silver nanoparticles in helicobacter pylori, helicobacter felis, and human lung (l132) and lung carcinoma a549 cells. *Nanoscale Res. Lett.* **2015**, *10*, 35. [CrossRef] [PubMed]
139. Zuberek, M.; Wojciechowska, D.; Krzyzanowski, D.; Meczynska-Wielgosz, S.; Kruszewski, M.; Grzelak, A. Glucose availability determines silver nanoparticles toxicity in HEPG2. *J. Nanobiotechnol.* **2015**, *13*, 72. [CrossRef] [PubMed]

140. Halliwell, B.; Clement, M.V.; Ramalingam, J.; Long, L.H. Hydrogen peroxide. Ubiquitous in cell culture and in vivo? *IUBMB Life* **2000**, *50*, 251–257. [CrossRef] [PubMed]
141. He, W.; Zhou, Q.; Yu, S.; Cai, D.; Wang, Q.; Zhang, X.; Huang, W.Q. Mechanism on atrial natriuretic peptide receptor in anti-anxiety with acupuncture based on its tranquilizing effect. *Zhongguo Zhen Jiu* **2015**, *35*, 101–104. [PubMed]
142. Hao, E.; Schatz, G.C. Electromagnetic fields around silver nanoparticles and dimers. *J. Chem. Phys.* **2004**, *120*, 357–366. [CrossRef] [PubMed]
143. Bohren, C.F.; Huffman, D.R. *Absorption and Scattering by a Sphere*; Wiley Online Library: New York, NY, USA, 1983.
144. Kreibig, U.; Vollmer, M. *Optical Properties of Metal Clusters*; Springer Science & Business Media: New York, NY, USA, 2013; Volume 25.
145. Hutter, E.; Fendler, J.H. Exploitation of localized surface plasmon resonance. *Adv. Mater.* **2004**, *16*, 1685–1706. [CrossRef]
146. Hecht, B.; Bielefeldt, H.; Novotny, L.; Inouye, Y.; Pohl, D. Local excitation, scattering, and interference of surface plasmons. *Phys. Rev. Lett.* **1996**, *77*, 1889. [CrossRef] [PubMed]
147. Jain, P.K.; Huang, X.; El-Sayed, I.H.; El-Sayed, M.A. Noble metals on the nanoscale: Optical and photothermal properties and some applications in imaging, sensing, biology, and medicine. *Acc. Chem. Res.* **2008**, *41*, 1578–1586. [CrossRef] [PubMed]
148. Schasfoort, R.B. *Handbook of Surface Plasmon Resonance*; Royal Society of Chemistry: Cambridge, UK, 2017.
149. Brongersma, M.L.; Halas, N.J.; Nordlander, P. Plasmon-induced hot carrier science and technology. *Nat. Nanotechnol.* **2015**, *10*, 25. [CrossRef] [PubMed]
150. Amendola, V.; Bakr, O.M.; Stellacci, F. A study of the surface plasmon resonance of silver nanoparticles by the discrete dipole approximation method: Effect of shape, size, structure, and assembly. *Plasmonics* **2010**, *5*, 85–97. [CrossRef]
151. Jacques, S.L. Optical properties of biological tissues: A review. *Phys. Med. Biol.* **2013**, *58*, R37. [CrossRef] [PubMed]
152. Evanoff, D.D.; Chumanov, G. Synthesis and optical properties of silver nanoparticles and arrays. *ChemPhysChem* **2005**, *6*, 1221–1231. [CrossRef] [PubMed]
153. Peiris, S.; McMurtrie, J.; Zhu, H.-Y. Metal nanoparticle photocatalysts: Emerging processes for green organic synthesis. *Catal. Sci. Technol.* **2016**, *6*, 320–338. [CrossRef]
154. Linic, S.; Aslam, U.; Boerigter, C.; Morabito, M. Photochemical transformations on plasmonic metal nanoparticles. *Nat. Mater.* **2015**, *14*, 567–576. [CrossRef] [PubMed]
155. Mukherjee, S.; Chowdhury, D.; Kotcherlakota, R.; Patra, S. Potential theranostics application of bio-synthesized silver nanoparticles (4-in-1 system). *Theranostics* **2014**, *4*, 316–335. [CrossRef] [PubMed]
156. Farrag, N.S.; El-Sabagh, H.A.; Al-mahallawi, A.M.; Amin, A.M.; AbdEl-Bary, A.; Mamdouh, W. Comparative study on radiolabeling and biodistribution of core-shell silver/polymeric nanoparticles-based theranostics for tumor targeting. *Int. J. Pharm.* **2017**, *529*, 123–133. [CrossRef] [PubMed]
157. Boca, S.C.; Potara, M.; Gabudean, A.M.; Juhem, A.; Baldeck, P.L.; Astilean, S. Chitosan-coated triangular silver nanoparticles as a novel class of biocompatible, highly effective photothermal transducers for in vitro cancer cell therapy. *Cancer Lett.* **2011**, *311*, 131–140. [CrossRef] [PubMed]
158. Kovács, D.; Igaz, N.; Keskeny, C.; Bélteky, P.; Tóth, T.; Gáspár, R.; Madarász, D.; Rázga, Z.; Kónya, Z.; Boros, I.M. Silver nanoparticles defeat p53-positive and p53-negative osteosarcoma cells by triggering mitochondrial stress and apoptosis. *Sci. Rep.* **2016**, *6*, 27902. [CrossRef] [PubMed]
159. Schrand, A.M.; Braydich-Stolle, L.K.; Schlager, J.J.; Dai, L.; Hussain, S.M. Can silver nanoparticles be useful as potential biological labels? *Nanotechnology* **2008**, *19*, 235104. [CrossRef] [PubMed]
160. Stensberg, M.C.; Wei, Q.; McLamore, E.S.; Porterfield, D.M.; Wei, A.; Sepulveda, M.S. Toxicological studies on silver nanoparticles: Challenges and opportunities in assessment, monitoring and imaging. *Nanomedicine* **2011**, *6*, 879–898. [CrossRef] [PubMed]
161. Tran, Q.H.; Le, A.-T. Silver nanoparticles: Synthesis, properties, toxicology, applications and perspectives. *Adv. Nat. Sci. Nanosci. Nanotechnol.* **2013**, *4*, 033001. [CrossRef]
162. Rahman, M.; Wang, J.; Patterson, T.; Saini, U.; Robinson, B.; Newport, G.; Murdock, R.; Schlager, J.; Hussain, S.; Ali, S. Expression of genes related to oxidative stress in the mouse brain after exposure to silver-25 nanoparticles. *Toxicol. Lett.* **2009**, *187*, 15–21. [CrossRef] [PubMed]

163. Sung, J.H.; Ji, J.H.; Park, J.D.; Yoon, J.U.; Kim, D.S.; Jeon, K.S.; Song, M.Y.; Jeong, J.; Han, B.S.; Han, J.H. Subchronic inhalation toxicity of silver nanoparticles. *Toxicol. Sci.* **2008**, *108*, 452–461. [CrossRef] [PubMed]
164. Van Aerle, R.; Lange, A.; Moorhouse, A.; Paszkiewicz, K.; Ball, K.; Johnston, B.D.; de-Bastos, E.; Booth, T.; Tyler, C.R.; Santos, E.M. Molecular mechanisms of toxicity of silver nanoparticles in zebrafish embryos. *Environ. Sci. Technol.* **2013**, *47*, 8005–8014. [CrossRef] [PubMed]
165. Munger, M.A.; Radwanski, P.; Hadlock, G.C.; Stoddard, G.; Shaaban, A.; Falconer, J.; Grainger, D.W.; Deering-Rice, C.E. In Vivo human time-exposure study of orally dosed commercial silver nanoparticles. *Nanomed. Nanotechnol. Biol. Med.* **2014**, *10*, 1–9. [CrossRef] [PubMed]

11

The Use of Artificial Gel Forming Bolalipids as Novel Formulations in Antimicrobial and Antifungal Therapy

Nathalie Goergen [1], Matthias Wojcik [1], Simon Drescher [2,3], Shashank Reddy Pinnapireddy [1], Jana Brüßler [1], Udo Bakowsky [1] and Jarmila Jedelská [1,*]

1 Department of Pharmaceutics and Biopharmaceutics, University of Marburg, 35037 Marburg, Germany
2 Institute of Pharmacy, Biophysical Pharmacy, Martin Luther University Halle-Wittenberg, 06120 Halle (Saale), Germany
3 Institute of Pharmacy, University of Greifswald, 17489 Greifswald, Germany
* Correspondence: jedelska@mailer.uni-marburg.de;

Abstract: The alarming growth of multi-drug resistant bacteria has led to a quest for alternative antibacterial therapeutics. One strategy to circumvent the already existing resistance is the use of photodynamic therapy. Antimicrobial photodynamic therapy (aPDT) involves the use of non-toxic photosensitizers in combination with light and in situ oxygen to generate toxic radical species within the microbial environment which circumvents the resistance building mechanism of the bacteria. Hydrogels are used ubiquitously in the biological and pharmaceutical fields, e.g., for wound dressing material or as drug delivery systems. Hydrogels formed by water-insoluble low-molecular weight gelators may potentially provide the much-needed benefits for these applications. Bolalipids are a superior example of such gelators. In the present work, two artificial bolalipids were used, namely PC-C32-PC and Me_2PE-C32-Me_2PE, which self-assemble in water into long and flexible nanofibers leading to a gelation of the surrounding solvent. The aim of the study was to create stable hydrogel formulations of both bolalipids and to investigate their applicability as a novel material for drug delivery systems. Furthermore, methylene blue—a well-known photosensitizer—was incorporated into the hydrogels in order to investigate the aPDT for the treatment of skin and mucosal infections using a custom designed LED device.

Keywords: hydrogel; drug delivery system; self-assembly; bolaform amphiphilic lipids; bolalipids; aerogel; chorioallantoic membrane model; antimicrobial photodynamic therapy

---

1. Introduction

Inappropriate use of antibiotics in humans and agriculture in recent decades has led to a rapid development of multi-drug resistant bacteria. According to WHO, antibiotic resistance is one of the biggest threats to global health, food security, and development, leading to longer hospital stays, higher medical costs and increased mortality [1]. Therefore, research into novel strategies to combat bacterial infections have become highly relevant. Photodynamic activity of chemical compounds towards bacterial microorganisms has been effective in the treatment of localized microbial infections [2]. The use of non-toxic photosensitizers in combination with light and in situ oxygen generates toxic radical species in the microbial environment [3,4]. Due to the unselective mechanism of action, antimicrobial photodynamic therapy (aPDT) has a broad spectrum of activity. In previous studies, it could be shown that antibiotic-resistant strains such as methicillin-resistant *Staphylococcus aureus* are as sensitive towards aPDT as non-resistant *Staphylococcus aureus* [4]. However, PDT is not only used in antibacterial research, but also in antifungal therapy [5,6]. In contrast to the PDT of tumors in which the photosensitizer is injected intratumorally or intravenously and is afterwards accumulated in the tumor tissue, the photosensitizer in aPDT is applied locally to the infected area, thereby making aPDT particularly suitable for the treatment of skin and soft tissue infections, such as burns or ulcus cruris [3,7].

For the local treatment, a drug delivery system (DDS) is necessary to deliver the drug in a controlled manner. Hydrogels have been used previously as DDS or wound dressing materials and possess most of the desirable characteristics [8–10]. They offer a moist wound environment, absorb blood and exudate and are suitable for cleansing of dry, sloughy or necrotic wounds by rehydrating dead tissues and enhancing the autolytic debridement [10]. Nevertheless, complications such as non-biodegradability, unfavorable mechanical properties or low biocompatibility are well-known limitations of the hydrogel technology in general [11].

Low biocompatibility is caused by the use of toxic cross-linkers or remaining unreacted monomers, oligomers and initiators of the hydrogel itself [12]. A broad variety of gelling agents have been described whereas low-molecular weight gelators have shown great potential as controlled DDS [13]. Within this expanding field of low-molecular weight gelators, lipids, which can self-assemble in hydrophilic media and thus form hydrogels, have garnered much interest [13]. A promising class among them are bipolar lipids, the so-called bolalipids. Bolalipids are defined as molecules that possess hydrophobic repeating units connecting hydrophilic head groups at the two ends of the hydrophobic core [14]. Both head groups can be identical (symmetric bolalipids) or they can differ in their size, charge, polarity and/or ability to (de) protonate (asymmetric bolalipids) [15–18]. Natural bolalipids originated from the membrane lipids of certain species of Archaea, especially from those of thermoacidophiles [19]. Archaea, apart from bacteria and eukaryotes, represent one of the three domains of life [20]. The organism Archaea thermoacidophiles is commonly found in exceptional ecological niches with high temperature of about 90 °C and a low pH of 2. These life circumstances result in the need of stable membranes, which make the bolalipids an interesting choice for new, innovative DDS. Previous work has shown that these naturally occurring lipids are well suitable to stabilize DDS [21–25].

Due to the fact, that the isolation of archaeal bolalipids from natural sources is expensive and often leads to a mixture of bolalipids with different alkyl chain pattern and head groups, artificial bolalipids offer an advantageous alternative [22,26,27]. A special class of artificial bolalipids, the single-chained ones, are able to form hydrogels by self-assembly [28]. This capacity is based on their ability to form an extended network of entangled helical nanofibers of 6–7 nm thickness depending on the concentration of bolalipid and the pH of the dispersion medium [28–30]. The self-assembly into nanofibers is mainly driven by hydrophobic (van-der-Waals) interactions of the long, single alkyl chain. In some cases, depending on the structure of the head group, these fibers are stabilized by hydrogen bonds. Finally, the fibers interact with the surrounding medium (water) also by means of hydrogen bonds, which leads to an efficient gelation of the solvent.

In the present work, we focused on two artificial bolalipids, namely PC-C32-PC and Me_2PE-C32-Me_2PE, which are composed of a long C32 alkyl chain and either two phosphocholine (PC) or dimethylphosphoethanolamine (Me_2PE) head groups. The chemical structures are depicted in Figure 1. Previous characterizations of the investigated bolalipids demonstrated gel formation with concentrations lower than 1 mg/mL [31,32] which makes them highly interesting as material for the use in novel DDS.

The aim of the study was to create stable formulations of both bolalipids and to investigate their applicability as a novel material for DDS. Furthermore, methylene blue (MB), a well-known photosensitizer [33–36] was incorporated into the formulations in order to consider the application of these formulations in aPDT for the treatment of skin and mucous infections.

For the characterization of all formulations, rotation viscometry as well as scanning electron microscopy was used. Drug release was performed using Franz diffusion cells. In addition to physical characterization of the bolalipid formulations, the biological aspects of DDS requirements were investigated. The ability of PC-C32-PC and Me_2PE-C32-Me_2PE to inhibit microbial growth of bacteria and fungi itself was examined by means of agar diffusion method [37,38]. To investigate the compliance on mucous tissue, the bolalipid formulations were topically applied on the chorioallantoic membrane (CAM) model and structural changes of the blood vessels were investigated [39].

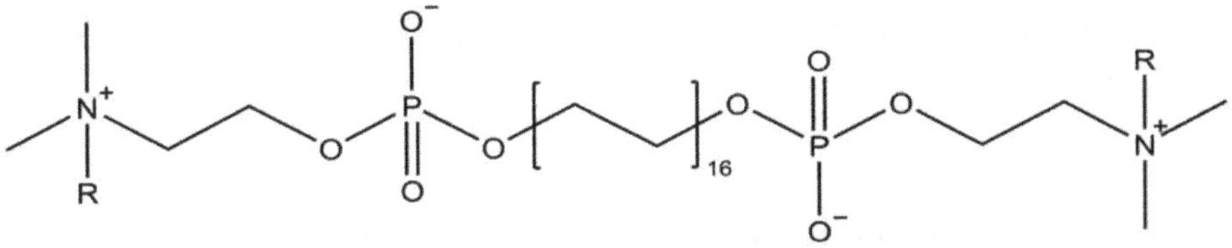

R = CH_3 (PC-C32-PC) R = H (Me_2PE-C32-Me_2PE)

Figure 1. Chemical structure of bolalipids PC-C32-PC and Me_2PE-C32-Me_2PE used in this study.

2. Materials and Methods

2.1. Materials

The bolalipids dotriacontane-1,1′-diylbis [2-(trimethylammino)ethyl phosphate] (PC-C32-PC) and dotriacontane-1,1′-diylbis [2-(dimethylammino)ethyl phosphate] (Me_2PE-C32-Me_2PE) were synthesized at the MLU Halle-Wittenberg (Halle, Germany) according to procedures described previously [40,41]. Sodium dodecyl sulfate and methylene blue were purchased from Carl Roth GmbH and Co. KG (Karlsruhe, Germany). Hydroxyethyl cellulose 300 (HEC 300; M_w ~ 807 g/mol) was obtained from Caesar and Loretz GmbH (Hilden, Germany). Physiological saline solution was purchased from B Braun (Melsungen, Germany). *Saccharomyces cerevisiae* were obtained from a retail outlet. Clinically isolated *Staphylococcus aureus* (ATCC 25923) was determined using MALDI Biotyper (Bruker Corporation, Billerica, MA, USA). Fertilized chicken eggs were obtained from Brormann GmbH (Rheda-Wiedenbrück, Germany). For all experiments ultrapure water from PURELAB®® flex 4 (ELGA LabWater, High Wycombe, UK) was used.

2.2. Preparation of Hydrogels and Aerogels

A defined amount of 5 mg/mL PC-C32-PC or Me_2PE-C32-Me_2PE was dissolved in ultrapure water in a 100 °C water bath. After cooling to room temperature, gelation occurred. For the release studies, MB was dissolved in the water prior to gelation. To compare the bolalipids with a commonly used hydrogel, 5 mg/mL HEC 300 dissolved in ultrapure water was used. To obtain aerogels, 75 μL of the hydrogels were pipetted into 96-well plates, frozen at −20 °C and transferred to a freeze dryer (ALPHA 1–4 LSC, Martin Christ Gefriertrocknungsanlangen GmbH, Osterode, Germany). The aerogels were stored under dry conditions after the preparation. For the rheological measurements, the aerogels were rehydrated in ultrapure water and stored at 37 °C.

2.3. Characterization

2.3.1. Rheological Characterization of Hydrogels and Rehydrated Aerogels

Rheometry was performed using a Haake™ Rotovisco 1 (Thermo Scientific, Karlsruhe, Germany) in the C/R ramp mode with cone/plate geometry of 60 mm in diameter and a slit of 0.54 mm. For each measurement, a sample volume of 2 mL was necessary to fill the slit. Before the measurement started, a recovery time of 10 min was applied after the slit size was reached. The recovery time was essential to make sure that the pre-stressed sample relaxed. The temperature was kept constant at 20 °C during the experiment, which was performed in triplicate for each substance.

2.3.2. Scanning Electron Microscopy (SEM) of Aerogels

To investigate the structure of bolalipid aerogels, SEM pictures were generated using Hitachi S-510 scanning electron microscope (Hitachi-High Technologies Europe GmbH, Krefeld, Germany) under a high vacuum of 4×10^{-6} mbar at 5 kV accelerating voltage and 30 μA emission current [42]. The aerogels as well as freeze-dried HEC 300 hydrogels were sputter coated with gold at 1.3×10^{-1} mbar vacuum under argon atmosphere for 1 min at 30 mA (Edwards S150, Edwards High Vacuum, Crawley, UK) [43]. This procedure ensures a sufficient conductivity of organic material, increases the signal of emitted electrons and leads to higher resolution of obtained pictures.

2.4. *Release Studies*

The release behaviors of bolalipid hydro- and aerogels were investigated using a vertical diffusion cell with a release area of approx. 180 mm^2 and a volume of 12 mL equipped with a 0.22 μm membrane filter. Acceptor chamber was filled with physiological buffer and the temperature was maintained at 37.8 °C [44]. As reference, HEC 300 containing the same concentration of gelling agent and drug was used. After placing the hydro- or aerogels into the donor chamber, samples were collected from the acceptor chamber at defined time points. The concentration of MB was calculated using microplate spectrometer (Multiskan™ GO, Thermo Scientific, Waltham, MA, USA) at a wavelength of 664 nm. The experiment was conducted with six diffusion cells for each formulation.

2.5. *Microbiology*

2.5.1. Antifungal Activity of PC-C32-PC and Me_2PE-C32-Me_2PE Hydro- or Aerogels

To investigate the antifungal effect of bolalipid hydrogels and aerogels, the agar diffusion test was used as described previously [37,38]. In brief, Mueller Hinton agar plates (BD GmbH, Heidelberg, Germany) were inoculated with a suspension of *Saccharomyces cerevisiae*. The samples containing PC-C32-PC or Me_2PE-C32-Me_2PE bolalipids were placed on the inoculated agar plates. After incubation overnight (Heraeus GmbH and Co. KG., Hanau, Germany) at 30 °C and 60% relative humidity, the antifungal activity was evaluated.

2.5.2. Antifungal Activity of Loaded PC-C32-PC and Me_2PE-C32-Me_2PE Aerogels by Means of PDT

Antifungal activity of bolalipid aerogels loaded with MB were investigated using PDT. The agar plates were inoculated in the same manner as described above (2.5.1). Then the loaded aerogels were placed on the inoculated agar plates. After an incubation time of 3 h, the complete agar plate was irradiated (λ_{ex} = 643 nm) using a custom designed LED device (Lumundus GmbH, Eisenach, Germany) for 20 min resulting in a radiation fluence of 26.88 J/cm^2. Further technical characteristics of the device were described before [45]. Non-irradiated, loaded bolalipid aerogels as well as empty aerogels and MB solution served as controls. Subsequently, the plates were returned into the incubator and incubated overnight at 30 °C and 60% relative humidity. After 18 h, the antifungal effect was evaluated. The experiments were performed in triplicate.

2.5.3. Antibacterial Activity of Loaded PC-C32-PC and Me_2PE-C32-Me_2PE Aerogels by Means of aPDT

The aPDT studies were carried out on clinically isolated *Staphylococcus aureus* using the agar diffusion test. Briefly, bacterial suspension was prepared performing the direct colony suspension method. Afterwards a sterile cotton swap was dipped into the suspension and the agar plates (BD Columbia agar, BD GmbH, Heidelberg, Germany) were inoculated. In a similar manner to the antifungal PDT experiments, the samples were placed on the surface of inoculated agar plates and after an incubation time of 3 h the whole area was irradiated (λ_{ex} = 643 nm) using the LED device (radiation fluence 26.88 J/cm^2). Non-irradiated, loaded bolalipid aerogels as well as empty aerogels were used as controls. Finally, the treated plates were returned to the incubator and incubated overnight at 37 °C and 5% CO_2. After 20 h, the antimicrobial effect was evaluated. The experiments were performed in triplicate.

2.6. Biocompatibility

To evaluate the biocompatibility of the bolalipid hydro- and aerogels, the CAM model was used. Upon delivery, fertilized chicken eggs were swabbed with 70% (*v*/*v*) ethanol and incubated at 37.8 °C and 60–70% relative humidity in a hatching incubator (Ehret KMB 6, Ehret GmbH, Emmendingen, Germany). Until egg development day (EDD) 4, the eggs were rotated all 4 h automatically. On EDD 4, a window (∅ 3 cm) at the broad pole was opened using a pneumatic egg opener (Schuett-Biotec GmbH, Göttingen, Germany). The eggs were then returned to the incubator [46].

2.6.1. Henn´s Egg Test on the Chorioallantoic Membrane (HET-CAM) of Hydrogels

On EDD 10, 300 µL of PC-C32-PC, Me_2PE-C32-Me_2PE or HEC 300 hydrogels were applied onto the CAM surface and observed under a stereomicroscope (Stemi 2000-C, Carl Zeiss Microscopy GmbH, Göttingen, Germany) at 13-fold magnification. Supplied shear stress during the pipetting procedure led to liquefaction of bolalipid hydrogels. As a positive control, 1% (*w*/*w*) sodium dodecyl sulfate (SDS) and as a negative control, physiological saline solution were used. Pictures were taken each minute beginning with the contact of the sample to the CAM surface up to 5 min using a digital camera connected to the stereomicroscope (Moticam 2000, Motic Deutschland GmbH, Wetzlar, Germany). Each image was captured using the Motic Image Plus 2.0 software, followed by calculation of the irritation score as described elsewhere previously [47]. The experiment was conducted with six eggs for each substance.

2.6.2. Modified HET-CAM Assay with Bolalipid Aerogels

To evaluate the long-term biocompatibility of bolalipid aerogels, PC-C32-PC or Me_2PE-C32-Me_2PE aerogels were carefully placed on the CAM surface at EDD 9. A daily analysis of the samples, vessel formation and health of the CAM surface was carried out at 13-fold magnification using a stereomicroscope [48,49]. Pictures were taken as described above. The experiment was performed with five eggs for each bolalipid aerogel.

3. Results and Discussion

The aim of the study was to develop a stable and applicable DDS for aPDT based on the bolalipids PC-C32-PC and Me_2PE-C32-Me_2PE. Previous characterizations were performed using 1 mg/mL bolalipid resulting in a low stability of the hydrogels of this concentration [31,32]. Expecting an increase in the macroscopic mechanical stability, for a perspective pharmaceutical application, the concentration of bolalipids was elevated to 5 mg/mL.

3.1. Characterization of Hydrogels and Aerogels

After dispersion of 5 mg/mL bolalipid (PC-C32-PC or Me_2PE-C32-Me_2PE) in ultrapure water, a hydrogel formation has been reported [28,30]. The hydrogels were thus characterized by rotational viscometry (Figure 2). The obtained rheological data were compared to those of 5 mg/mL HEC 300 hydrogels as a reference. The measurements revealed that the viscosity of bolalipid hydrogels decreased at minimal shear forces. The low stability of these hydrogels in contrast to HEC 300 could be explained with weak interactions between the hydrophobic chains of the bolalipids (van-der-Waals only) and fewer amount of hydrogen bonds between the nanofibers [50]. Minimal shear forces thus led to a disintegration of the weakly bond nanofibers. This disintegration goes along with the rapid decrease of the viscosity and loss of the gel structure.

To optimize the stability of the obtained bolalipid hydrogels, the incorporated mobile phase was sublimated using a conventional freeze dryer. All samples were lyophilized under the same conditions. During this process, the hydrogels were transformed into bolalipid aerogels. These more stable and applicable DDS were characterized by SEM (Figure 3). Whereas obtained bolalipid aerogels retained a porous appearance (Figure 3a,b), the HEC 300 formulation displayed a compact appearance

(Figure 3c). Due to the porous structures of the bolalipid aerogels, they were able to reform hydrogels in situ after addition of liquid.

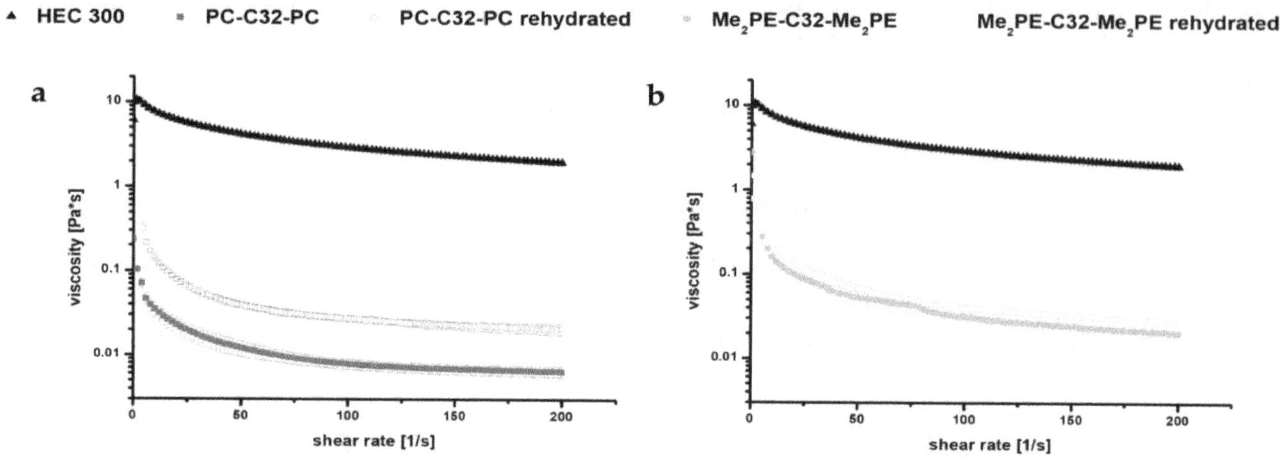

Figure 2. Rheological measurements of 5 mg/mL (**a**) PC-C32-PC and (**b**) Me_2PE-C32-Me_2PE bolalipid hydrogels and rehydrated aerogels, respectively, compared to HEC 300 hydrogels.

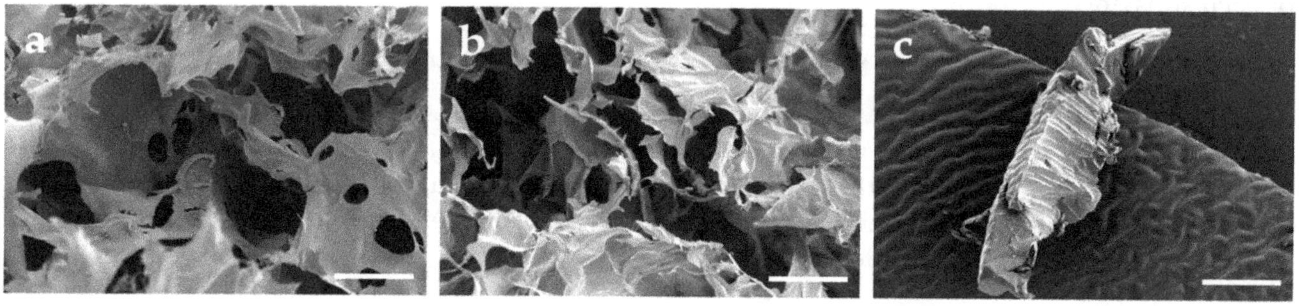

Figure 3. SEM images of (**a**) PC-C32-PC aerogel, (**b**) Me_2PE-C32-Me_2PE aerogel, and (**c**) freeze-dried HEC 300 hydrogel. Scale bar represents 100 μm.

The rheological behavior of rehydrated bolalipid aerogels was compared with the rheological properties of the bolalipid hydrogels. Obtained data indicate a slightly different behavior of rehydrated PC-C32-PC aerogel compared to its hydrogel. The rehydrated aerogel displayed a low increase of viscosity. In the case of Me_2PE-C32-Me_2PE, the rehydrated aerogel showed nearly the same rheological characteristics as compared to its hydrogel (see Figure 2).

3.2. Release Studies

A suitable and controlled drug release is an essential part of a DDS. The drug release rate depends on several factors, e.g., application site, porosity and degradation of DDS as well as exposed surface area. The ability of hydrogel systems to release incorporated substances has been extensively reported and mathematically described in the last years [51–53]. Recent research suggests three types of release: diffusion-controlled, chemically-controlled or swelling-controlled. However, all systems are mainly based on the diffusion of the therapeutic agent out of the bulk system. Furthermore, the phenomenon of diffusion is closely connected to the structure of the material through which the diffusion takes place [12].

In the present study, MB was used as a model drug. MB has several indications in medicine; it has been used to treat methemoglobinemia, malaria and urinary tract infections. During the last two decades, MB has attracted interest as a photosensitizer especially in cancer research [35,36,54]. Recently, MB has become increasingly important in antimicrobial studies [54,55]. An amount of 3.8 mg/mL of MB was distributed in the hydrogels. The results of the release studies are plotted in Figure 4.

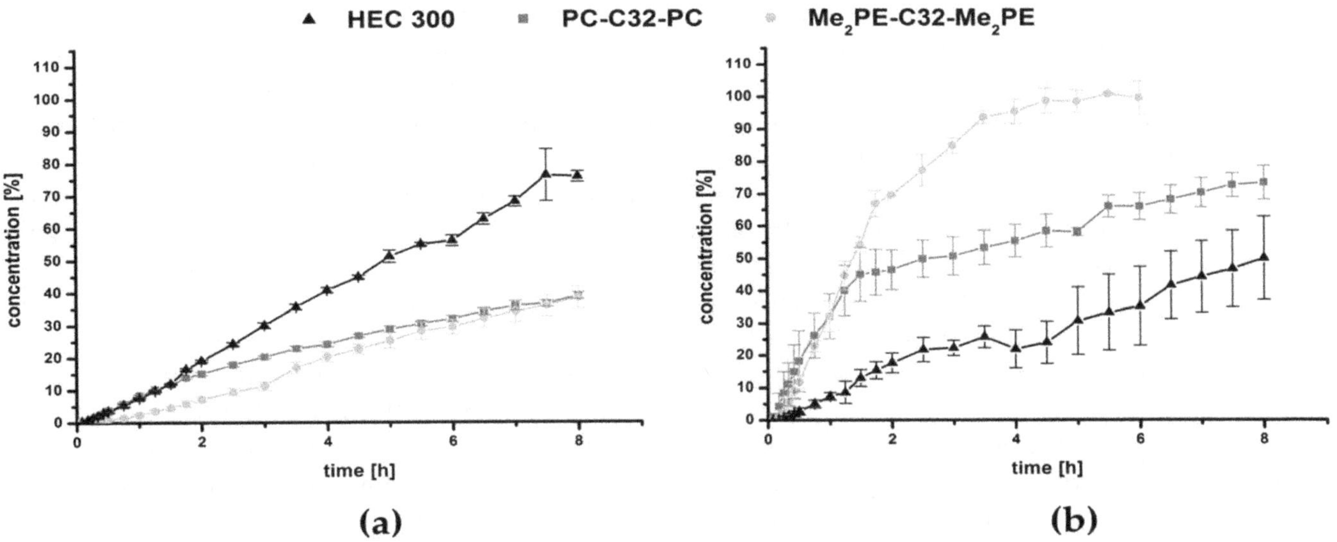

Figure 4. Drug release of (**a**) hydrogels and (**b**) aerogels using PC-C32-PC, Me_2PE-C32-Me_2PE and HEC 300, respectively.

Over the time period of 8 h, both bolalipid hydrogels released less than 40% of MB, while the reference with the same amount of gelling agent HEC 300 released approximately 75% (Figure 4a). This property could be explained by the structure of the bolalipid hydrogel: The hydrogel is formed due to the entanglement of nanofibers built up by the bolalipids [28,29]. Within these nanofibers, the bolalipid molecules are arranged side-by-side but twisted relative to each other due to the bulky PC or Me_2PE headgroup compared to the small cross-sectional area of one single alkyl chain. This twist leads to a helical superstructure of the nanofibers with hydrophobic grooves that are exposed to the surrounding water [56]. Hydrophobic and amphiphilic substances can now interact with these grooves, which was previously shown for cholesterol [57], phospholipids such as dipalmitoylphosphatidylcholine [58], and the fluorescence probe bis-ANS [59]. It is therefore conceivable that also MB, carrying a phenothiazine core, interacts with these hydrophobic grooves of the bolalipid nanofibers. In contrast, HEC 300 is a nonionic and hydrophilic gelling agent, which is not able to form hydrophobic interactions. Hence, the release of MB is lower and slower when bolalipid hydrogels are compared to the HEC 300 hydrogel. Comparing both bolalipids, the release of Me_2PE-C32-Me_2PE was slightly lower than those of PC-C32-PC. This is due to the ability of Me_2PE-C32-Me_2PE to form additional hydrogen bond to MB, using the proton at the quarternary amine, which is absent in PC-C32-PC bolalipid.

The release profile changed dramatically after the lyophilization process. In Figure 4b, the results showed a burst release of all bolalipid aerogels in contrast to the freeze-dried HEC 300, which displayed approximately a linear release rate. Within the first 1.5 h, the release rate of both bolalipid aerogels presented nearly the same behavior because it was mainly controlled by the fast diffusion of the MB out of the bolalipid aerogel framework. The water influx into the aerogels led to the formation of hydrogels. For PC-C32-PC, this re-forming could be observed within a few hours; whereas in the case of Me_2PE-C32-Me_2PE aerogels, it took several days to transform to a hydrogel again. The release from the PC-C32-PC aerogel seemed to be swelling-controlled after 1.5 h. For the Me_2PE-C32-Me_2PE aerogel, the release remained very fast after 1.5 h, indicating a rapid diffusion of the drug out of the aerogel. Comparing both bolalipid aerogels with lyophilized HEC 300, a higher amount of released MB was measured. Since the release rate from aerogels is determined by several factors, such as the interaction of MB with the gelling agent in the dry state and the velocity of the water influx into the aerogel (and the re-formation of the hydrogel), an interpretation of the data is difficult. Nevertheless, to explain this release behavior, the following scenario is conceivable. As mentioned before, hydrophobic interactions between MB and the hydrophobic grooves of the bolalipid nanofibers led to the slow release of MB from the bolalipid hydrogels. These hydrophobic interactions consist of an enthalpic contribution (van-der-Waals interactions) and an entropic contribution, i.e., the release of bound water molecules. In the case of an aerogel, the entropic contributions to the hydrophobic interactions are missing, since no water is present in the aerogel. Hence, the remaining van-der-Waals interactions between MB and the bolalipid aerogel are much weaker compared to the hydrogen bond interactions between MB and the HEC 300 aerogel, leading to a faster release of MB from the bolalipid aerogels. The higher release rate from Me_2PE-C32-Me_2PE aerogel compared to the PC-C32-PC counterpart could be explained by the slower influx of water. Furthermore, the structure of the obtained bolalipid aerogels was completely different when compared to the lyophilized HEC 300 hydrogel. Both bolalipid aerogels showed a high number of pores (Figure 3a,b) whereas no pores could be found in the HEC 300 sample (Figure 3c), which led to higher exposed area of the aerogel framework to the surrounding medium. This could explain the different release behaviors of the freeze-dried systems. Additionally, the different sizes of the error bars plotted in the graphs (Figure 4) could be elucidated with the fact that the drug release rate is strongly dependent on the exposed area of the DDS to the acceptor medium: Hydrogels are viscous and hence spread quickly over the entire area of the donor chamber, whereas the aerogels change their contact area quite slowly and differently for each sample leading to larger error bars.

3.3. *Microbiology*

Antimicrobial resistance is not a new phenomenon, but the impact of antibiotics to kill bacteria efficiently has dramatically decreased during the last years [60,61]. The ability of bacteria to develop appropriate resistance against a high amount of antibiotics in short time led to challenges in antimicrobial therapy. An antimicrobial activity of the DDS itself, would offer huge benefits. We investigated the ability of both bolalipids to inhibit the growth of fungi as well as bacteria, using different methods.

3.3.1. Antifungal Activity of PC-C32-PC and Me_2PE-C32-Me_2PE Hydro- or Aerogels

Previous studies have shown that PC-C22-PC (Irlbacholine), a bolalipid with shorter alkyl chain, which can be found in *Irlbachia alata* and *Anthocleista djalonensis*, is effective against the fungus *Trichophyton rubrum* and other fungal infections [62,63]. To investigate the antifungal activity of both bolalipid hydro- and aerogels, the agar diffusion test [37,38] was performed. *Saccharomyces cerevisiae* was used as model yeast. To compare the ability of the formulations to inhibit the growth of the model yeast, aerogels as well as hydrogels (75 μL) were applied on inoculated agar plates. After 24 h, fungal growth on the agar plate was observed. While PC-C32-PC hydrogel spread out to a broad shape (Figure 5a1), Me_2PE-C32-Me_2PE hydrogel retained more or less its original form (Figure 5a2). Comparing the aerogel-formulations of both lipids, in the case of the PC-C32-PC, a fast rehydration to hydrogel took place (Figure 5b1), whereas the Me_2PE-C32-Me_2PE aerogel was not able to reform hydrogel during the incubation time. However, in all cases, the inhibition zone was not evident. This indicates that the examined bolalipids itself did not possess any antifungal activity.

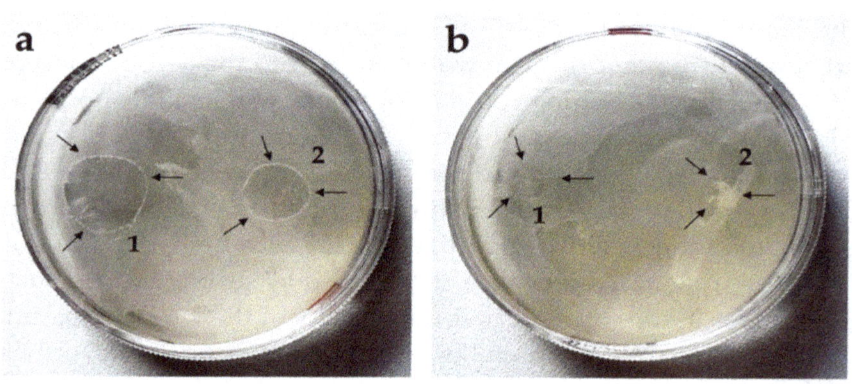

Figure 5. Agar diffusion test on *Saccharomyces cerevisiae*. Arrows indicate the bolalipid (**a**) hydrogels and (**b**) aerogels of (1) PC-C32-PC and (2) Me_2PE-C32-Me_2PE.

3.3.2. Antifungal Activity of Loaded PC-C32-PC and Me_2PE-C32-Me_2PE Aerogels by Means of PDT

Superficial skin mycosis is one of the most frequent diseases in human beings which is mainly caused by dermatophytes which exhibit increasing rates of resistant strains [5,6]. The appearance of drug resistant strains is more and more frequent in immunocompromised individuals such as high-risk groups, e.g., HIV+ and cancer patients undergoing chemotherapy [5]. In dermatology, PDT has proven to be a useful treatment for a variety of selected inflammatory diseases [3,5] as well as fungal infections [6]. Previous studies demonstrated that *Candida albicans* and dermatophytes were effectively killed by MB solution in combination with light. *Saccharomyces cerevisiae* was chosen as model yeast to investigate the antifungal activity of both bolalipid aerogels. The results are summarized in Table 1. Non-irradiated methylene blue released from the aerogels did not affect the growth of the yeast significantly. Irradiation resulted in an occurrence of a characteristic area with absence of yeast growth. Yeasts incubated with unloaded aerogels showed natural growth regardless of irradiation (Supplementary Figure S1).

Table 1. Results of size measurements of the inhibition zones in mm (mean value).

Bolalipid	Sample	Non-Irradiated [mm]	Irradiated [mm]
PC-C32-PC	aerogel	4.5	4.7
	aerogel containing MB	5.3	13.7
Me_2PE-C32-Me_2PE	aerogel	4.0	4.7
	aerogel containing MB	6.7	15.3

3.3.3. aPDT with PC-C32-PC and Me_2PE-C32-Me_2PE Aerogels Containing Methylene Blue

As reported previously, *Staphylococcus aureus* is almost the universal cause of furuncles, carbuncles and skin abscesses and are worldwide the most commonly identified agent responsible for skin and soft tissue infection [64]. Earlier studies have shown that MB in combination with light reduced bacterial growth. In some clinical cases, an effective PDT using MB as a photosensitizer for skin ulcers could be demonstrated. This kind of therapy led to clinical and microbial cure with no significant adverse effects [54]. According to the data obtained from release studies and the antifungal activity tests, we decided to use only bolalipid aerogels loaded with MB for the aPDT experiment. Based on the data of Tardivo et al. the fluence was set to 26.88 J/cm^2 [35].

From the results (Figure 6) it is clearly evident that MB affected the growth of *Staphylococcus aureus*. In the case of non-irradiated agar plates (Figure 6a1,b1), the zone with absence of bacterial growth occurred in the immediate surrounding of the aerogel. In the case of irradiated plates, more extensive effect was observed (Figure 6a2,b2). As expected, bacteria incubated with unloaded aerogels exhibited normal growth regardless of irradiation, thus demonstrating that light source alone had no toxic effect (Supplementary Figure S2). Comparing the size of the inhibition zone of both irradiated bolalipids, Me_2PE-C32-Me_2PE demonstrated a slightly larger zone of inhibition to that of PC-C32-PC, which could be explained by the release profile of the bolalipid aerogels (Figure 4b). As mentioned before, Me_2PE-C32-Me_2PE showed a higher burst release comparing to PC-C32-PC. During the incubation time of 3 h, more MB was released out of the Me_2PE-C32-Me_2PE aerogel resulting in a higher aPDT effect.

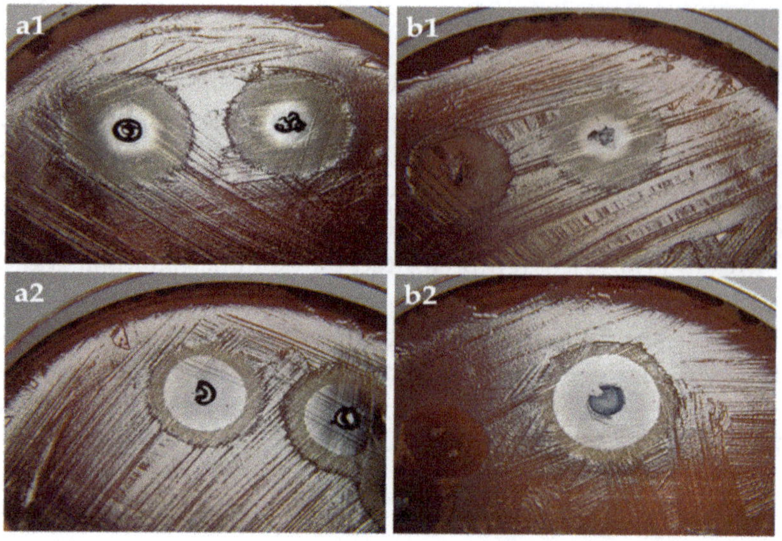

Figure 6. (**a**) PC-C32-PC and (**b**) Me_2PE-C32-Me_2PE aerogel containing MB on *Staphylococcus aureus*. (1) non-irradiated and (2) irradiated samples. The size of the inhibition zones of irradiated samples ranged between 13 mm and 17 mm.

3.4. *Biocompatibility*

As mentioned before, aPDT is well suitable for the treatment of skin, soft tissue and mucosal infections [3,7]. Therefore, DDS used for aPDT should exhibit a favorable biocompatibility. Preclinical assays applying mammalian models are still time-consuming and controversial [65]. Conventional in vivo tests are time- and labor-intensive as well as expensive. The CAM model allows an uncomplicated, economical and fast procedure with results comparable to mammalian models [66].

3.4.1. HET-CAM of Bolalipid Hydrogels

Mucosa compatibility study of hydrogels was performed using HET-CAM test [67], which replaced the Draize rabbit eye test [68]. During the experiment, the occurrence of hemorrhage, coagulation and lysis was monitored, and the irritation scores (IS) were determined. The results of HET-CAM assay, shown in Figure 7 indicated no irritation potential of PC-C32-PC and Me_2PE-C32-Me_2PE, respectively. During the treatment with 1% (*w*/*w*) SDS solution (positive control; Figure 7a), CAM displayed multiple injuries resulting in an IS of 18.7 in average corresponding to "strong irritation assessment". In contrast, an IS of 0 for each egg treated with both bolalipid hydrogels (Figure 7c,d) as well as physiological saline solution (negative control; Figure 7b), indicated "practically no" irritation assessment [69].

The PC-C32-PC bola lipid showed a remarkable characteristic on CAM surface: With progressing time, an increased rigidity of the applied dispersion was observed, which resulted in white streaks and opalescence as shown in Figure 7c2. This characteristic did not influence the vessels on the CAM surface. During the observation time of 5 min, this behavior did not occur in the case of the Me_2PE-C32-Me_2PE bolalipid.

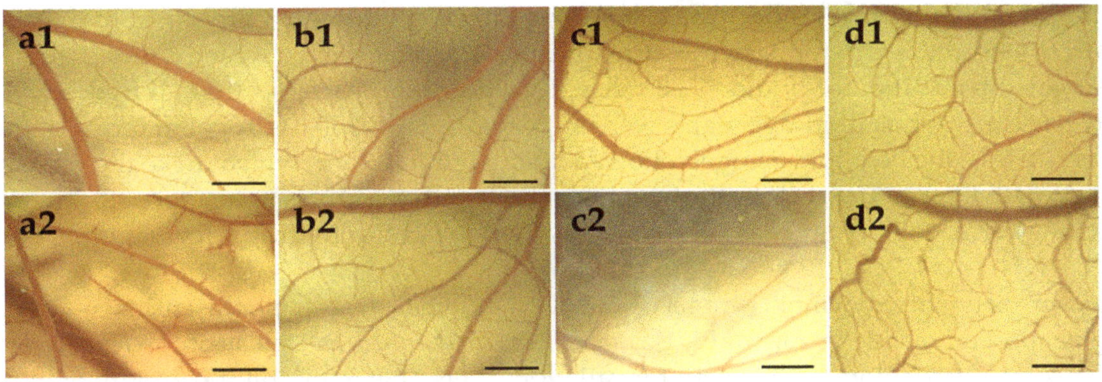

Figure 7. Stereomicroscopic images of chorioallantoic membrane (CAM) on egg development day (EDD) 10 (1) before and (2) 5 min after the treatment with (**a**) 1% (*w*/*w*) sodium dodecyl sulfate (SDS) solution, (**b**) physiological saline solution, (**c**) PC-C32-PC hydrogel and (**d**) Me_2PE-C32-Me_2PE hydrogel. Scale bar represents 1 mm.

3.4.2. HET-CAM of Bolalipid Aerogels

Biocompatibility of bolalipid aerogels was investigated in long-term CAM assay. Beginning with EDD 9, the occurrence of hemorrhage, lysis, coagulation or angiogenesis was monitored daily until EDD 14. During the rehydration process of bolalipid aerogels, and the thereto related osmotic suction, micro vessels in the capillary plexus could be damaged.

As shown in Figure 8, both bolalipid aerogels showed no irritation. It is clearly visible that PC-C32-PC aerogel rehydrated to hydrogel immediately after the placement on the CAM surface, while Me_2PE-C32-Me_2PE aerogels needed several days. The gelation process is indicated by arrows in Figure 8: It began from the border of bolalipid aerogels and progressed to the center of it. The different gelation processes of both bolalipids could be explained again with the chemical structure of PC-C32-PC and Me_2PE-C32-Me_2PE. As assumed before, due to hydrogen bond mediated stabilization of the head groups in the Me_2PE-C32-Me_2PE bolalipid aerogel, less hydrogen bonds can be assembled to the surrounding fluid.

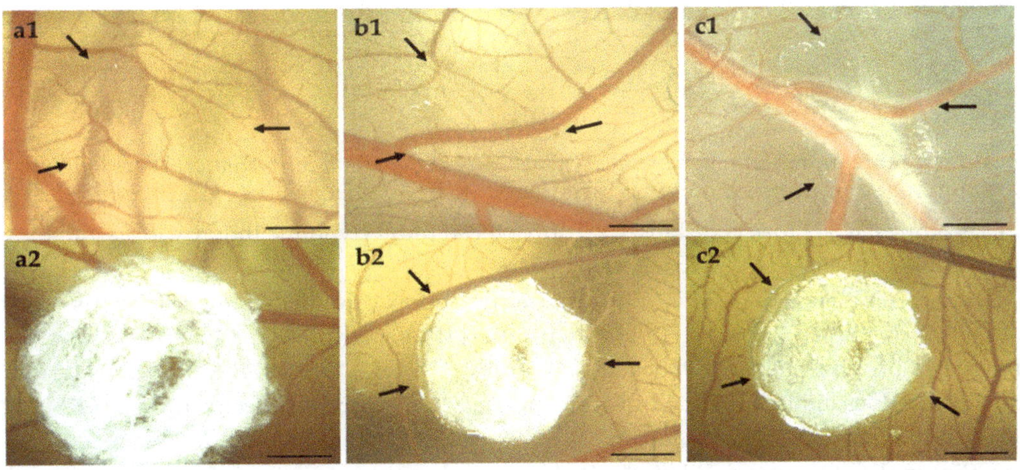

Figure 8. Stereomicroscopic images of CAM on (**a**) EDD 9, (**b**) EDD 12, and (**c**) EDD 14. The arrows indicate hydrogel formation of (1) PC-C32-PC aerogel and (2) Me_2PE-C32-Me_2PE aerogel. Scale bar represents 1 mm.

4. Conclusions

The aim of the study was to create stable formulation of both bolalipids and to investigate their suitability as a novel material for a drug delivery system (DDS). It was detectable that the stability of the self-assembled hydrogels decreased with minimal shear forces. With the help of sublimation in a conventional freeze-drier, it was possible to create stable aerogels, which could be transformed into hydrogels by addition of liquid. The release studies demonstrated that all hydrogels showed sustained release, but bolalipid hydrogels were superior to HEC 300 hydrogel in terms of the release time. Nevertheless, the bolalipid aerogels showed a high burst release, which make them unsuitable as DDS in their native form. Combining the benefits of both systems seems to be more effective. Aerogels possess a long-term stability and easy-to-handle system for in situ hydrogel formation.

However, using these bolalipid aerogels that have methylene blue—a photosensitizer—incorporated, antimicrobial photodynamic therapy (aPDT) of *Staphylococcus aureus* as well as of *Saccharomyces cerevisiae* could be successfully demonstrated. Both formulations were able to inhibit the growth of bacteria and yeast. However, the treatment with light using the custom designed LED device led to an additional antimicrobial effect of bolalipid aerogels.

In the biocompatibility studies on the chorioallantoic membrane (CAM) surface, both bolalipid formulations showed an excellent biocompatibility and thus making them a potential material for DDS. Furthermore, in the biocompatibility studies on CAM surface of the hydrogels, it was clearly evident that both bolalipid hydrogels, especially PC-C32-PC, show a high solidification capacity under body temperature conditions.

These results make the PC-C32-PC and Me_2PE-C32-Me_2PE bolalipids an interesting novel material for DDS with a potential for the application in aPDT for the treatment of skin and mucosal infections.

Author Contributions: Conceptualization: J.J., U.B.; Methodology: N.G., S.D.; Investigations: N.G., J.J., M.W., J.B.; Writing—original draft: N.G., J.J., J.B.; Resources: U.B.; Writing—review and editing: S.D., S.R.P. All authors agree with the final version of the manuscript. The authors declare that the content of this paper has not been published or submitted for publication elsewhere.

Acknowledgments: The authors would like to express their gratitude towards Erika Czyžová and Jan Němec (Department of Microbiology, Nemocnice Šumperk, Czech Republic) for their outstanding support and technical assistance as well as Lumundus GmbH (Eisenach, Germany) for the development of the customer designed LED device used in this study.

References

1. World Health Organization. *Antimicrobial Resistance: Global Report on Surveillance*; World Health Organization: Geneva, Switzerland, 2014.
2. Maisch, T.; Szeimies, R.M.; Jori, G.; Abels, C. Antibacterial photodynamic therapy in dermatology. *Photochem. Photobiol. Sci.* **2004**, *10*, 907–917. [CrossRef] [PubMed]
3. Dai, T.; Huang, Y.Y.; Hamblin, M.R. Photodynamic therapy for localized infections—State of the art. *Photodiagn. Photodyn. Ther.* **2009**, *6*, 170–188. [CrossRef] [PubMed]
4. Wainwright, M.; Phoenix, D.A.; Laycock, S.L.; Wareing, D.R.A.; Wright, P.A. Photobactericidal activity of phenothiazinium dyes against methicillin-resistant strains of Staphylococcus aureus. *FEMS Microbiol. Lett.* **1998**, *160*, 177–181. [CrossRef] [PubMed]
5. Calzavara-Pinton, P.G.; Venturini, M.; Sala, R. A comprehensive overview of photodynamic therapy in the treatment of superficial fungal infections of the skin. *J. Photochem. Photobiol. B Biol.* **2005**, *78*, 1–6. [CrossRef] [PubMed]
6. Baltazar, L.M.; Ray, A.; Santos, D.A.; Cisalpino, P.S.; Friedman, A.J.; Nosanchuk, J.D. Antimicrobial photodynamic therapy: An effective alternative approach to control fungal infections. *Front. Microbiol.* **2015**, *6*, 202. [CrossRef] [PubMed]

7. Akilov, O.E.; Kosaka, S.; O'Riordan, K.; Hasan, T. Photodynamic therapy for cutaneous leishmaniasis: The effectiveness of topical phenothiaziniums in parasite eradication and Th1 immune response stimulation. *Photochem. Photobiol. Sci.* **2007**, *6*, 1067–1075. [CrossRef]
8. Lin, C.C.; Metters, A.T. controlled release formulations: Network design and mathematical modeling. *Adv. Drug Deliv. Rev.* **2006**, *58*, 1379–1408. [CrossRef]
9. Caló, E.; Khutoryanskiy, V.V. Biomedical applications of hydrogels: A review of patents and commercial products. *Eur. Polym. J.* **2015**, *65*, 252–267. [CrossRef]
10. Boateng, J.S.; Matthews, K.H.; Stevens, H.N.; Eccleston, G.M. Wound healing dressings and drug delivery systems: A review. *J. Pharm. Sci.* **2008**, *97*, 2892–2923. [CrossRef]
11. Ullah, F.; Othman, M.B.H.; Javed, F.; Ahmad, Z.; Akil, H.M. Classification, processing and application of hydrogels: A review. *Mater. Sci. Eng. C* **2015**, *57*, 414–433. [CrossRef]
12. Peppas, N.A.; Bures, P.; Leobandung, W.; Ichikawa, H. Hydrogels in pharmaceutical formulations. *Eur. J. Pharm. Biopharm.* **2000**, *50*, 27–46. [CrossRef]
13. Bhattacharya, S.; Acharya, S.G. Impressive gelation in organic solvents by synthetic, low molecular mass, self-organizing urethane amides of L-phenylalanine. *Chem. Mater.* **1999**, *11*, 3121–3132. [CrossRef]
14. Fuhrhop, J.H.; Wang, T. Bolaamphiphiles. *Chem. Rev.* **2004**, *104*, 2901–2938. [CrossRef] [PubMed]
15. Nuraje, N.; Bai, H.; Su, K. Bolaamphiphilic molecules: Assembly and applications. *Prog. Polym. Sci.* **2013**, *38*, 302–343. [CrossRef]
16. Graf, G.; Drescher, S.; Meister, A.; Garamus, V.M.; Dobner, B.; Blume, A. Tuning the aggregation behaviour of single-chain bolaamphiphiles in aqueous suspension by changes in headgroup asymmetry. *Soft Matter* **2013**, *9*, 9562–9571. [CrossRef] [PubMed]
17. Drescher, S.; Lechner, B.D.; Garamus, V.M.; Almásy, L.; Meister, A.; Blume, A. The headgroup (a) symmetry strongly determines the aggregation behavior of single-chain phenylene-modified bolalipids and their miscibility with classical phospholipids. *Langmuir* **2014**, *30*, 9273–9284. [CrossRef] [PubMed]
18. Markowski, T.; Drescher, S.; Förster, G.; Lechner, B.D.; Meister, A.; Blume, A.; Dobner, B. Highly asymmetrical glycerol diether bolalipids: Synthesis and temperature-dependent aggregation behavior. *Langmuir* **2015**, *31*, 10683–10692. [CrossRef] [PubMed]
19. Gulik, A.; Luzzati, V.; De Rosa, M.; Gambacorta, A. Structure and polymorphism of bipolar isopranyl ether lipids from archaebacteria. *J. Mol. Biol.* **1985**, *182*, 131–149. [CrossRef]
20. Woese, C.R. Bacterial evolution. *Microbiol. Rev.* **1987**, *51*, 221.
21. Mahmoud, G.; Jedelská, J.; Strehlow, B.; Bakowsky, U. ether lipids derived from thermoacidophilic archaeon Sulfolobus acidocaldarius for membrane stabilization of chlorin e6 based liposomes for photodynamic therapy. *Eur. J. Pharm. Biopharm.* **2015**, *95*, 88–98. [CrossRef]
22. Engelhardt, K.H.; Pinnapireddy, S.R.; Baghdan, E.; Jedelská, J.; Bakowsky, U. Transfection studies with colloidal systems containing highly purified bipolar tetraether lipids from *Sulfolobus acidocaldarius*. *Archaea* **2017**, *2017*, 12. [CrossRef] [PubMed]
23. Mahmoud, G.; Jedelská, J.; Strehlow, B.; Omar, S.; Schneider, M.; Bakowsky, U. Photo-responsive tetraether lipids based vesicles for prophyrin mediated vascular targeting and direct phototherapy. *Colloids Surf. B Biointerfaces* **2017**, *159*, 720–728. [CrossRef] [PubMed]
24. Plenagl, N.; Duse, L.; Seitz, B.S.; Goergen, N.; Pinnapireddy, S.R.; Jedelska, J.; Brüßler, J.; Bakowsky, U. Photodynamic therapy–hypericin tetraether liposome conjugates and their antitumor and antiangiogenic activity. *Drug Deliv.* **2019**, *26*, 23–33. [CrossRef] [PubMed]
25. Plenagl, N.; Seitz, B.S.; Reddy Pinnapireddy, S.; Jedelská, J.; Brüßler, J.; Bakowsky, U. Hypericin loaded liposomes for anti-microbial photodynamic therapy of gram-positive bacteria. *Phys. Status Solidi A* **2018**, *215*, 1700837. [CrossRef]
26. Jacquemet, A.; Barbeau, J.; Lemiègre, L.; Benvegnu, T. Archaeal tetraether bipolar lipids: Structures, functions and applications. *Biochimie* **2009**, *91*, 711–717. [CrossRef] [PubMed]
27. De Rosa, M.; Gambacorta, A. The lipids of archaebacteria. *Progr. Lipid Res.* **1988**, *27*, 153–175. [CrossRef]
28. Köhler, K.; Förster, G.; Hauser, A.; Dobner, B.; Heiser, U.F.; Ziethe, F.; Blume, A. Self-assembly in a bipolar phosphocholine–water system: The formation of nanofibers and hydrogels. *Angewandte Chem. Int. Ed.* **2004**, *43*, 245–247. [CrossRef]

29. Köhler, K.; Förster, G.; Hauser, A.; Dobner, B.; Heiser, U.F.; Ziethe, F.; Richter, W.; Steiniger, F.; Drechsler, M.; Stettin, H.; et al. Temperature-dependent behavior of a symmetric long-chain bolaamphiphile with phosphocholine headgroups in water: From hydrogel to nanoparticles. *J. Am. Chem. Soc.* **2004**, *126*, 16804–16813. [CrossRef]
30. Köhler, K.; Meister, A.; Förster, G.; Dobner, B.; Drescher, S.; Ziethe, F.; Richter, W.; Steiniger, F.; Drechsler, M.; Hause, G.; et al. Conformational and thermal behavior of a pH-sensitive bolaform hydrogelator. *Soft Matter* **2006**, *2*, 77–86. [CrossRef]
31. Graf, G.; Drescher, S.; Meister, A.; Dobner, B.; Blume, A. Self-assembled bolaamphiphile fibers have intermediate properties between crystalline nanofibers and wormlike micelles: Formation of viscoelastic hydrogels switchable by changes in pH and salinity. *J. Phys. Chem. B* **2011**, *115*, 10478–10487. [CrossRef]
32. Meister, A.; Bastrop, M.; Koschoreck, S.; Garamus, V.M.; Sinemus, T.; Hempel, G.; Drescher, S.; Dobner, B.; Richtering, W.; Huber, K.; et al. Structure-property relationship in stimulus-responsive bolaamphiphile hydrogels. *Langmuir* **2007**, *23*, 7715–7723. [CrossRef]
33. Tatsuta, M.; Okuda, S.; Tamura, H.; Taniguchi, H. Endoscopic diagnosis of early gastric cancer by the endoscopic congo red-methylene blue test. *Cancer* **1982**, *50*, 2956–2960. [CrossRef]
34. Wainwright, M.; Crossley, K.B. Methylene blue-a therapeutic dye for all seasons? *J. Chemother.* **2002**, *14*, 431–443. [CrossRef] [PubMed]
35. Tardivo, J.P.; Del Giglio, A.; de Oliveira, C.S.; Gabrielli, D.S.; Junqueira, H.C.; Tada, D.B.; Severino, D.; Baptista, M.S. Methylene blue in photodynamic therapy: From basic mechanisms to clinical applications. *Photodiagn. Photodyn. Ther.* **2005**, *2*, 175–191. [CrossRef]
36. Koch, W.H.; Bass, G.E. Sodium azide affects methylene blue concentration in Salmonella typhimurium and Saccharomyces cerevisiae. *Photochem. Photobiol.* **1984**, *39*, 841–845. [CrossRef] [PubMed]
37. Balouiri, M.; Sadiki, M.; Ibnsouda, S.K. Methods for in vitro evaluating antimicrobial activity: A review. *J. Pharm. Anal.* **2016**, *6*, 71–79. [CrossRef]
38. Arikan, S.; Paetznick, V.; Rex, J.H. Comparative evaluation of disk diffusion with microdilution assay in susceptibility testing of caspofungin against Aspergillus and Fusarium isolates. *Antimicrob. Agents Chemother.* **2002**, *46*, 3084–3087. [CrossRef]
39. Ribatti, D.; Nico, B.; Vacca, A.; Roncali, L.; Burri, P.H.; Djonov, V. Chorioallantoic membrane capillary bed: A useful target for studying angiogenesis and anti-angiogenesis in vivo. *Anat. Rec. An Off. Publ. Am. Assoc. Anat.* **2001**, *264*, 317–324. [CrossRef]
40. Drescher, S.; Meister, A.; Blume, A.; Karlsson, G.; Almgren, M.; Dobner, B. General synthesis and aggregation behaviour of a series of single-chain 1, ω-Bis (phosphocholines). *Chem. A Eur. J.* **2007**, *13*, 5300–5307. [CrossRef]
41. Meister, A.; Drescher, S.; Garamus, V.M.; Karlsson, G.; Graf, G.; Dobner, B.; Blume, A. Temperature-dependent self-assembly and mixing behavior of symmetrical single-chain bolaamphiphiles. *Langmuir* **2008**, *24*, 6238–6246. [CrossRef]
42. Vögeling, H.; Duse, L.; Seitz, B.S.; Plenagl, N.; Wojcik, M.; Pinnapireddy, S.R.; Bakowsky, U. Multilayer bacteriostatic coating for surface modified titanium implants. *Phys. Stat. Solidi A* **2018**, *215*, 1700844. [CrossRef]
43. Pinnapireddy, S.R.; Duse, L.; Strehlow, B.; Schäfer, J.; Bakowsky, U. Composite liposome-PEI/nucleic acid lipopolyplexes for safe and efficient gene delivery and gene knockdown. *Colloids Surf. B Biointerfaces* **2017**, *158*, 93–101. [CrossRef] [PubMed]
44. Chanmugam, A.; Langemo, D.; Thomason, K.; Haan, J.; Altenburger, E.A.; Tippett, A.; Zortman, T.A. Relative temperature maximum in wound infection and inflammation as compared with a control subject using long-wave infrared thermography. *Adv. Skin Wound Care* **2017**, *30*, 406–414. [CrossRef] [PubMed]
45. Duse, L.; Pinnapireddy, S.R.; Strehlow, B.; Jedelská, J.; Bakowsky, U. Low level LED photodynamic therapy using curcumin loaded tetraether liposomes. *Eur. J. Pharm. Biopharm.* **2018**, *126*, 233–241. [CrossRef] [PubMed]
46. Tariq, I.; Pinnapireddy, S.R.; Duse, L.; Ali, M.Y.; Ali, S.; Amin, M.U.; Goergen, N.; Jedelská, J.; Bakowsky, U. Lipodendriplexes: A promising nanocarrier for enhanced gene delivery with minimal cytotoxicity. *Eur. J. Pharm. Biopharm.* **2019**, *135*, 72–82. [CrossRef] [PubMed]

47. Lüring, C.; Kalteis, T.; Wild, K.; Perlick, L.U.; Grifka, J. Gewebetoxizität lokaler Anästhetika im HET-CAM-Test. *Der Schmerz* **2003**, *17*, 185–190. [PubMed]
48. Hobzova, R.; Hampejsova, Z.; Cerna, T.; Hrabeta, J.; Venclikova, K.; Jedelska, J.; Bakowsky, U.; Bosakova, Z.; Lhotka, M.; Vaculin, S.; et al. Poly (d, l-lactide)/polyethylene glycol micro/nanofiber mats as paclitaxel-eluting carriers: Preparation and characterization of fibers, in vitro drug release, antiangiogenic activity and tumor recurrence prevention. *Mater. Sci. Eng. C* **2019**, *98*, 982–993. [CrossRef] [PubMed]
49. Ribatti, D.; Nico, B.; Vacca, A.; Presta, M. The gelatin sponge–chorioallantoic membrane assay. *Nat. Protoc.* **2006**, *1*, 85. [CrossRef]
50. Blume, A.; Drescher, S.; Meister, A.; Graf, G.; Dobner, B. Tuning the aggregation behaviour of single-chain bolaphospholipids in aqueous suspension: From nanoparticles to nanofibres to lamellar phases. *Faraday Discuss.* **2013**, *161*, 193–213. [CrossRef]
51. Dash, S.; Murthy, P.N.; Nath, L.; Chowdhury, P. Kinetic modeling on drug release from controlled drug delivery systems. *Acta Pol. Pharm* **2010**, *67*, 217–223.
52. Langer, R.; Peppas, N. Chemical and physical structure of polymers as carriers for controlled release of bioactive agents: A review. *J. Macromol. Sci. Rev. Macromol. Chem. Phys.* **1983**, *23*, 61–126. [CrossRef]
53. Amsden, B. Solute diffusion within hydrogels. Mechanisms and models. *Macromolecules* **1998**, *31*, 8382–8395. [CrossRef]
54. Aspiroz, C.; Sevil, M.; Toyas, C.; Gilaberte, Y. Photodynamic therapy with methylene blue for skin ulcers infected with *Pseudomonas aeruginosa* and *Fusarium* spp. *Actas Dermo Sifiliogr.* **2017**, *108*, e45–e48. [CrossRef] [PubMed]
55. Schick, E.; Riick, A.; Boehncke, W.H.; Kaufmann, R. Topical photodynamic therapy using methylene blue and 5-aminolaevulinic acid in psoriasis. *J. Derm. Treat.* **1997**, *8*, 17–19. [CrossRef]
56. Meister, A.; Drescher, S.; Mey, I.; Wahab, M.; Graf, G.; Garamus, V.M.; Blume, A. Helical nanofibers of self-assembled bipolar phospholipids as template for gold nanoparticles. *J. Phys. Chem. B* **2008**, *112*, 4506–4511. [CrossRef]
57. Blume, A.; Drescher, S.; Graf, G.; Koehler, K.; Meister, A. Self-assembly of different single-chain bolaphospholipids and their miscibility with phospholipids or classical amphiphiles. *Adv. Colloid Interface Sci.* **2014**, *208*, 264–278. [CrossRef] [PubMed]
58. Meister, A.; Köhler, K.; Drescher, S.; Dobner, B.; Karlsson, G.; Edwards, K.; Blume, A. Mixing behaviour of a symmetrical single-chain bolaamphiphile with phospholipids. *Soft Matter* **2007**, *3*, 1025–1031. [CrossRef]
59. Kordts, M.; Kerth, A.; Drescher, S.; Ott, M.; Blume, A. The cmc-value of a bolalipid with two phosphocholine headgroups and a C24 alkyl chain: Unusual binding properties of fluorescence probes to bolalipid aggregates. *J. Colloid Interface Sci.* **2017**, *501*, 294–303. [CrossRef]
60. Maisch, T. Resistance in antimicrobial photodynamic inactivation of bacteria. *Photochem. Photobiol. Sci.* **2015**, *14*, 1518–1526. [CrossRef]
61. Jindal, A.K.; Pandya, K.; Khan, I.D. Antimicrobial resistance: A public health challenge. *Med. J. Armed Forces India* **2015**, *71*, 178–181. [CrossRef]
62. Bierer, D.E.; Gerber, R.E.; Jolad, S.D.; Ubillas, R.P.; Randle, J.; Nauka, E.; Latour, J.; Dener, J.M.; Fort, D.M.; Kuo, J.E.; et al. Isolation, structure elucidation, and synthesis of irlbacholine, 1, 22-Bis [[[2-(trimethylammonium) ethoxy] phosphinyl] oxy] docosane: A novel antifungal plant metabolite from Irlbachia alata and Anthocleista djalonensis. *J. Org. Chem.* **1995**, *60*, 7022–7026. [CrossRef]
63. Lu, Q.; Ubillas, R.P.; Zhou, Y.; Dubenko, L.G.; Dener, J.M.; Litvak, J.; Phuan, P.-W.; Flores, M.; Ye, Z.; Gerber, E.; et al. Synthetic analogues of irlbacholine: A novel antifungal plant metabolite isolated from *Irlbachia alata*. *J. Nat. Prod.* **1999**, *62*, 824–828. [CrossRef] [PubMed]
64. McCaig, L.F.; Mc Donald, L.C.; Mandal, S.; Jernigan, D.B. *Staphylococcus aureus*-associated skin and soft tissue infections in ambulatory care. *Emerg. Infect. Dis.* **2006**, *12*, 1715–1723. [CrossRef] [PubMed]
65. Hendriksen, C.F. Replacement, reduction and refinement alternatives to animal use in vaccine potency measurement. *Expert Rev. Vaccines* **2009**, *8*, 313–322. [CrossRef] [PubMed]
66. Nowak-Sliwinska, P.; Segura, T.; Iruela-Arispe, M.L. The chicken chorioallantoic membrane model in biology, medicine and bioengineering. *Angiogenesis* **2014**, *17*, 779–804. [CrossRef] [PubMed]
67. Steiling, W.; Bracher, M.; Courtellemont, P.; De Silva, O. The HET–CAM, a useful in vitro assay for assessing the eye irritation properties of cosmetic formulations and ingredients. *Toxicol. In Vitro* **1999**, *13*, 375–384. [CrossRef]

68. Spielmann, H.; Kalweit, S.; Liebsch, M.; Wirnsberger, T.; Gerner, I.; Bertram-Neis, E.; Steiling, W. Validation study of alternatives to the Draize eye irritation test in Germany: Cytotoxicity testing and HET-CAM test with 136 industrial chemicals. *Toxicol. In Vitro* **1993**, *7*, 505–510. [CrossRef]
69. Luepke, N.P. Hen's egg chorioallantoic membrane test for irritation potential. *Food Chem. Toxicol.* **1985**, *23*, 287–291. [CrossRef]

12

Easy Synthesis and Characterization of Holmium-Doped SPIONs

Magdalena Osial, Paulina Rybicka, Marek Pękała, Grzegorz Cichowicz, Michał K. Cyrański and Paweł Krysiński *

Faculty of Chemistry, University of Warsaw, Pasteura 1 Street, 02-093 Warsaw, Poland; magdalena@osial.eu (M.O.); p.rybicka@student.uw.edu.pl (P.R.); pekala@chem.uw.edu.pl (M.P.); gcichowicz@chem.uw.edu.pl (G.C.); mkc@chem.uw.edu.pl (M.K.C.)
* Correspondence: pakrys@chem.uw.edu.pl;

Abstract: The exceptional magnetic properties of superparamagnetic iron oxide nanoparticles (SPIONs) make them promising materials for biomedical applications like hyperthermia, drug targeting and imaging. Easy preparation of SPIONs with the controllable, well-defined properties is a key factor of their practical application. In this work, we report a simple synthesis of Ho-doped SPIONs by the co-precipitation route, with controlled size, shape and magnetic properties. To investigate the influence of the ions ratio on the nanoparticles' properties, multiple techniques were used. Powder X-ray diffraction (PXRD) confirmed the crystallographic structure, indicating formation of an Fe_3O_4 core doped with holmium. In addition, transmission electron microscopy (TEM) confirmed the correlation of the crystallites' shape and size with the experimental conditions, pointing to critical holmium content around 5% for the preparation of uniformly shaped grains, while larger holmium content leads to uniaxial growth with a prism shape. Studies of the magnetic behaviour of nanoparticles show that magnetization varies with changes in the initial Ho^{3+} ions percentage during precipitation, while below 5% of Ho in doped Fe_3O_4 is relatively stable and sufficient for biomedicine applications. The characterization of prepared nanoparticles suggests that co-precipitation is a simple and efficient technique for the synthesis of superparamagnetic, Ho-doped SPIONs for hyperthermia application.

Keywords: superparamagnetic iron oxide nanoparticles; SPIONs; rare-earth doping; holmium; endoradiotherapy

---

1. Introduction

In recent years, magnetic nanoparticles like magnetite (Fe_3O_4) have allowed for significant progress in the field of drug delivery and cancer treatment [1,2]. Efforts focused on the rapid development and study of magnetic iron-oxide-based nanoparticles have drastically increased, especially in the case of their applications in oncology [3], where highly efficient carcinogenic cell destruction is needed.

Nanosized iron oxide exhibits a wide range of magnetic properties depending on the shape, size and chemical composition of the particles. Magnetite nanoparticles ranging from a few nanometers up to 100 nm are very attractive in a wide array of modern scientific fields, such as nanotechnology [4–6] biotechnology [7], MRI contrast agents [8], magnetic separation and immobilization [9] etc. These nanomaterials can also be effective for medical applications including bioimaging [10] and biosensing in diagnostics (theranostics) [11,12], controlled drug delivery and cancer therapeutics [13–16]. Several excellent reviews have been published on the synthesis, functionalization and application of magnetic nanoparticles [17,18].

Much of the literature focuses on the medical application of nanoparticles based on the superparamagnetic iron oxide nanoparticles SPIONs because of their easy synthesis, stability and biocompatibility [19–21]. Due to their biocompatibility, they are already used in clinical trials [22,23]. A very interesting prospect is to enhance their size-dependent properties like low toxicity, facile synthesis [24], surface-to-volume ratio, superparamagnetism [25,26] and affect the magnetic interactions through doping the core of nanoparticles with different metal ions. Usually transition metals are effective dopants, changing the magnetic properties of iron oxide nanoparticles [27,28]. Whilst doping of magnetite with lanthanides such as Ho, Gd, Tb, as well as other metals, e.g., Re, Y, is common and simple in principle, establishing the synthesis procedure with controlled shape, size and magnetic properties is difficult [10,15,16]. Lanthanide-doped nanoparticles can be directed to the tumour tissues with the help of an external magnet. Thus, they can serve not only as drug carriers in targeted drug delivery or magnetic hyperthermia, but also in so-called endoradiotherapy. The latter feature can be easily implemented by replacing the "cold" atoms of lanthanides in the superparamagnetic core with their "hot" nuclei, emitting soft β(-) radiation suitable for the internal radiotherapy, localized directly within the tumour. Thus, these nanoparticles can be used simultaneously in targeted drug delivery, hyperthermia and endoradiotherapy. Moreover, the amount of radionuclides per single nanoparticle greatly exceeds the amount of radionuclides per single molecule found in radiopharmaceuticals being currently used in radiotherapies. Therefore, such multifunctional nanoparticles may become indispensable in many areas of modern medicine. For that application the lanthanides of ionic radius matching the SPIONs crystal lattice and high magnetic moment have to be chosen. The spinel structure in magnetite-based nanoparticles of formula MFe_2O_4, where Fe^{3+} ions occupy octahedral sites [29] and divalent metal ions M such as Fe^{2+}, Ni^{2+}, etc. occupy the tetrahedral positions in the crystal [30], can be modified through the substitution of the Fe^{3+} with different trivalent ions. Substitution with ions with an ionic radius similar to Fe^{3+} (0.785 Å) [31] does not affect the magnetic behaviour of the doped SPIONs significantly, while the incorporation of lanthanide ions like Ho^{3+} (1.01 Å) [32] with a large radius, ca. 30% larger than Fe^{3+}, may lead to core anisotropy, crystallographic lattice alterations and a decrease in the magnetic properties due to the Fe(III) and Ho(III) ionic radii mismatch [33,34].

The influence of the incorporation of lanthanide ions into the core of SPIONs is still poorly understood. We are aware of the fact that the largest, octahedral site of the magnetite lattice can accommodate cations up to ca. 85–90 pm radius, and there is a large ionic radii mismatch for Ho^{3+} (104 pm) as compared to Fe^{3+} (78.5 pm) ions that are to be replaced in this lattice. However, the literature data [35] and our results for SPIONs modified with Tb (106 pm) [33] indicate that such replacement is possible, at least for terbium cations, requiring local lattice distortion and favouring incorporation of these ions into octahedral and surface sites. On the other hand, most ferrites are ferrimagnetic, i.e., part of magnetic moments of the constituent ions are antiparallel, partially compensating for the overall magnetic moment of SPIONs. Therefore, the introduction of lanthanide metal ions of different ionic radii than Fe^{3+} may alter the crystallographic structure, resulting in an increase of unpaired spins and enhancing the saturation magnetization. This behaviour would be very advantageous for a drug delivery system based on SPIONs.

Since the properties of magnetic nanoparticles are strongly related to their shape and size, various methods and synthetic conditions are directed towards control over their chemical composition, morphology of formed crystallites, degree of agglomeration and magnetic properties.

The literature refers to co-precipitation, the microemulsions polyol process, solvothermal and sonochemical techniques as suitable solutions for the preparation of iron-oxide-based nanoparticles dispersed in water [36–38]. Among the many SPIONs synthetic procedures, co-precipitation is a promising technique due to its simplicity and productivity. The conditions of synthesis like ion concentration, pH of the solution as well as duration of synthesis and heat treatment are crucial to determine the physicochemical properties of SPIONs.

In this paper, we report on the morphology and magnetic and structural properties of Ho-doped iron oxide magnetic nanoparticles synthesized by the co-precipitation method from a solution containing different molar concentrations of all ions forming the nanoparticle core. To avoid elimination by clearance organs, the hydrodynamic diameter of the nanoparticles should remain in the range of 10–100 nm [16]. Therefore, we focused on nanoparticles that were uniform in size, with a hydrodynamic diameter below 100 nm. Holmium dopant was chosen since it can be easily replaced by its ^{166}Ho radionuclide emitting β(-) "soft radiation suitable for targeted endoradiotherapy" and due to its high magnetic moment (~10.6 μ_B) [39], which is expected to enhance a magnetization of ferrites studied. On the other hand, the atomic size mismatch is found to distort the atomic lattice and weaken the magnetic properties.

2. Materials and Methods

Iron (II) chloride tetrahydrate $FeCl_2 \cdot 4H_2O$ puriss p.a. ≥99% (RT), iron (III) chloride hexahydrate $FeCl_3 \cdot 6H_2O$ Aldrich ACS reagent 97% were supplied from Sigma-Aldrich, Germany, holmium (III) chloride hexahydrate $HoCl_3 \cdot 6H_2O$ 99.9% trace metals was obtained from Sigma-Aldrich, 25% ammonia solution NH_4OH was supplied from CHEMPUR, Poland. All chemicals were of analytical grade standards and used as received. Deionized water with resistivity 18.2 MΩ cm at 25 °C was obtained using the Milli-Q ultra-pure water filtering system (Merck, Darmstadt, Germany). Successfully prepared SPIONs were modified with 3-phosphonopropionic acid obtained from Sigma-Aldrich with 94% grade acid with the use of analytical-grade NaOH from CHEMPUR, Poland.

SPIONs were synthesized by the co-precipitation technique in aqueous media containing different batches of ions having a molar percentage of Ho(III) vs. total iron content of 1%, 2.5%, 5%, 7.5% and 10%. The required amounts of salts were dissolved in a beaker to reach the complete dissolution of 87.5 mL solution with pH around 1.9 and molarity 0.1 M of the $FeCl_2 \cdot 4H_2O$, 0.1 M of the $FeCl_3 \cdot 6H_2O$ and $HoCl_3 \cdot 6H_2O$ in amounts from 1–10% instead of Fe^{3+} ions. The solution was stirred mechanically for 10 min at a rate of 500 rpm (chosen as the minimum to obtain a stable vortex), and after that the ammonia was added drop by drop to the solution, and stirred for an additional 30 min. During the addition of ammonia the solution turned black, indicating the formation of a suspension with nanoparticles (see Figure 1). The schematic reaction taking place during synthesis is presented as follows:

$$xFe^{3+} + (2-x)Ho^{3+} + Fe^{2+} + 8OH^- \rightarrow Ho_{(2-x)}Fe_xFeO_4 + 4H_2O.$$

After 30 min the beaker with suspension was left on the magnet for an additional 30 min for sedimentation, and suspended nanoparticles were washed with water and acetone alternatively to remove the residual NH_4OH and all unreacted compounds.

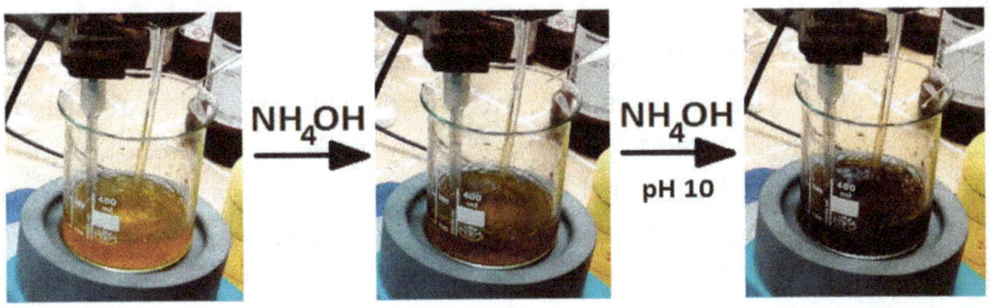

Figure 1. Image of the co-precipitation of Ho-doped ferrite nanoparticles under NH_3 addition.

Nanoparticles were stabilized with 3-phosphonopropionic acid (CEPA), where 20 mg of CEPA were used per 1 mg of nanoparticles. The SPIONs were suspended in water, and then a CEPA solution with a pH of ~5 (set by the addition of an appropriate amount of 0.1 M NaOH) was added dropwise with mechanical stirring. After CEPA addition into the SPIONs suspension, the solution was continuously stirred for the next 30 min and the suspension of nanoparticles stabilized with CEPA was washed several times with water to remove any unreacted products.

Transmission electron microscopy images were recorded using EF-TEM, Zeiss Libra 120 Plus, Stuttgart, Germany microscope operating at 120 kV. Samples were prepared from the sonicated aqueous suspensions and a drop was placed on the copper grid covered with formvar/carbon layer and dried in air. Dynamic light scattering (DLS) was used as a complementary technique to analyse the size of nanoparticles. Measurements were carried out with Malvern Instruments Zetasizer Nano ZS, Malvern, United Kingdom. The powder X-ray diffraction patterns were recorded with a powder diffraction X-ray diffractometer (PXRD) Bruker D8 Discover, Massachusets, USA operating with Debye–Scherrer geometry with Cu Kα radiation with line λ = 1.540598 Å and a scan rate of 1° per minute in 0.012° steps covering the 2θ angle range from 20° to 130°. Measurements were performed at RT. The X-ray photoelectron spectroscopy (XPS) measurements were performed using PHI 5000 VersaProbe (ULVAC-PHI) spectrometer, Gothenburg, Sweden with monochromatic Al Kα radiation (hν = 1486.6 eV) from X-ray source operating at 100 μm spot size, 25 W and 15 kV. XPS data were analysed with CasaXPS software ver. 2.3.16, Wimslow, United Kingdom. The binding energy values were calibrated and normalized to the C 1s peak at 284.8 eV. The magnetic behaviour of samples was verified with a QD vibrating sample magnetometer VSM over the magnetic field range from −2.0 T to +2.0 T in the temperature from 100 K to 300 K stabilized to accuracy of about 0.01 K. Magnetization and coercive fields were measured with accuracy better than 1%. Thermogravimetric analysis (TGA) was performed with TGA Q50 (TA Instruments), New Castle, USA, under nitrogen.

3. Results

SPIONs were synthesized through the co-precipitation method, which is a widely used technique for the preparation of SPIONs from aqueous solutions [40,41]. To verify how changes in the holmium doping affect the shape, size, crystallinity and magnetic properties of the synthesized SPIONs, multiple techniques were used. The magnetic properties of the superparamagnetic core are affected by size and shape. Smaller SPIONs with a high surface area to volume ratio yield smaller mass magnetization than larger SPIONs due to the increased contribution of the surface anisotropic layer decreasing the overall magnetization. This is usually explained in terms of a core-shell model, where the magnetically dead layer, strains and distortions at the surface are claimed to be responsible for the particle size effects [42]. Therefore, in order to elucidate only the effects of holmium doping on the magnetic behaviour of SPIONs, we have chosen a synthetic procedure yielding SPIONs of low size distributions and good crystallinity. The controlled size distribution is also beneficial from the point of view of their prospective medical applications, as discussed in Section 1.

3.1. Morphology Studies

The changes of morphology of SPIONs under Ho doping were studied with TEM. The images obtained by TEM reveal the differences in the morphology for nanoparticles with various concentrations of Ho^{3+} vs. Fe^{3+} used during the synthesis. The high level of aggregation observed on the presented images is caused by sample preparation for TEM analysis: the ethanol suspension is placed on the TEM grids and during the solvent evaporation the nanoparticles aggregate (the Marangoni effect). The literature attributes the dependence of morphology to the experimental conditions, indicating the formation of nanoparticles (SPIONs) having spherical [43], quasi-spherical [44], and even octahedral [45] shapes. As can be seen in Figure 2, the aggregates of undoped nanoparticles (a), doped with 1% (b), and 2.5% (c) of holmium have a spherical shape with an average diameter of about 10–15 mm, whereas higher doping results in an irregular axial growth of the crystals and an increase of the grain size up to 30–40 nm. Spherical particles, similar to pristine magnetite nanoparticles (Figure 2a), are formed when holmium doping does not exceed 2.5%, only slightly affecting the crystal structure of nanoferrites. Exceeding the critical value of the holmium dopant in the ferrite lattice stimulates the crystal growth in one direction. Particles shown in

Figure 2a,b appear to be monodispersed, and of similar morphology. Typical histogram exemplifying the size distribution of nanoparticles for Fe_3O_4@2.5%Ho, is shown in Figure 3, below.

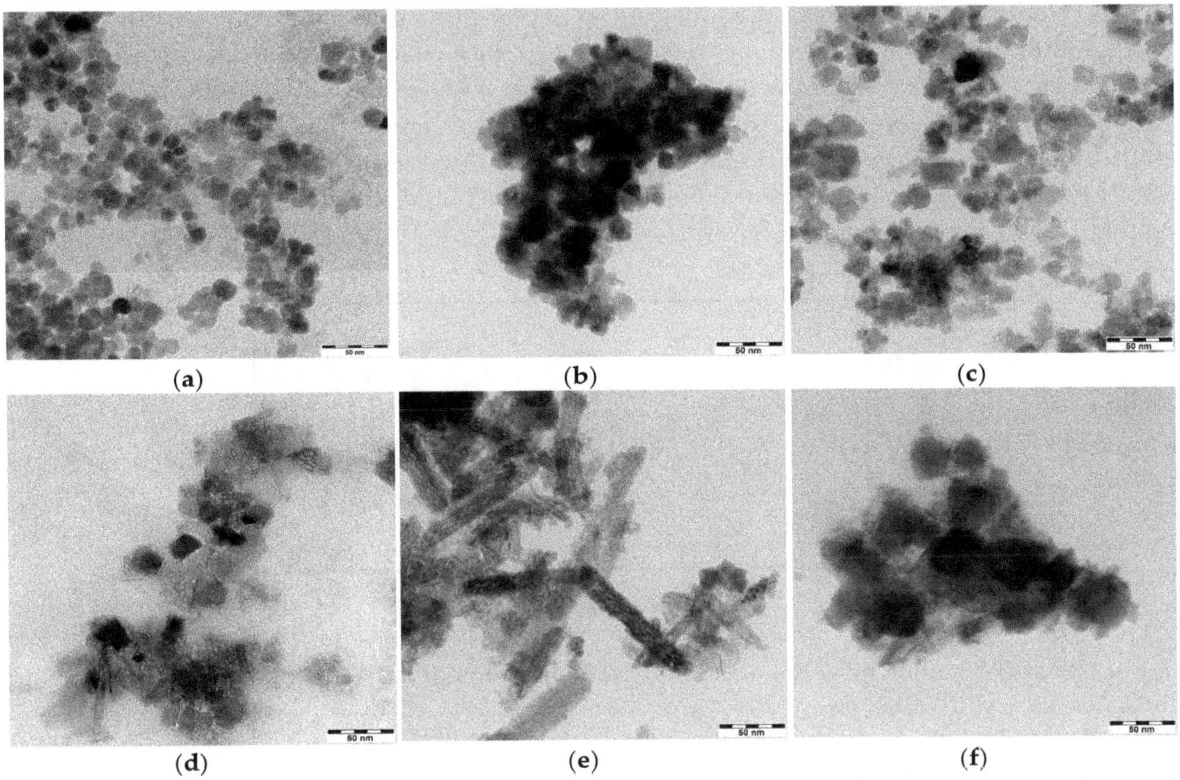

Figure 2. TEM images of (**a**) undoped iron oxide SPIONs, and doped with (**b**) 1%; (**c**) 2.5%; (**d**) 5%; (**e**) 7.5%; (**f**) 10% of holmium obtained by co-precipitation (scale bar: 50 nm).

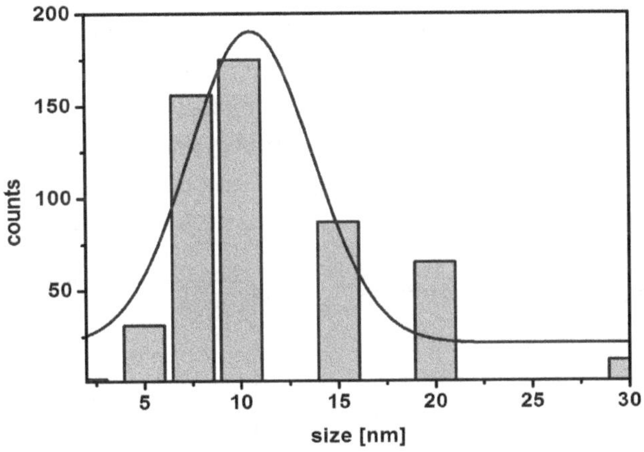

Figure 3. Histogram for Fe_3O_4@2.5%Ho.

3.2. Size Distribution and Zeta Potential Studies

The size distribution of all samples was also investigated by means of dynamic light scattering (DLS) in an aqueous dispersion. Likewise assessed from the TEM analysis, the size of the investigated SPIONs is similar; however, SPIONs are not stabilized with any organic shell, and therefore they tend to precipitate spontaneously within a few minutes. Therefore, we stabilized them with a CEPA shell.

As can be seen in Figure 4, the size of the unmodified SPIONs containing 2.5% of holmium is ca. 89 nm in diameter, while after modification of their surface with CEPA this value is lower by ca.

20 nm. A lower diameter of SPIONs covered with CEPA suggests that they are more dispersed than the unmodified ones. In comparison to the TEM analysis, the diameter value for uncovered SPIONs is higher because DLS reports the hydrodynamic diameter including the solvation shell of SPIONs agglomerate, whereas TEM images show only the solid core of nanoparticles. To confirm if unmodified SPIONs agglomerate, the zeta potential corresponding to the surface potential was measured. The zeta potential value for uncovered SPIONs suspended in water is about −2.7 mV, while after covering with CEPA the zeta potential value is about −32.5 mV. SPIONs covered with CEPA are stable at pH 7 for more than a week, while non-covered tend to aggregate spontaneously.

This behaviour suggests the presence of strong electric charges on the SPIONs covered with CEPA, keeping all SPIONs away from each other.

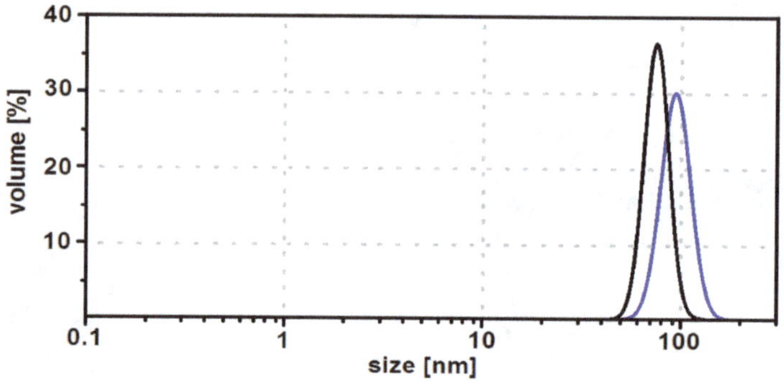

Figure 4. Size distribution by volume for Fe_3O_4@2.5%Ho unmodified (blue curve) and modified with CEPA (black curve).

3.3. *Thermogravimetric Analysis*

The TGA analysis of nanoparticles doped with 1% and 2.5% of holmium and surface-modified with 3-phosphoropropionic acid was carried out in the range from ambient temperature to 600 °C with a heating rate of 10 °C/min under the nitrogen atmosphere. The TG curves indicate a total weight loss of Fe_3O_4@2.5%Ho nanoparticles due to the decomposition of the organic material from the surface of nanoparticles. On the basis of the thermograms presented in Figure 5, the quantity of 3-phosphoropropionic acid was evaluated. The organic shell constitutes ca. 7.5% for Fe_3O_4@1%Ho and 9% for Fe_3O_4@2.5%Ho of the conjugate mass, which gives 0.075 mg ($4.9 \cdot 10^{-7}$ mol) per 1 mg of Fe_3O_4@1%Ho SPIONs, and 0.09 mg ($5.8 \cdot 10^{-7}$ mol) per 1 mg of Fe_3O_4@2.5%Ho SPIONs. Based on the zeta potential studies, it is seen that such an amount of CEPA is sufficient to stabilize SPIONs.

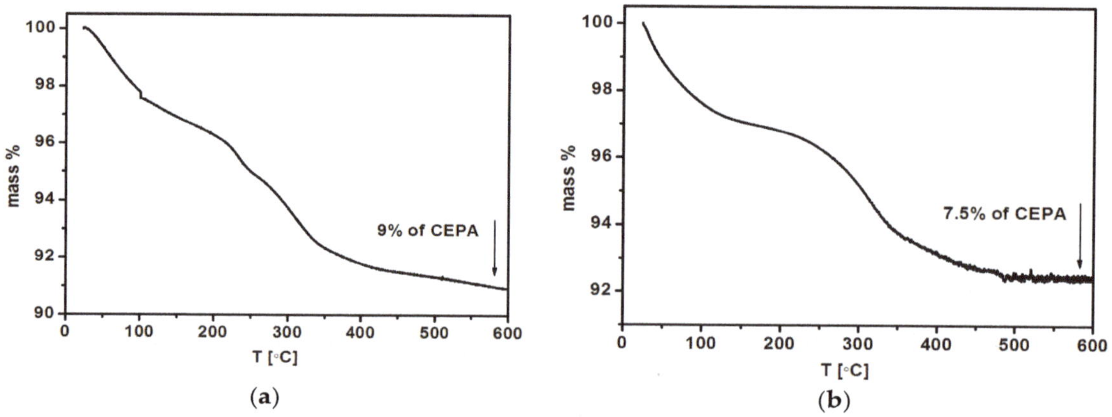

Figure 5. Thermograms of the SPIONs modified with 3-phosphoropropionic acid: (**a**) Fe_3O_4@1%Ho@CEPA, and (**b**) Fe_3O_4@2.5%Ho@CEPA.

3.4. Crystallographic Structure

Powder diffraction patterns were recorded with a powder diffraction X-ray diffractometer (PXRD) operating with Debye–Scherrer geometry and Cu Kα radiation with line λ = 1.540598 Å. Measurements were performed at RT and a scan rate of 1° per minute in 0.012° steps, covering the 2θ angle range from 20° to 130°. For nanoparticles containing 1–10 at. % of holmium, the diffraction patterns consist of a series of peaks, whose positions reveal the Fe_3O_4 phase (*JCPDS* file, No. 19-0629 for magnetite) (see Figure 6). Due to the high iron content in the crystals, the X-ray fluorescence is revealed as a noisy background in all recorded patterns. Synthesized nanoparticles have a high surface-to-volume ratio, crystal strains and surface defects, which contributes to the full width at half maximum (FWHM) of the reflexes. Their small size also correlates to the relatively broad shape of these patterns. According to the literature, the experimental conditions influence the crystal structure of prepared nanoparticles as well as other properties [46].

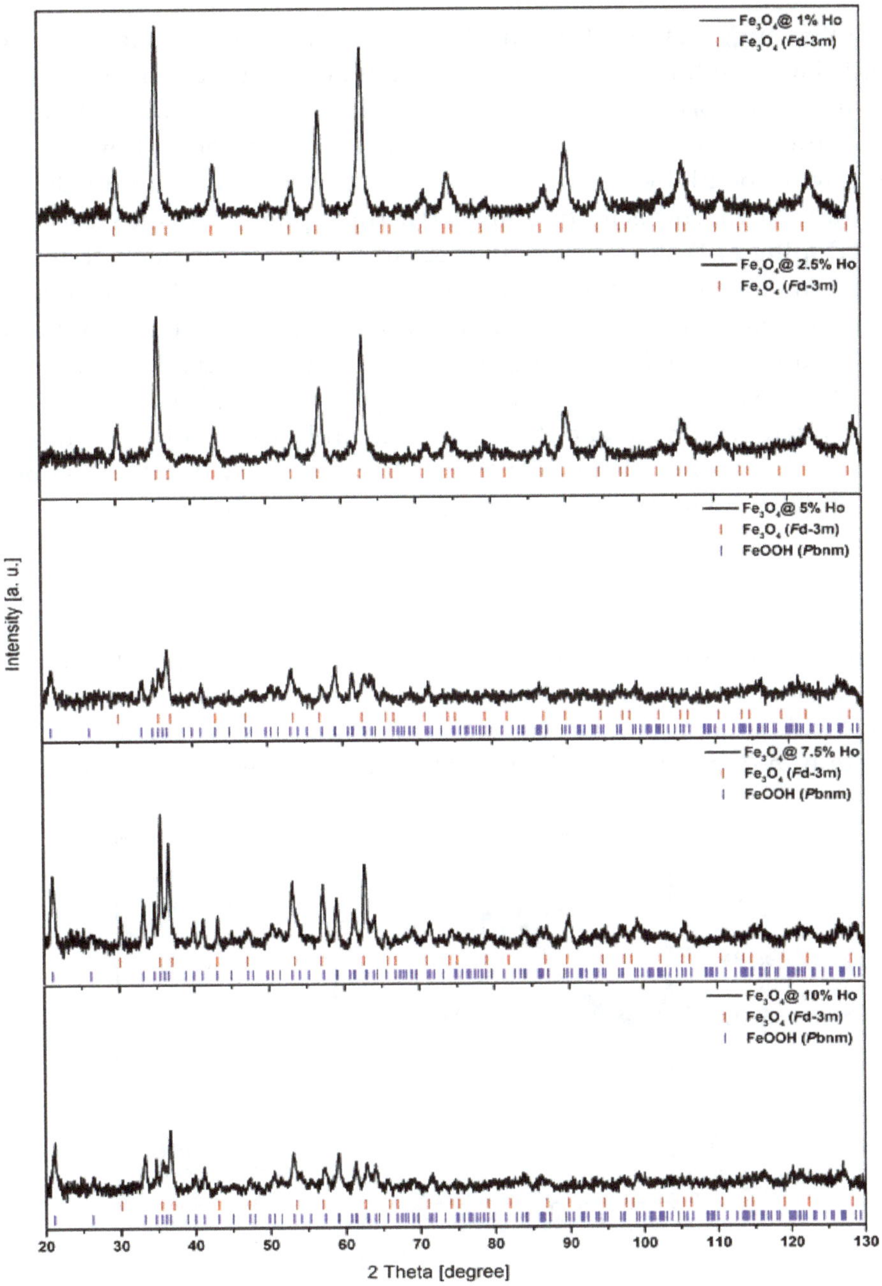

Figure 6. PXRD patterns of undoped and Ho-doped nanoferrite crystallites.

Samples doped with 1 at. % and 2.5 at. % holmium reveal reflexes characteristic of the *Fd*-3 m space group with single phase composition, while increasing holmium doping leads to poorer crystallinity and the additional formation of *P*bnm space group of goethite: α-FeOOH. The PXRD patterns explain the sudden change of crystal shape presented in the TEM images (see Figure 2), where crystallites with irregular shape appear. Line broadening in the recorded XRD patterns enables the calculation of the crystal size based on the Scherrer formula [47] and subsequent comparison to the TEM results. The average crystallite size in pure Fe_3O_4 is about 10 nm, while the size of the doped SPIONs increases to ca. 17 ± 2 nm (below 5% doping), which correlates with the TEM studies. The appearance of goethite with a 5–10% doping level leads to the poorer crystallinity and increasing amorphism of the obtained precipitate. Additionally, the shape of SPIONs is elongated due to the presence of FeOOH, which appears within this doping in the crystallites and, contrary to Fe_3O_4, crystallizes as a rhombic structure. [48]. In accordance with the literature [39], we do not observe a separate phase of Ho_2O_3.

The literature [35] suggests that lanthanide ions are incorporated into the octahedral sites of the crystallographic lattice, while such a replacement of Fe^{3+} with larger ions can cause a distortion of the lattice. Within this work we replaced Fe^{3+} having an ionic radius about 78.5 p, with Ho^{3+} ions, which are around 30% larger (~101 pm). The diffraction patterns show that the crystallinity is poorer for samples with the highest holmium content. Doping above 5% leads to polycrystallinity, and randomly distributed vacancies in the spinel structure appear. Drastic lattice deformation occurs with 5% holmium doping at Fe_3O_4 crystal. It is obvious that within such changes of the structure, the morphology of formed nanoparticles and magnetic properties should also change. We are inclined to assign the observed changes to the fact that at this doping level the amount of Ho is too large to be accommodated within the *Fd*-3m space group. As a consequence, this may lead to the observed polycrystallinity of SPIONs. Nevertheless, these results show that, up to a given doping level, Ho^{3+} ions can be incorporated within magnetite crystallites and not merely adsorb onto the surface of SPIONs. Such adsorption will not lead to lattice distortions. However, we cannot exclude at least partial adsorption on Ho^{3+} ions onto a well-developed surface of SPIONs.

3.5. XPS Analysis

In addition to the XRD studies, X-ray photoelectron spectroscopy was applied to investigate the chemical composition of the formed nanoparticles with 2.5% holmium doping. For this purpose, the analysis of the binding energy of Ho 4d and Fe 2p regions was carried out. The overall survey spectrum of the holmium-doped iron oxide nanoparticles is presented in Figure 7.

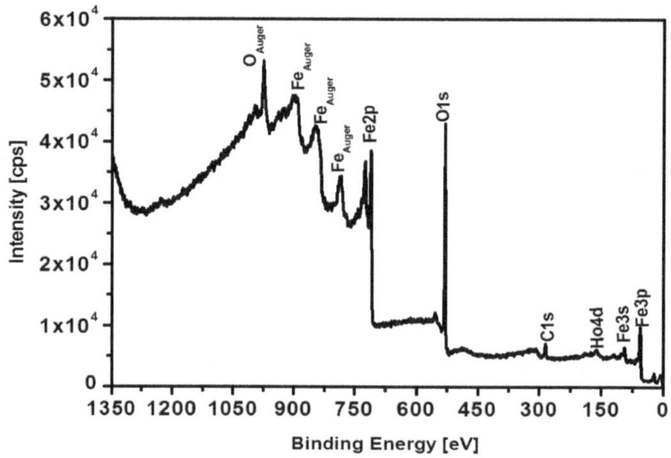

Figure 7. XPS survey spectrum of Fe_3O_4@2.5 at. % Ho nanoparticles.

Figure 8a,b shows the indicative regions of Fe 2p and Ho 4d binding energies, respectively, with deconvolution. As can be seen in Figure 8a, the spectrum can be fit to the doped iron oxide, where the peak positions of the Fe $2p_{3/2}$ and Fe $2p_{1/2}$ corresponding to the Fe^{3+} octahedral species [49] are located at binding energy 710.4 eV and 723.9 eV, respectively. The peak at 710.4 eV can be deconvoluted into two peaks: Fe^{2+} $2p_{3/2}$ and $Fe^{3+}2p_{3/2}$, respectively, ascribed to magnetite, but the precise deconvolution depends largely upon the model used [50]. The presence of satellite peaks at 718.7 eV and 732.5 eV may originate from the high-spin Fe^{2+} $2p_{3/2}$ shake-up. [50].

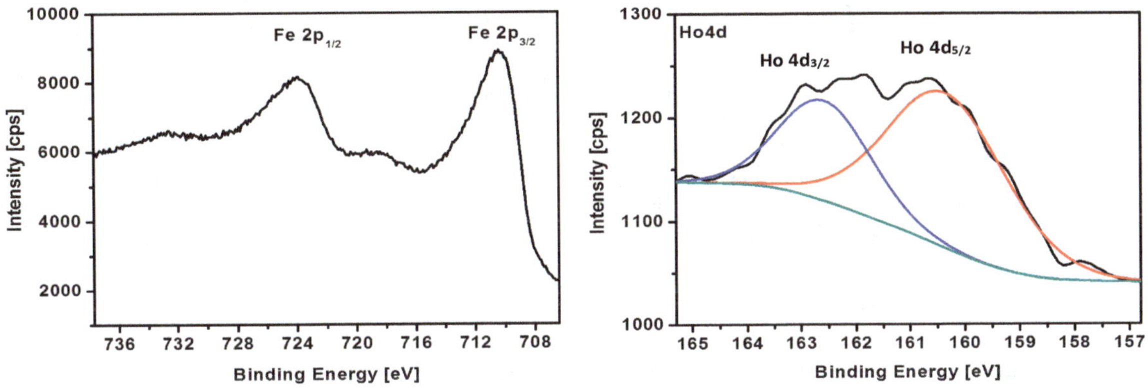

(a) (b)

Figure 8. XPS spectra of (**a**) Fe 2p and (**b**) Ho 4d region for Fe_3O_4@2.5%Ho SPIONs.

The experimental results are similar to the literature data for iron at different oxidation states [51]. Figure 8b presents the peaks at binding energies 160.5 eV and 162.7 eV, characteristic to Ho^{3+} $4d_{5/2}$/ and $4d_{3/2}$, indicating that holmium has been incorporated into the crystal lattice of iron oxide [52]. Due to the low amount of holmium in our samples, these peaks are of low intensity; therefore, their further analysis can be inaccurate.

3.6. Magnetic Analysis

Magnetic measurements of the ferrite-based nanoparticles were performed in a broad range of the applied magnetic field. Magnetization of the SPIONs studied increases abruptly in magnetic fields up to about 300 Oe and then approaches saturation at both 100 K and 300 K (Figure 9). The corresponding values of magnetization are lower for the 300 K isotherm than for the 100 K one. This magnetization decrease is consistent with a magnetization description given by the Brillouin function, which predicts magnetization suppression caused by the rising temperature [42,53,54]. The saturation magnetization M_s measured at 100 K for the pure Fe_3O_4 nanoparticles is found to be 83 emu/g, which is close to the value obtained for the undoped bulk magnetite. The magnetization value of nanoparticles depends on the experimental conditions during synthesis [54,55]. The M_s magnetization decreases down to 65 emu/g with the rise in temperature from 100 to 300 K (see Figure 9). The magnetization at both 100 K and 300 K decreases gradually when Ho doping rises from 1% to 10%. For 1% of Ho doping, only a slight M_s reduction is observed. The saturation magnetization, M_s, of SPIONs doped with 2.5% being about 50 emu/g at 300 K is sufficient for magnetic separation under the applied external magnetic field (see Figure 9); however, subsequent doping above 2.5% of holmium leads to a decrease in the magnetization and degradation of the superparamagnetic properties, which is not satisfactory from a biomedical point of view.

The more detailed inspection of magnetization hysteresis loops in weak fields (Figure 10) allows us to determine the coercive field H_c. At a temperature of 300 K, the coercive fields are equal 15 Oe and 10 Oe for the pure magnetite and SPIONs with 1% of Ho, respectively. Such a low coercive field (H_c) as well as the shape of the magnetization curve are the characteristic features of superparamagnetic materials. The coercive field also remains low for the 2.5% and 5% doping, whereas H_c increases for 7.5% and 10% doping (Figure 11). On the other hand, one may notice the remarkably larger H_c values ranging between about 60 and 120 Oe, when the SPIONs studied become ferromagnetic at 100 K (Figure 11) [56].

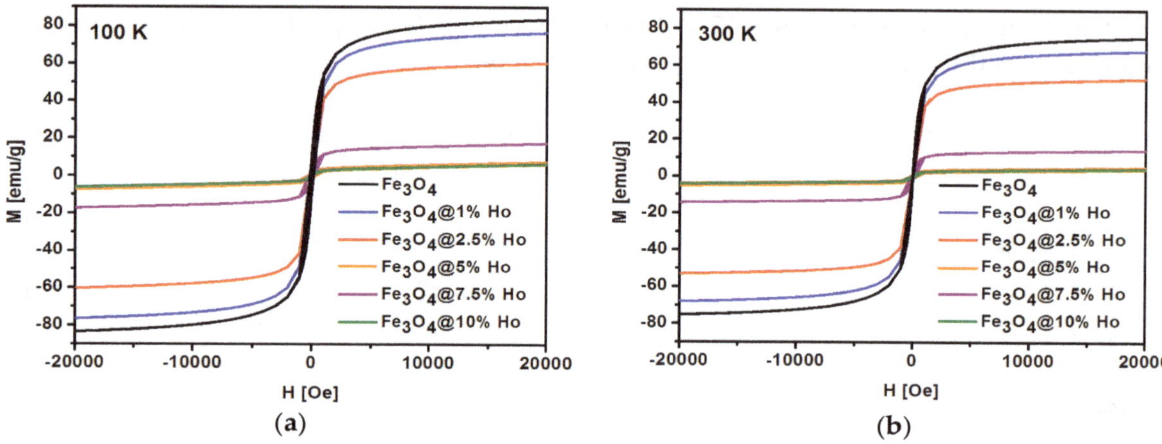

Figure 9. Magnetization isotherms for SPIONs with different Ho content measured at (**a**) 100 K and (**b**) 300 K.

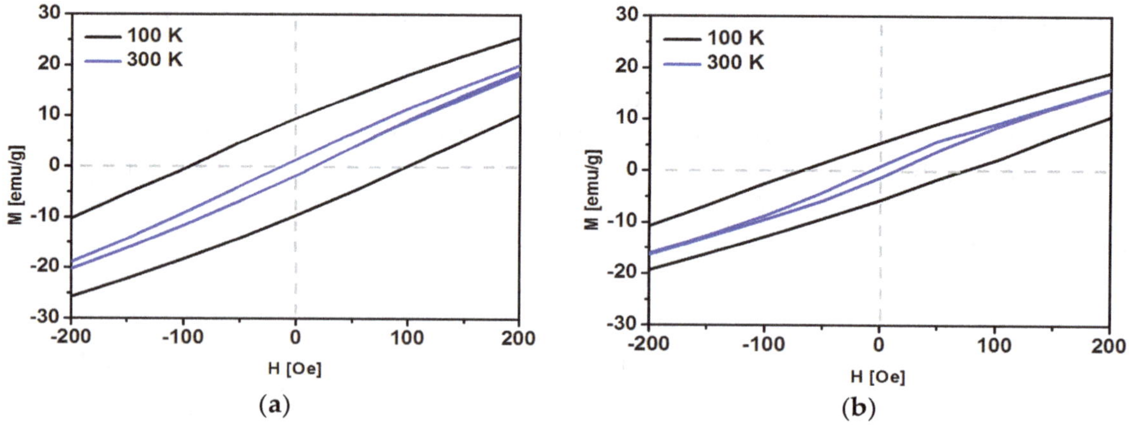

Figure 10. Magnetization loops K for (**a**) Fe_3O_4, (**b**) Fe_3O_4@1% Ho registered at 100 K and 300 K from −200 Oe to 200 Oe.

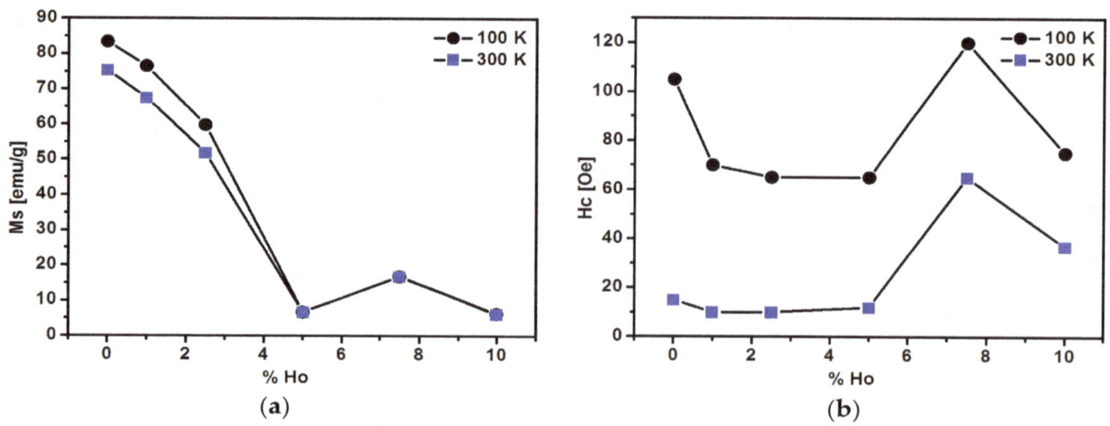

Figure 11. Values of (**a**) saturation magnetization at 20.000 Oe and (**b**) coercive field as a function of holmium content in SPIONs measured at 100 K and 300 K. Error bars are smaller than the data symbols.

A depletion of magnetic properties is observed for the higher holmium content. The saturation magnetization M_S drops when Ho doping is above 2.5% (Figure 11). This is accompanied by an increase in the coercive field H_c above 5% of Ho. The observed changes may be due to several reasons. The crystallographic lattice is found to be distorted at an Ho content exceeding 2.5%, as discussed in chapter 3.4. Crystallographic Structure.

It is also observed that the grains start to deviate from a spherical shape. Moreover, the doped ferrites become multiphasic as the additional α-FeOOH goethite phase appears in the NPs. This goethite phase is known to contain vacancies, which enhance the coercivity fields [57]. Thus, the magnetization results correlate well with the crystallographic data (vide supra).

The observed degradation of magnetic properties of studied ferrites is consistent with a two-phase approach of the so-called core-shell model, which is commonly used in analysis of fine structured materials [54]. The magnetic and electrical properties of transition-metal-based oxides are known to be strongly affected by various types of structural and chemical disorder [54,58–60]. The level of disorder may be accounted for by the volume fraction of disordered phase contained in the solid. In the polycrystalline and nanocrystalline solids a mean size of grains/crystallites is on the order of micrometers or tens of nanometers, respectively.

The surface layer/shell of grains and crystallites contains a material that is strongly structurally disordered as compared to the inner core of crystallites, which preserves the long-range translational symmetry characteristic of the bulk material. The thickness of the surface layer/shell extends from one to about a few nanometers and weakly depends on preparation method [43]. Thus, the volume fraction of a surface shell is known to increase abruptly when grain sizes are reduced down to the nanometer range [48,49,54]. In a rough approximation, the surface shell is often assumed to be nonmagnetic or weakly magnetic. Therefore, the magnetization of a nanostructured solid becomes suppressed as compared to the bulk material of the same chemical composition. In order to enhance their magnetization, materials like magnetite are doped with e.g., rare earth ions bearing a large magnetic moment. This approach may be successful to some extent since the atomic size mismatch between Fe and rare earth atoms starts to distort the atomic lattice and deplete the magnetic parameters. Finally, the magnetic properties of the doped ferrites studied in this work result from two competing factors: the atomic size mismatch and the high magnetic moment of Ho ions.

The magnetic properties of prepared SPIONs are stable. The dependence of magnetization in the Zero-Field-Cooled (ZFC) and Field-Cooled (FC) modes in the applied DC field of 100 Oe was measured versus temperature range from 60 to 350 K (Figure 12). The FC magnetization varies only weakly in the temperature range studied. The ZFC magnetization is a monotonically increasing function of temperature; however, the ZFC maximum related to the blocking temperature T_B, may be located above 350 K. The shape of the ZFC curve may be due to the relatively broad grain size distribution.

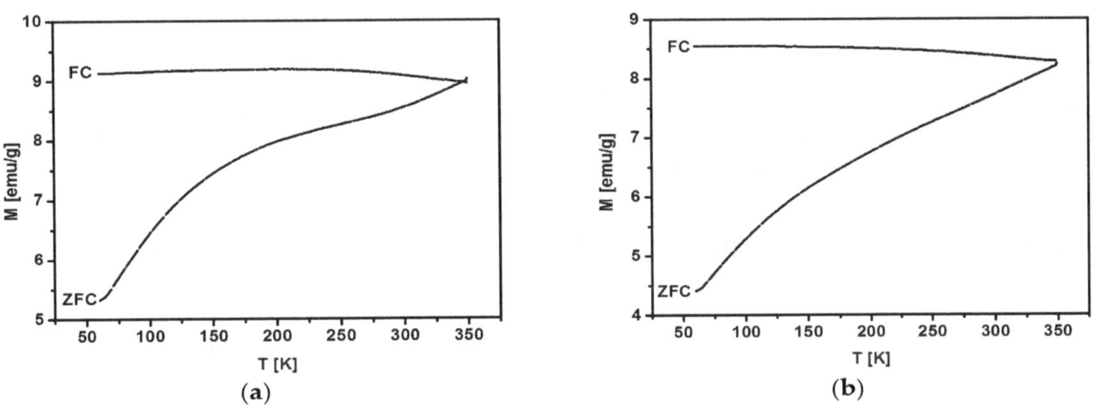

Figure 12. Temperature dependence of ZFC and FC magnetization at 100 Oe for nanoparticles doped with (**a**) 1% and (**b**) 2.5% of holmium.

4. Discussion

The aim of this work was to introduce a simple approach to incorporate the lanthanide, Ho^{3+}, ions into the ferrite oxide nanoparticles through the co-precipitation synthesis at room temperature, forming Ho-doped multifunctional SPIONs for their further modifications for biomedical applications. SPIONs doped with holmium were successfully synthesized in conditions enabling us to control their properties, such as shape, size, magnetization and structure. We have found that 2.5% molar of holmium in the ferrite-based SPIONs is maximal value yielding SPIONs with homogeneous phase and high magnetization above 60 emu/g. Undoped and 1–2.5% Ho-doped samples have a size ranging from a few to 20 nm in diameters, whereas further increase in the holmium content causes the growth of their size and irregular shape of the grains. We also observed an unusual drop in the magnetic properties at 5% of holmium in SPIONs, which we are inclined to assign to the size mismatch of Ho^{3+} and Fe^{3+} ions, leading to crystal lattice strain, defects in the structure and the formation of the goethite phase. The conclusion on the formation of α-FeOOH in the synthesized nanoparticles is additionally supported by the appearance of coercivity under the influence of an external magnetic field. XPS analysis confirmed the presence of holmium-doped iron oxide SPIONs. In contrast to the heterogeneous samples, SPIONs doped with 1–2.5% reveal superparamagnetic behaviour at room temperature and XRD patterns confirm that they maintain a homogeneous phase with well-formed crystallites. As they are synthesized, SPIONs tend to aggregate in the aqueous media. Subsequent modification with a CEPA organic shell stabilizes the suspension due to the electrostatic repulsion of negatively charged carboxylic groups of 3-phosphoropropionic acid shell. Further studies will attempt to implement the replacement of "cold" atoms of Ho in the superparamagnetic core with its ^{166}Ho radionuclide, emitting "soft" $\beta(-)$ radiation limited only to the distance of several millimeters, for the multiplied therapeutic effect of endoradiotherapy and magnetic hyperthermia.

5. Conclusions

In summary, using an efficient co-precipitation technique we obtained and characterized SPIONs doped with holmium. Taking into account their physicochemical properties, the superparamagnetic SPIONs doped with 1–2.5% holmium can be used for biomedical applications. The incorporation of such an amount of lanthanide is optimal for maintaining high magnetization and the homogeneous crystal structure of SPIONs, as a core SPIONs for modification with organic linkers and antitumor drugs. SPIONs prepared via the proposed route have great potential application in the biomedical field.

6. Patents

Application no. P-424901.

Author Contributions: M.O. and P.K. conceived and designed the experiments; M.O. and P.R. synthesized nanoparticles and performed DLS measurements/analysis, M.O. measured TGA and modified nanoparticles, M.P. performed/interpreted magnetometry experiments, G.C. and M.K.C. performed/interpreted XRD experiments, M.O. and P.K. analysed the data and wrote the paper.

Acknowledgments: Thanks to Marcin Pisarek, PhD (Polish Academy of Science in Warsaw), for carrying out the XPS measurements and analysis.

References

1. Wu, M.; Huang, S. Magnetic nanoparticles in cancer diagnosis, drug delivery and treatment (Review). *Mol. Clin. Oncol.* **2017**, *7*, 738–746. [CrossRef] [PubMed]

2. Brzozowska, M.; Krysinski, P. Synthesis and functionalization of magnetic nanopartciles with covalently bound electroactive compound doxorubicine. *Electrochim. Acta* **2009**, *54*, 5065–5070. [CrossRef]

3. Banobre-López, M.; Teijeiro, A.; Rivas, J. Magnetic nanoparticles-based hyperthermia for cancer treatment. *Rep. Pract. Oncol. Radiother.* **2013**, *18*, 397–400. [CrossRef] [PubMed]

4. Tsuotoaka, T. Frequency dispersion of complex permeability in Mn-Zn and Ni-Zn spinel ferrites and their composite materials. *J. Appl. Phys.* **2003**, *93*, 2789–2796. [CrossRef]

5. Hartshorne, H.; Backhouse, C.J.; Lee, W.E. Ferrofluid-based microchip pump and valve. *Sens. Actuators B* **2004**, *99*, 592–600. [CrossRef]

6. Condomitti, U.; Almeida, S.N.; Silveira, A.T., Jr.; de Melo, F.; Toma, H.E. Green Processing of Strategic Elements Based on Magnetic Nanohydrometallurgy. *J. Baz. Chem. Soc.* **2018**, *29*, 948–959. [CrossRef]

7. Bucak, S.; Jones, D.A.; Laibinis, P.E.; Hatton, T.A. Protein separations using colloidal magnetic nanoparticles. *Biotechnol. Prog.* **2003**, *19*, 477–484. [CrossRef] [PubMed]

8. Li, Z.; AdYi, P.W.; Sun, Q.; Lei, H.; Zhao, H.L.; Zhu, H.Z.; Smith, S.C.; Lan, M.B.; Lu, G.Q. Ultrasmall Water-Soluble and Biocompatible Magnetic Iron Oxide Nanoparticles as Positive and Negative Dual Contrast Agents. *Funct. Mater.* **2012**, *22*, 2387–2393. [CrossRef]

9. Zhou, L.; He, B.; Zhang, F. Facile one-pot synthesis of iron oxide nanoparticles cross-linked magnetic poly(vinyl alcohol) gel beads for drug delivery. *ACS Appl. Mater. Interfaces* **2012**, *4*, 192–199. [CrossRef] [PubMed]

10. Kim, J.; Piao, Y.; Hyeon, T. Multifunctional nanostructured materials for multimodal imaging, and simultaneous imaging and therapy. *Chem. Soc. Rev.* **2009**, *38*, 372–390. [CrossRef] [PubMed]

11. Zhang, W.; Li, X.; Zou, R.; Wu, H.; Shi, H.; Yu, S.; Liu, Y. Multifunctional glucose biosensors from Fe_3O_4 nanoparticles modified chitosan/graphene nanocomposites. *Sci Rep.* **2015**, *5*, 11129. [CrossRef] [PubMed]

12. Li, X.; Wen, F.; Creran, B.; Jeong, Y.; Zhang, X.; Rotello, V.M. Colorimetric protein sensing using catalytically amplified sensor arrays. *Small* **2012**, *8*, 3589–3592. [CrossRef] [PubMed]

13. Zhang, Q.; Liu, J.; Yuan, K.; Zhang, Z.; Zhang, X.; Fang, X. A multi-controlled drug delivery system based on magnetic mesoporous Fe_3O_4 nanopaticles and a phase change material for cancer thermo-chemotherapy. *Nanotechnology* **2017**, *28*, 405101. [CrossRef] [PubMed]

14. Chen, F.H.; Gao, Q.; Ni, J.Z. The grafting and release behavior of doxorubincine from Fe_3O_4@SiO_2 core–shell structure nanoparticles via an acid cleaving amide bond: the potential for magnetic targeting drug delivery. *Nanotechnology* **2008**, *19*, 165103. [CrossRef] [PubMed]

15. Pugazhendhi, A.; Edison, T.; Nesakumar, J.I.; Karuppusamy, I.; Brindhadevi, K. Inorganic nanoparticles: A potential cancer therapy for human welfare. *Int. J. Pharm.* **2018**, *539*, 104–111. [CrossRef] [PubMed]

16. Kievit, F.M.; Zhang, M. Surface engineering of iron oxide nanoparticles for targeted cancer therapy. *Acc. Chem. Res.* **2011**, *44*, 853–862. [CrossRef] [PubMed]

17. Safarik, I.; Baldikova, E.; Prochazkova, J.; Safarikova, M.; Pospiskova, K. Magnetically Modified Agricultural and Food Waste: Preparation and Application. *J. Agric. Food Chem.* **2018**, *66*, 2538–2552. [CrossRef] [PubMed]

18. Cardoso, V.F.; Francesko, A.; Ribeiro, C.; Bañobre-López, M.; Martins, P.; Lanceros-Mendez, S. Advances in Magnetic Nanopartciles for Biomedical Applications. *Adv. Healthc. Mater.* **2017**, *7*, 1–35. [CrossRef]

19. Cortajarena, A.L.; Ortega, D.; Ocampo, S.M.; Gonzalez-García, A.; Couleaud, P.; Miranda, R.; Belda-Iniesta, C.; Ayuso-Sacido, A. Engineering iron oxide nanoparticles for clinical settings. *Nanobiomedicine* **2014**, *1*, 2. [CrossRef]

20. Stamopoulos, D.; Manios, E.; Gogola, V.; Niarchos, D.; Pissas, M. On the biocompatibility of Fe_3O_4 ferromagnetic nanoparticles with human blood cells. *J. Nanosci. Nanotechnol.* **2010**, *10*, 6110–6115. [CrossRef] [PubMed]

21. Li, L.; Jiang, W.; Luo, K.; Song, H.; Lan, F.; Wu, Y.; Gu, Z. Superparamagnetic iron oxide nanoparticles as MRI contrast agents for non-invasive stem cell labeling and tracking. *Theranostics* **2013**, *3*, 595–615. [CrossRef] [PubMed]

22. Maier-Hauff, K.; Ulrich, F.; Nestler, D.; Niehoff, H.; Wust, P.; Thiesen, B.; Orawa, H.; Budach, V.; Jordan, A. Efficacy and safety of intratumoral thermotherapy using magnetic iron-oxide nanoparticles combined with external beam radiotherapy on patients with recurrent glioblastoma multiforme. *J. Neuro-Oncol.* **2011**, *103*, 317–324. [CrossRef] [PubMed]

23. Maier-Hauff, K.; Rothe, R.; Scholz, R.; Gneveckow, U.; Thiesen, B.; Feussner, A.; Deimling, A.; Waldoefner, N.; Felix, R.; Jordan, A. Intracranial thermotherapy using magnetic nanoparticles combined with external beam radiotherapy: Results of a feasibility study on patients with glioblastoma multiforme. *J. Neuro-Oncol.* **2007**, *81*, 53–60. [CrossRef] [PubMed]
24. Hasany, S.; Ahmed, I.; Rajan, J.; Rehman, A. Systematic review of the preparation techniques of iron oxide magnetic nanoparticles. *Nanosci. Nanotechnol.* **2012**, *2*, 148–158. [CrossRef]
25. Huber, D.L. Synthesis, properties, and applications of iron nanoparticles. *Small* **2005**, *1*, 482–501. [CrossRef] [PubMed]
26. De Cuyper, M.; Joniau, M. Magnetoliposomes. Formation and structural characterization. *Eur. Biophys. J.* **1988**, *15*, 311–319. [CrossRef] [PubMed]
27. De Silva, C.R.; Smith, S.; Shim, I.; Pyun, J.; Gutu, T.; Jiao, J.; Zheng, Z. Lanthanide(III)-Doped Magnetite Nanoparticles. *J. Am. Chem. Soc.* **2009**, *131*, 6336–6337. [CrossRef] [PubMed]
28. Petran, A.; Radu, T.; Borodi, G.; Nan, A.; Suciu, M.; Turcu, R. Effects of rare earth doping on multi-core iron oxide nanoparticles properties. *Appl. Surf. Sci.* **2018**, *428*, 492–499. [CrossRef]
29. Kanasamy, G.; Maity, D. Recent advances in superparamagnetic iron oxide nanoparticles (SPIONs) for in vitro and in vivo cancer nanotheranostics. *Int. J. Pharm.* **2015**, *496*, 191–218. [CrossRef] [PubMed]
30. Raana, G.; Johri, U.C. A study on structural and magnetic properties of Ni-substituted magnetite nanopartciles. *J. Alloys Compd.* **2013**, *577*, 376–381. [CrossRef]
31. Mariotto, G.; Murphy, S.; Berdunov, N.; Ceballos, S.F.; Shvets, I.V. Influence of Ca and K on the reconstruction of the Fe_3O_4(001) surface. *Surf. Sci.* **2004**, *564*, 79–86. [CrossRef]
32. Webelements. Available online: https://www.webelements.com/holmium/atom_sizes.html (accessed on 16 May 2018).
33. Rekorajska, A.; Cichowicz, G.; Cyranski, M.K.; Grden, M.; Pekala, M.; Blanchard, G.J.; Krysinski, P. Synthesis and Characterization of Tb-Doped Nanoferrites. *ChemNanoMat* **2018**, *4*, 231–242. [CrossRef]
34. Chaturvedi, S.; Rabindranath, B.; Sathe, V.; Kulkarni, S.; Singh, S. Holmium induced enhanced functionality at room temperature and structural phase transition at high temperature in bismuth ferrite nanopartciles. *J. Mater. Chem. C* **2016**, *4*, 780–792. [CrossRef]
35. Rice, K.P.; Russek, S.E.; Geiss, R.H.; Shaw, J.M.; Usselman, R.J.; Evarts, E.R.; Silva, T.J.; Nembach, H.T.; Arenholtz, E.; Idzerda, Y.U. Temperature-dependent structure of Tb-doped magnetite nanoparticles. *Appl. Phys. Lett.* **2015**, *106*, 062409. [CrossRef]
36. Wu, W.; He, Q.; Jiang, C. Magnetic Iron Oxide Nanoparticles: Synthesis and Surface Functionalization Strategies. *Nanoscale Res. Lett.* **2008**, *3*, 397–415. [CrossRef] [PubMed]
37. Laurent, S.; Forge, D.; Port, M.; Roch, A.; Robic, C.; Elst, L.V.; Muller, R.N. Magnetic Iron Oxide Nanoparticles: Synthesis, Stabilization, Vectorization, Physicochemical Characterizations, and Biological Applications. *Chem. Rev.* **2008**, *108*, 2064–2110. [CrossRef] [PubMed]
38. Mamani, J.B.; Costa-Filho, A.J.; Cornejo, D.R.; Vieira, E.D.; Gamarra, L.F. Synthesis and characterization of magnetite nanoparticles coated with lauric acid. *Mater. Charact.* **2013**, *81*, 28–36. [CrossRef]
39. Bloemen, M.; Vandendriessche, S.; Goovaerts, V.; Brullot, W.; Vanbel, M.; Carron, S.; Geukens, N.; Parac-Vogt, T.; Verbiest, T. Synthesis and characterization of holmium-doped iron oxide nanopartciles. *Materials* **2014**, *7*, 1154–1164. [CrossRef] [PubMed]
40. Thanh, N.T.K.; Maclean, N.; Mahiddine, S. Mechanisms of nucleation and growth of nanoparticles in solution. *Chem. Rev.* **2014**, *114*, 7610–7630. [CrossRef] [PubMed]
41. Vikram, S.; Dhakshnamoorthy, M.; Vasanthakumari, R.; Rajamani, A.R.; Rangarajan, M.; Tsuzuki, T. Tuning the magnetic properties of iron oxide nanoparticles by a room-temperature. *J. Nanosci. Nanotechnol.* **2015**, *15*, 3870–3878. [CrossRef] [PubMed]
42. Baaziz, H.; Tozri, A.; Dhahri, E.; Hlil, E.K. Effect of particle size reduction on the structural, magnetic properties and the spin excitations in ferromagnetic insulator $L_{0.9}Sr_{0.1}MnO_3$ nanoparticles. *Ceram Int.* **2015**, *41*, 2955–2962. [CrossRef]
43. Ozel, F.; Kockar, H. Growth and characterizations of magnetic nanoparticles under hydrothermal conditions: Reaction time and temperature. *J. Magn. Mater.* **2015**, *373*, 213–216. [CrossRef]
44. Klein, S.; Sommer, A.; Distel, L.V.R.; Hazemann, J.-L.; Kröner, W.; Neuhuber, W.; Müller, P.; Proux, O.; Kryschi, C. Superparamagnetic iron oxide nanoparticles as novel X-ray enhancer for low-dose radiation therapy. *J. Phys. Chem. B* **2014**, *118*, 6159–6166. [CrossRef] [PubMed]

45. Li, W.P.; Liao, P.Y.; Su, C.H.; Yeh, C.S. Formation of oligonucleotide-gated silica shell-coated Fe_3O_4–Au core–shell nanotrisoctahedra for magnetically targeted and near-infrared light-responsive theranostic platform. *J. Am. Chem. Soc.* **2014**, *136*, 10062–10075. [CrossRef] [PubMed]
46. Serna, C.J.; Bødker, F.; Mørup, S.; Morales, M.P.; Sandiumenge, F.; Veintemillas Verdaguer, S. Spin frustration in maghemite nanoparticles. *Solid State Commun.* **2001**, *118*, 437–440. [CrossRef]
47. Hummer, D.H.; Heaney, P.J.; Post, J.E. In situ observations of particles size evolution during the hydrothermal crystallization of TiO_2: A time-resolved synchrotron SAXS and WAXS study. *J. Cryst. Growth* **2012**, *344*, 51–58. [CrossRef]
48. Li, D.; Hu, X.; Sun, Y.; Su, S.; Xia, A.; Ge, H. Geothite (α-FeOOH) nanopowders synthesized via a surfactant-assisted hydrothermal method: Morphology, magnetic properties and conversion to rice-like α-Fe_2O_3 after annealing. *RSC Adv.* **2015**, *5*, 27091–27096. [CrossRef]
49. Wilson, D.; Langell, M.A. XPS analysis of oleylamine/oleic acid capped Fe_3O_4 nanoparticles as a function of temperature. *Surf. Sci.* **2014**, *303*, 6–13. [CrossRef]
50. Grosvenor, A.P.; Kobe, B.A.; Biesinger, M.C.; McIntyre, N.S. Investigation of multiplet splitting of Fe 2p XPS spectra and bonding in iron compounds. *Surf. Interface Anal.* **2004**, *36*, 1564–1574. [CrossRef]
51. Yamashita, T.; Hayes, P. Analysis of XPS spectra of Fe^{2+} and Fe^{3+} ions in oxide materials. *Appl. Surf. Sci.* **2008**, *254*, 2441–2449. [CrossRef]
52. Fan, Z.; Wu, T.; Xu, X. Synthesis of reduced grapheme oxide as a platform for loading β-$NaYF_4$:Ho^{3+}@TiO_2 based on an advanced visible light-driven photocatalyst. *Sci. Rep.* **2017**, *7*, 13833. [CrossRef] [PubMed]
53. Coey, J.M.D. *Magnetism and Magnetic Materials*; Cambridge University Press: Cambridge, UK, 2010.
54. Baaziz, W.; Pichon, B.P.; Fleutot, S.; Liu, Y.; Lefevre, C.; Greneche, J.M.; Toumi, M.; Mhiri, T.; Begin-Colin, S. Magnetic iron oxide nanoparticles: reproducible tuning of the size and nanosized-dependent composition, defects, and spin canting. *J. Phys. Chem. C* **2014**, *118*, 3795–3810. [CrossRef]
55. Ho, D.; Sun, X.; Sun, S. Monodisperse magnetic nanoparticles for theranostic applications. *Acc. Chem. Res.* **2011**, *44*, 875–882. [CrossRef] [PubMed]
56. Köferstein, R.; Walther, T.; Hesse, D.; Ebbinghaus, S.G. Preparation and characterization of nanosized magnesium ferrite powders by starch-gel process and corresponding ceramics. *J. Mater. Sci.* **2013**, *48*, 6509–6518. [CrossRef]
57. Lee, G.H.; Kim, S.H.; Choi, B.J.; Huh, S.H. Magnetic Properties of needle-like α-FeOOH and γ-FeOOH nanopartciles. *J. Korean Phys. Soc.* **2004**, *45*, 1019–1024. [CrossRef]
58. Veverka, P.; Kaman, O.; Knížek, K.; Novák, P.; Maryško, M.; Jirák, Z. Magnetic properties of rare-earth-doped $La_{0.7}Sr_{0.3}MnO_3$. *J. Phys. Condensed Matter* **2017**, *29*, 035803. [CrossRef] [PubMed]
59. Markovich, V.; Fita, I.; Wisniewski, A.; Mogilyansky, D.; Puzniak, R.; Titelman, L.; Martin, C.; Gorodetsky, G. Size effect on the magnetic properties of antiferromagnetic $La_{0.2}Ca_{0.8}MnO_3$ nanoparticles. *Phys. Rev. B* **2010**, *81*, 094428. [CrossRef]
60. Curiale, J.; Granada, M.; Troiani, H.E.; Sánchez, R.D.; Leyva, A.G.; Levy, P.; Samwer, K. Magnetic dead layer in ferromagnetic manganite nanoparticles. *Appl. Phys. Lett.* **2009**, *95*, 043106. [CrossRef]

13

Syringeable Self-Organizing Gels that Trigger Gold Nanoparticle Formation for Localized Thermal Ablation

Sonia Cabana-Montenegro [1], Silvia Barbosa [2], Pablo Taboada [2], Angel Concheiro [1] and Carmen Alvarez-Lorenzo [1,*]

1 Departamento de Farmacología, Farmacia y Tecnología Farmacéutica, R+D Pharma Group (GI-1645), Facultad de Farmacia and Health Research Institute of Santiago de Compostela (IDIS), Universidade de Santiago de Compostela, 15782 Santiago de Compostela, Spain; scabmon@gmail.com (S.C.-M.); angel.concheiro@usc.es (A.C.)

2 Área de Física de la Materia Condensada, Facultad de Física, Universidade de Santiago de Compostela, 15782 Santiago de Compostela, Spain; silvia.barbosa@usc.es (S.B.); pablo.taboada@usc.es (P.T.)

* Correspondence: carmen.alvarez.lorenzo@usc.es;

Abstract: Block copolymer dispersions that form gels at body temperature and that additionally are able to reduce a gold salt to nanoparticles (AuNPs) directly in the final formulation under mild conditions were designed as hybrid depots for photothermal therapy. The in situ gelling systems may retain AuNPs in the application zone for a long time so that localized elevations of temperature can be achieved each time the zone is irradiated. To carry out the work, dispersions were prepared covering a wide range of poloxamine Tetronic 1307:gold salt molar ratios in NaCl media (also varying from pure water to hypertonic solution). Even at copolymer concentrations well above the critical micelle concentration, the reducing power of the copolymer was maintained, and AuNPs were formed in few hours without extra additives. Varying the copolymer and NaCl concentrations allowed a fine tuning of nanoparticles' shape from spherical to triangular nanoplates, which determined that the surface plasmon resonance showed a maximum intensity at 540 nm or at 1000 nm, respectively. The information gathered on the effects of (i) the poloxamine concentration on AuNPs' size and shape under isotonic conditions, (ii) the AuNPs on the temperature-induced gelling transition, and (iii) the gel properties on the photothermal responsiveness of the AuNPs during successive irradiation cycles may help the rational design of one-pot gels with built-in temperature and light responsiveness.

Keywords: in situ gelling systems; photo-thermal therapy; gold reduction; localized heating effect; irradiation cycles; syringeable implant

---

1. Introduction

Gold nanoparticles (AuNPs) are receiving a great deal of attention because of their capability to perform as theranostic agents [1–5]. Their localized surface plasmon resonance (LSPR) allows for efficient conversion of radiation energy into heat, increasing the temperature of the surroundings remarkably but reversibly. Tuning the shape of AuNPs' selective light absorption in the wavelength range of the first biological window is possible [6]. Moreover, AuNPs can be easily decorated with therapeutic molecules, shielding coatings, and specific cell ligands to combine passive and active targeting [7]. All of these properties are particularly suitable to provide chemotherapy and phototherapy (including thermal ablation) synergisms in the eradication of tumor cells and pathogen microorganisms [8–11].

Most research in the field has been focused on the intravenous administration of AuNPs for cancer therapy. However, relatively rapid clearance of AuNPs from the bloodstream and accumulation in the liver and spleen hampers the distribution towards the target site and obligates the administration of repeated injections [12,13]. Intratumoral injection of AuNPs has been also proposed as a way to solve some physiological barriers and concentrate the nanoparticles in the affected tissue [14]. In this case, precise positioning of the AuNPs nearby the affected cells is difficult, which, in turn, hinders the attainment of predictable/reproducible levels of attached therapeutic agents and temperature. To overcome this problem, implantable solid depots with dimensions similar to those of brachytherapy seeds were designed recently [15]. In that case, poly(ethylene oxide) (PEO)-coated spherical AuNPs (ranging from 5 to 50 nm) were encapsulated in calcium alginate rods (0.8 mm diameter $\times$ 4 mm length) to be administered using a pre-loaded needle approach. The calcium alginate rods provided sustained release of the AuNPs in the tumor tissue. Also, lately, it has been demonstrated that integration of AuNPs in polymer systems that cause the AuNPs to assembly in vivo forming large supramolecular structures allows the LSPR peaks to be tuned towards the near-infrared (NIR) window in biological tissue (650–1350 nm) for more efficient cancer photothermal therapy and imaging [16,17].

The aim of the present work was to design in situ gelling systems from block copolymers that can transform a gold salt into AuNPs directly in the final injectable formulation and then self-assemble under physiological conditions to render a gel depot that allows repeated photothermal therapy cycles in the injection site. The overall purpose is to simplify the development (in one step under mild conditions) of gel depots containing AuNPs that can fully develop their photothermal properties without loss of efficiency after several light irradiations. Relevantly, since there is no covalent grafting of the composite components, gel erosion in vivo after treatment would cause the dissociation of the assemblies and thus the release of single AuNPs avoiding compromise their clearance from the body [16,17]. Poly(ethylene oxide)-poly(propylene oxide)-poly(ethylene oxide), PEO–PPO–PEO, block copolymers (namely poloxamers) have been shown able to trigger gold reduction under certain conditions without the need for strong reductant agents and providing a stabilizing shell [18,19]. The size of the obtained AuNPs can be tuned by changing the molecular weight and concentration of the poloxamer, preferably below the critical micelle concentration (CMC). The reducing power of PEO blocks causes nuclei formation to occur quite rapidly, while the stabilizing contribution of PPO blocks adsorbed on the nuclei makes the subsequent growth more slowly [20]. Compared to the linear poloxamer copolymers, the X-shaped poloxamines formed by four arms of PEO–PPO blocks linked by an ethylenediamine group may offer additional features [21–23]. The presence of the tertiary amines cause the copolymer to exhibit both temperature and pH responsiveness [24–27]. Moreover, the amine groups may contribute to further binding and reduction of gold ions, while the looser self-assembly of the copolymer may expedite the growth of the nanoparticles. These features may allow for more precise regulation of the kinetic and thermodynamic parameters involved in AuNP formation, which, in turn, should facilitate fine tuning of the shape of the nanoparticles [21]. So far, most studies have been carried out with low molecular weight PEO–PPO–PEO copolymers at concentrations below or close to those typical of micelle formation, where the predominant species are unimers or single micelles. Differently, the purpose of our work was to use a biocompatible poloxamine of relatively high molecular weight (Tetronic 1307, T1307) covering concentrations up to those suitable for forming aqueous micellar dispersions that, once injected, can undergo the sol-to-gel transition at the physiological temperature. T1307 is formed by four arms of PEO–PPO blocks (72 EO units and 23 PO units, each arm) connected to a central ethylenediamine group [24]. A gold salt was added to the poloxamine dispersions at two different concentrations, and the spontaneous formation of nanoparticles without the addition of other reagents was monitored. Since syringeable formulations should be isotonic, the effects of the ionic strength on the size and shape of the AuNPs formed were also investigated. Compared to solid depots, in situ gelling systems can perfectly fill gaps in tumor resection areas (covering tumor borders) or form soft depots in tumor or infected tissues. Thus, it can be hypothesized that the obtained in situ formed gold-reductant gels may retain the AuNPs in the application site for a prolonged amount of time for full exploitation of their light-induced heating. Rational design requires an insight to be gained into the effects of (i) the poloxamine concentration on AuNPs' size and shape, (ii) AuNPs on the temperature-induced gelling transition, and (iii) the gel properties on the responsiveness of the AuNPs. All these issues were investigated herein in detail.

2. Materials and Methods

2.1. Materials

Tetronic 1307 (T1307; molecular weight 18,000; PEO content 70 wt%) was supplied by BASF Corporation (Mount Olive, NJ, USA) and used as received. Hydrogen tetrachloroaurate(III) ($HAuCl_4$) and sodium chloride (NaCl) were from Sigma Aldrich (St Louis, MO, USA) and used without further purification. Distilled water was used for all experiments. All other reagents were analytical grade.

2.2. Gel Preparation and Nanoparticles Formation

T1307 solutions (0.25, 1, 5, 10, 15, 20, and 30 mM) were prepared in water and in 0.154 or 1.0 M NaCl aqueous medium by mixing under magnetic stirring in an ice-water bath. Aliquots of each T1307 solution (2 mL) in every medium were placed in glass vials. Then, $HAuCl_4$ aqueous solution (0.2 mL; 0.5 or 5 mM) was added to the vials and mixed with vortex for 2 min. After that, solutions were kept in the fridge for 4 hours. The final $HAuCl_4$ concentration was 0.05 or 0.5 mM. The systems were designed as T1307(x)/Au(y), where x and y represent the concentration (mM) of each component. Before measurements, all T1307/Au dispersions were stored for 24 h at 20 °C. The pH was recorded for all dispersions.

2.3. Nanoparticle Characterization

The UV-Vis spectra of T1307/Au dispersions were recorded in the 400 to 1100 nm range (Agilent 8453, Frankfurt am Main, Germany). The morphology of the nanoparticles was visualized in a scanning transmission electron microscope (STEM). Drops (5 µL) of T1307 dispersions with AuNPs were placed on grids covered with Fomvar film. After 30 s, the excess was carefully removed with a tip of filter paper. The samples were observed both with and without staining (with phosphotungstic acid) using a ZEISS UltraPlus FESEM apparatus fitted with a STEM detector (Oberkochen, Germany). Hydrodynamic particle size and zeta potential were measured in triplicate at room temperature using a Malvern Nano ZS (Worcestershire, UK) instrument. Before measurements, all solutions were sonicated for three minutes at room temperature to break up weak agglomerates. Thermal gravimetric analysis (TGA) was performed using a Discovery TGA 55 (TA Instruments, New Castle, DE, USA) and the sample dispersion was heated up to 450 °C at 10 °C/min and then was kept isothermal at 450 °C for 1 min.

2.4. Rheology

The storage or elastic (G′) and the loss or viscous (G″) moduli of T1307 (10, 15, and 20 mM)/Au (0.05 or 0.5 mM) dispersions in water and in 0.154 and 1 M NaCl aqueous medium were evaluated, at least in duplicate, using a Rheolyst AR-1000N rheometer equipped with an AR2500 data analyzer, a Peltier plate, and a cone with 6 cm diameter (TA Instruments, Hertfordshire, UK). To determine the influence of temperature on both moduli, tests were carried out at 5 rad/s from 15 to 45 °C with a heating rate of 2 °C/min.

2.5. Photothermal Measurements

Aliquots (2.2 mL) of T1307 (10, 15, and 20 mM)/Au (0.05 or 0.5 mM) dispersions were placed in 24-well plates and kept at 37 °C (using a temperature-controlled plate). The wells were irradiated with a 980 nm laser (Apollo Instruments, Inc. S10-976-1, Irvine, CA, USA) with a spot size of 1 cm^2 and power of 0.5, 1, and 2 W/cm^2 for 20 min at a distance of 8 cm from the laser. Temperature elevation was registered in the dispersion with a thermocouple (XS Instruments 3JKT, Carpi MO, Italy). Two independent experiments were carried out for each composition. Additionally, T1307 (15 and 20 mM)/Au (0.05 or 0.5 mM) dispersions were subjected to three successive irradiation cycles (8–12 min) at power densities of 0.5 and 2 W/cm^2, and the temperature was recorded during the whole process.

3. Results and Discussion

3.1. Reduction of $AuCl_4^-$ Ions and Formation of Gold Nanoparticles

A first aim of this work was to elucidate whether the high molecular weight poloxamine T1307 is able to induce the reduction of gold ions under mild conditions, even when the copolymer concentration is well above the CMC and in the absence of any other chemicals, in order to preserve the previously demonstrated high biocompatibility of this block copolymer dispersions [25,28,29]. In the case of poloxamers, it has been shown that both the size and shape of metal nanoparticles are determined by competition between nucleation (metal ion reduction in bulk) and growth (metal ion reduction on nuclei) processes, which are controlled by the amphiphilic character of the block copolymer [19]. PEO blocks form crown ether-like domains that bind and reduce $AuCl_4^-$ ions, which triggers the formation of AuNPs. PPO blocks mediate copolymer adsorption onto the nanoparticles' surfaces. This results in competition between $AuCl_4^-$ ion reduction in the bulk solution and on the particle surface, which, in turn, leads to an enhancement of the number of particles or an increase in particle size, respectively [18].

The formation of AuNPs in the presence of T1307 in media of different NaCl concentrations was monitored by recording the UV-visible spectrum. The gold salt was added at two different concentrations (0.05 and 0.5 mM final concentration) to T1307 (0.25, 1, 5, 10, 15, 20, and 30 mM) dispersions prepared in water and in 0.154 and 1.0 M NaCl aqueous mediums. The NaCl concentration was chosen to be the isotonic value (0.154 M) or a hypertonic value (1.0 M) that is still tolerable if small volumes are injected [30]. We have previously shown that increasing the NaCl concentration from 0 to 1 M notably decreases the CMC of T1307 (from 1% to 0.1%, i.e., from 0.55 to 0.05 mM); namely, the salt facilitates the copolymer self-assembly and also diminishes the gelling temperature [31]. Therefore, the use of NaCl may also help to elucidate whether the reducing power of the copolymer after self-assembly in micelles is similar to that of the unimers free in the medium.

Interestingly, mixing T1307 and gold salt caused the initially yellowish dispersions (the color of the starting $HAuCl_4$ solution) to begin to exhibit the typical pink-red characteristic color of AuNP formation after few hours of incubation (Figure 1). Nevertheless, relevant differences were observed as a function of T1307, gold, and NaCl concentrations. It should be noted that a further increase in $HAuCl_4$ up to 10 mM prevented AuNP formation, probably because the strongly acidic pH of the system ($\cong$2.0) and the lack of sufficient T1307 to trigger the reduction process. Interestingly, when T1307 (1 and 10 mM) containing 10 mM $HAuCl_4$ dispersions were diluted with the corresponding T1307 solution, the reduction phenomenon was triggered similarly to the systems initially prepared with less gold salt. This opens the possibility of preparing the T1307/gold salt dispersions in advance, and then the moment at which the reduction (i.e., AuNPs\ formation) should occur may be regulated by adding more copolymer. Relevantly, poloxamine dispersions in water had slightly alkaline pH, and when mixed with the diluted $HAuCl_4$ solutions, the pH of the dispersions was in the 6.3 to 7.6 range, which is perfectly suitable for injectable systems.

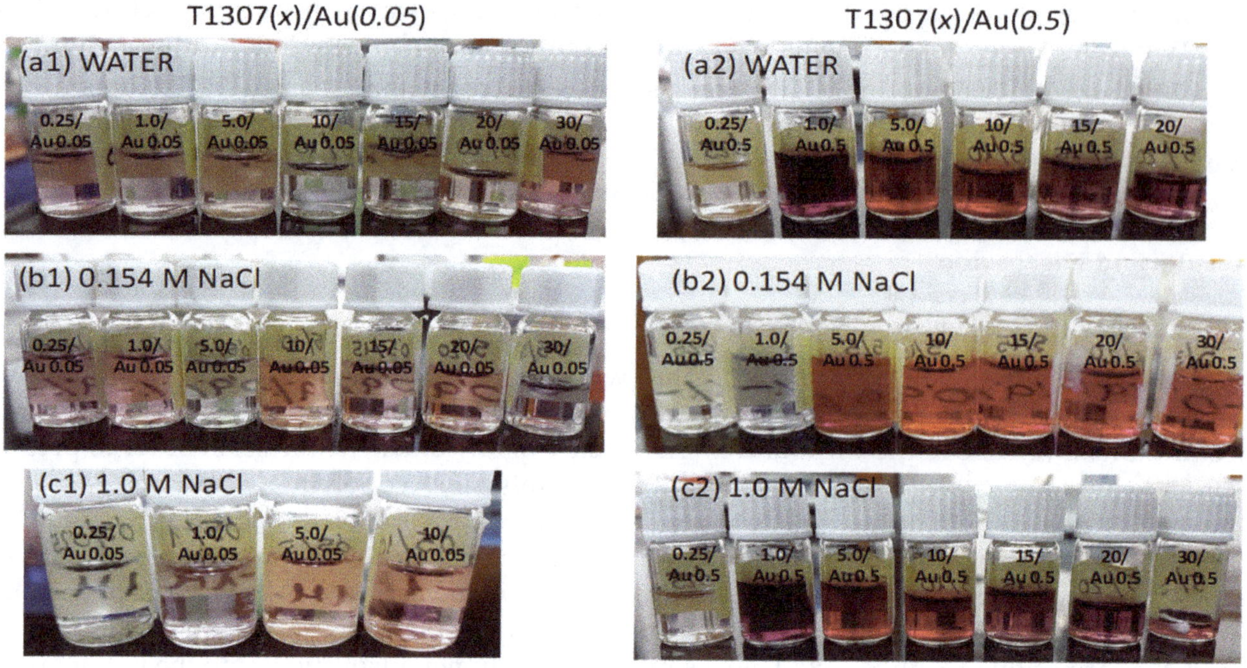

Figure 1. Appearance of T1307/$HAuCl_4$ dispersions in water (**a1**,**a2**) or NaCl 0.154 M (**b1**,**b2**) and 1.0 M (**c1**,**c2**) medium after incubation for 4 h at 4 °C. The systems were designed as T1307 (*x*)/Au (*y*) where *x* and *y* represent the concentration (mM) of each component.

Diluted T1307 dispersions (concentration < 10 mM) in water prepared with the lower concentration in gold salt (0.05 mM) showed LPSR peaks centered at ~540 nm, which is typical of the LSPR of spherical AuNPs (Figure 2a1). Differently, after increasing the T1307 concentration, the LSPRs were centered at ~1000 nm, which corresponds to the in-plane resonance of the triangular planar objects [21]; namely, gold nanoplates had been formed (as confirmed below with STEM images). A similar result was observed when the gold salt was added at a ten times higher concentration (Figure 2a2). Spherical gold nanoparticles predominated in dispersions with a T1307 concentration below 10 mM; meanwhile, the LSPR of gold nanoplates was evident for higher T1307 concentrations. The T1307 10 mM concentration seems to be a threshold value; namely, this concentration triggered the rapid formation of nanoplates when 0.05 mM $HAuCl_4$ was added, but it was insufficient in the presence of 0.5 mM $HAuCl_4$. Indeed, nanosphere LSPR predominated, and only a minor shoulder typical of nanoplates was recorded for T1307 (10 mM)/Au (0.5) in water (Figure 2a2). In a previous work, spherical AuNPs (6–7 nm in diameter) were also reported to be formed using Pluronic L121 (10 mM)/Au (0.25 mM) in water, but nanoplate formation did not occur [19]. In contrast, a low molecular weight poloxamine T904 (MW 6700 Da) triggered the formation of gold triangular and hexagonal nanoplates (174 nm size) at low molar ratio (e.g., T904 (1.5)/Au (0.5)), but after increasing the copolymer concentration, there was a decrease in the number of nanoplates and for T904 (6–140)/Au (0.5), nearly perfect Au nanospheres (up to 40 nm in size) were formed [21]. These shape and size changes recorded for T904 were attributed to the fact that the nanoplate formation benefit from a slow Au (III) to Au (0) reduction rate, which is favored under mild reducing conditions. It has been hypothesized that the selective adsorption of the poloxamine on {111} crystallographic planes of the growing AuNPs due to their lowest energy hinders the growth on these planes and promotes anisotropic growth along the {110} plane, which favors the formation of (111) bounded structures as thin nanoplates [21]. In the case of T1307/Au dispersions, the formation of nanoplates may be favored by the fact that the reaction rate occurred at 4 °C, differently to the incubation at room temperature, or even at a higher temperature, as applied in other protocols [19,21]. Indeed, it was previously observed that heating at up to 70 °C favors rapid and full conversion in spherical nanoparticles [19,21].

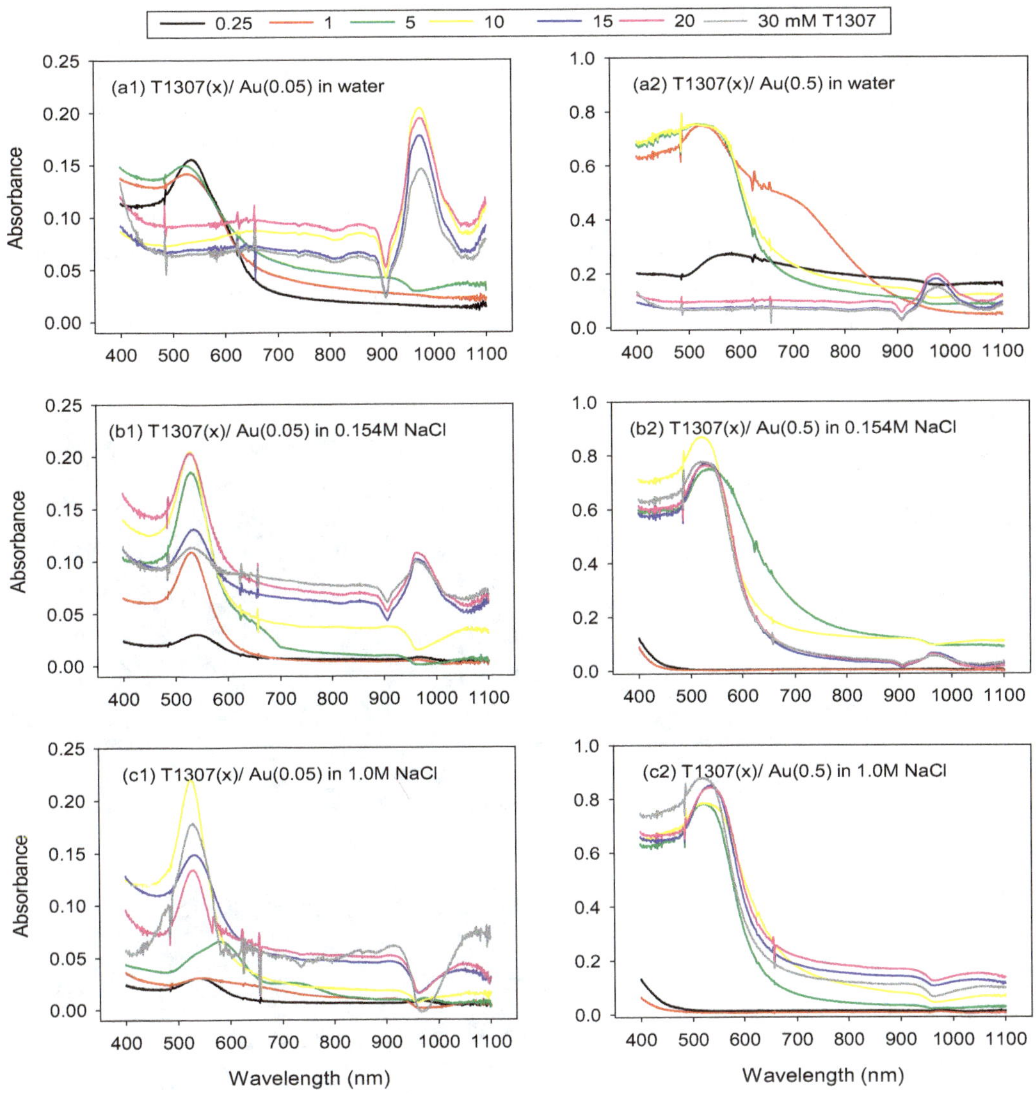

Figure 2. Absorption spectrum of T1307 (0.25, 1, 5, 10, 15, 20, and 30 mM)/Au (0.05 and 0.5 mM) dispersions prepared in (**a**) water, (**b**) 0.154 M NaCl, and (**c**) 1.0 M NaCl aqueous medium. Plots on the left refer to systems prepared with 0.05 mM $HAuCl_4$, and plots on the right refer to those prepared with 0.5 mM $HAuCl_4$.

Interestingly, the LSPR spectra provided evidence that the addition of NaCl favors nanosphere formation in detriment of nanoplates. In 0.154 M NaCl medium, all T1307 dispersions mixed with the lowest $HAuCl_4$ concentration tested led to nanospheres (absorption peak centered in ~540 nm) and the presence of nanoplates was also evident at 15 to 30 mM for T1307 (absorption peak at ~1000 nm) (Figure 2b1). A further increase in $HAuCl_4$ concentration (Figure 2b2) revealed that the lowest T1307 concentrations (0.25 and 1 mM) did not trigger significant reduction (as also observed in Figure 1b2); an intermediate T1307 concentration (5–10 mM) favored nanosphere formation; and a further increase in T1307 (15–30 mM) facilitated the coexistence of both nanospheres and nanoplates. Similar results were obtained in 1.0 M NaCl medium, but the LSPR peak of nanoplates attenuated even more (Figure 2c1,c2). It has been previously shown that NaCl causes poloxamers and poloxamines (including T1307) to become more hydrophobic and thus more prone to self-assemble into unimodal micelles [31,32]. Therefore, although Cl^- ions have been reported to favor nanoplate formation because of specific adsorption onto crystal facets [33], the decrease in T1307 CMC should result in less unimers being available for reduction and a faster transfer of gold ions into the micelles with the subsequent formation of spherical nanoparticles [21].

3.2. *AuNP Morphology: STEM and DLS*

Scanning transmission electron microscopy (STEM) images allowed visualization of both micelles and AuNPs (Figure 3). Phosphotungstic acid staining provided evidence that the micelles become larger when the NaCl concentration increases (as observed, e.g., for T1307 (10)/Au (0.05) in 1M NaCl) as confirmed by DLS. Both spherical particles and nanoprisms or triangular plates coexisted in the T1307 (10)/Au (0.05) in 0.154 M NaCl, in good agreement with the LSPR spectrum recorded. Interestingly, the AuNPs seem to be encapsulated in the copolymer aggregates and different morphologies of gold particles even coexisted close each other (see insert showing triangles and spheres). Increasing the copolymer and $HAuCl_4$ concentration led to gold nanoprisms with sizes predominantly between 140 and 200 nm, also in good agreement with the LSPR spectrum.

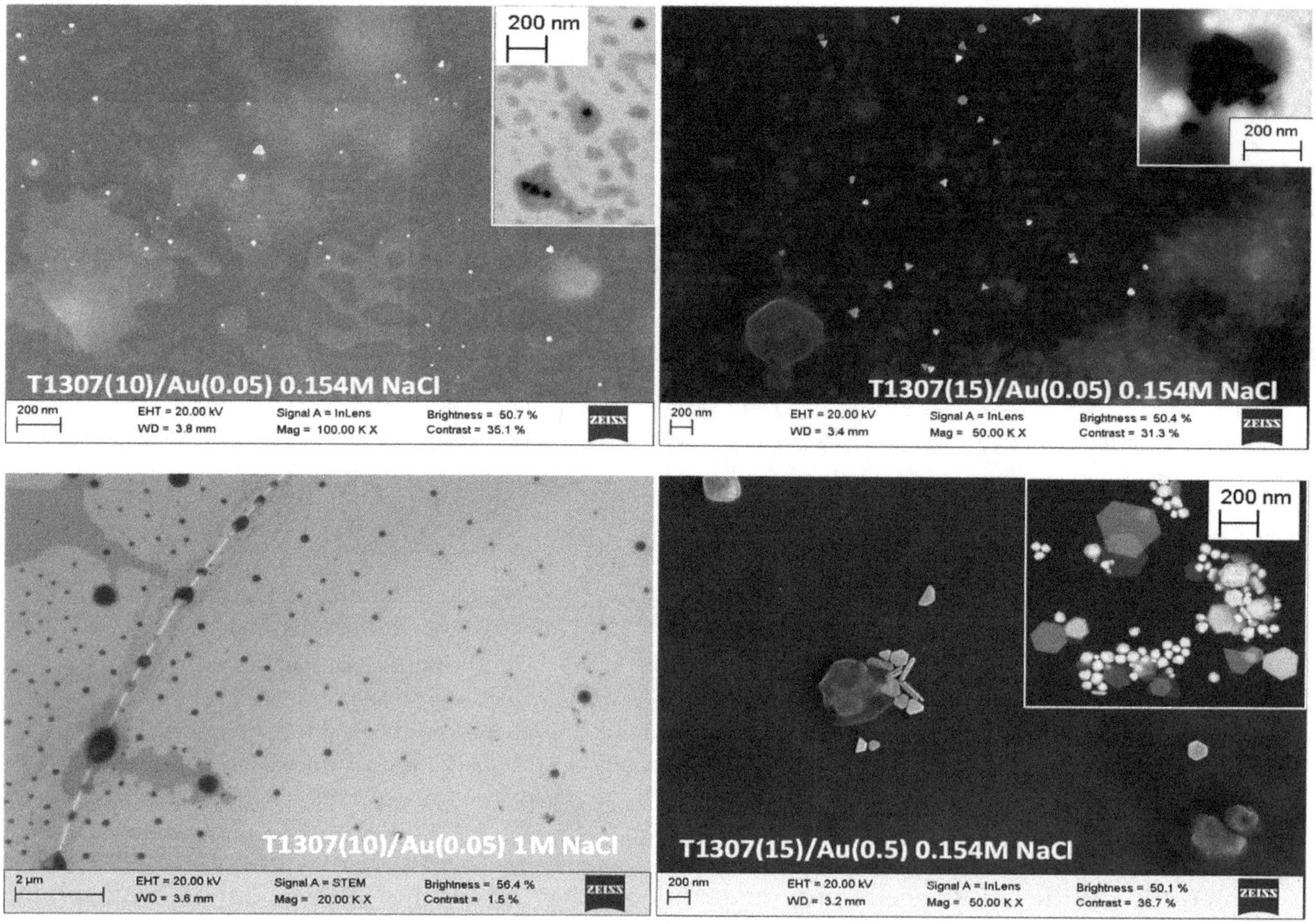

Figure 3. STEM micrographs of T1307 (x mM)/Au (y mM) dispersions prepared in different media and observed using various detectors (micrographs on the left were recorded using phosphotungstic acid staining, while those on the right were taken without staining).

The values of hydrodynamic particle size obtained from DLS measurements for T1307/Au dispersions in water and in salt solutions are listed in Table 1. In general terms, the size of the copolymer–AuNP aggregates increased when the copolymer and/or NaCl concentration increased. As observed before, poloxamine aggregation is favored in the presence of NaCl due to a salting-out effect that makes the copolymer become more hydrophobic [31]. This increase in size was particularly evident for T1307 concentrations close to the CMC (0.25–1 mM). The larger sizes recorded for T1307 10 mM systems prepared in 0.154 and 1 M NaCl may be due to the combination of several AuNPs in each copolymer aggregate, as suggested by the STEM images.

Table 1. Hydrodynamic diameter (nm) recorded at room temperature using DLS for copolymer/gold aggregates formed in T1307/Au dispersions in water or NaCl medium.

$[AuCl_4]$ mM	[T1307] mM	Ø (nm) in H_2O	Ø (nm) in 0.154 M NaCl	Ø (nm) in 1 M NaCl
0.05	0.25	2.34 (0.24)	75.8 (21.2)	12.95 (1.63)
	1	35.99 (2.47)	83.6 (21.5)	113.6 (31.2)
	5	68.43 (7.01)	125.9 (23.9)	238.6 (60.5)
	10	116.5 (15.57)	325.8 (65.0)	742.1 (81.9)
0.5	0.25	14.28 (1.01)	102.0 (19.3)	94.5 (20.0)
	1	36.07 (7.93)	194.1 (44.5)	268.5 (58.1)
	5	94.46 (20.02)	284.0 (61.7)	157.3 (62.0)
	10	187.6 (19.89)	466.6 (72.3)	725.8 (98.1)

3.3. Photothermal Measurements

To evaluate the hyperthermia potential of the AuNPs spontaneously formed in the gelling dispersions, the temperature increase generated during NIR laser irradiation (980 nm) was recorded while maintaining the dispersions in a pre-tempered environment of 37 °C to mimic physiological conditions. The photothermal efficiency was tested using T1307 (10, 15, and 20 mM)/Au (0.05 and 0.5 mM) dispersions in water, and in 0.154 M and 1 M NaCl media, a few hours after the in situ formation of the nanoparticles (i.e., after 4 h storage at 4 °C). These dispersions were irradiated for 20 min at 0.5, 1, and 2 W/cm^2 power densities. Previously, 20 mM T1307 dispersions (without gold salt) in water and in 0.154 M and 1 M NaCl media were irradiated at 0.5 and 2 W/cm^2 in order to record the temperature increase of the background, which was 0.4 °C in the first 5 min and 1.1 °C after 30 min of irradiation. Increases of temperature recorded for the systems containing the nanoparticles are shown in Figures 4 and 5 without correction of the background temperature.

After modifying the concentration of the block copolymer in the dispersion, the photothermal responsiveness varied. T1307 (10 mM)/Au (0.5 mM) dispersions in water achieved the maximum temperature elevation when the laser was applied for 20 min at 0.5, 1, and 2 W/cm^2 (Figure 4a). An increase in the copolymer concentration gave rise to a modification in the photothermal responsiveness. The increase in temperature after 20 min of irradiation at 2 W/cm^2 in T1307 (15 mM)/Au (0.5 mM) dispersions in 1 M NaCl medium was 8.4 °C higher (i.e., up to 23.4 °C) than that achieved in the dispersions of the same composition prepared in water (i.e., 15 °C) (Figure 4b). The temperature of T1307 (20 mM)/Au (0.5 mM) dispersions in 0.154 M NaCl increased to 18.9 °C after 5 min of irradiation with the highest power density, and it increased to 23.6 °C after 20 min (Figure 4c). After irradiating for 5 min at the maximum power density, all dispersions achieved a temperature that surpasses the required threshold for the thermal ablation of cancer cells with temperature elevations above 42 °C [34].

Overall, the increases in temperature (with respect a basal value of 37 °C) of 15–20 °C in isotonic medium when irradiated with NIR light of very mild intensity (1 W/cm^2; typical power densities tested are in 1 to 100 W/cm^2 range [35,36]) can be considered remarkable and are in good agreement with the formation of non-spherical gold nanostructures. It should be noted that assuming 100% conversion of gold salt into AuNPs, the concentration in gold nanostructures in the T1307/Au 0.05 and 0.5 M dispersions would be 9.85 and 98.5 µg/mL, respectively. These values are in good agreement with the chart residue of the systems recorded by TGA at 450 °C.

It has been previously reported that hybrid polymer AuNPs (15.6 µg/mL) in the form of spheres (12 nm), stars (50 nm), and rods (50 nm) caused increases in temperature of 5, 13, and 18 °C, respectively, upon 1.34 W/cm^2 light irradiation (continuous wave, λ = 725–2500 nm), which was explained by the progressive shift of the LSPR spectra towards the NIR region [6]. A temperature increase of 10 °C has been reported for pH-induced aggregated gold nanospheres (individual size 33 nm) at 20 µg/mL upon 13.9 W/cm^2 light irradiation (808 nm) [16]. The increase in thermal efficiency observed when the T1307 concentration increased from 10 to 30 mM for a fixed power density (e.g., 1 W/cm^2) could be related to the fact that, as discussed below, the T1307 10 mM dispersions did not form gels in this range of temperatures, or the gels formed were weak, whereas T1307 15 mM underwent gelling when heating, and T1307 20 mM were already gels at the basal temperature of the study. In this regard, it has been previously observed that temperature-responsive hybrid elastin-like polypeptide/AuNPs at 120 µg/mL did not show photothermal effects at low temperatures (individual size 30 nm), but caused an increase in temperature of 20–30 °C (irradiation conditions: 808 nm, 1.0 W/cm^2, 4 min) when they were previously heated (at 30 °C) to form aggregates (940 nm) [17]. Similarly, a clustering effect may be involved in T1037 dispersions under gelling conditions.

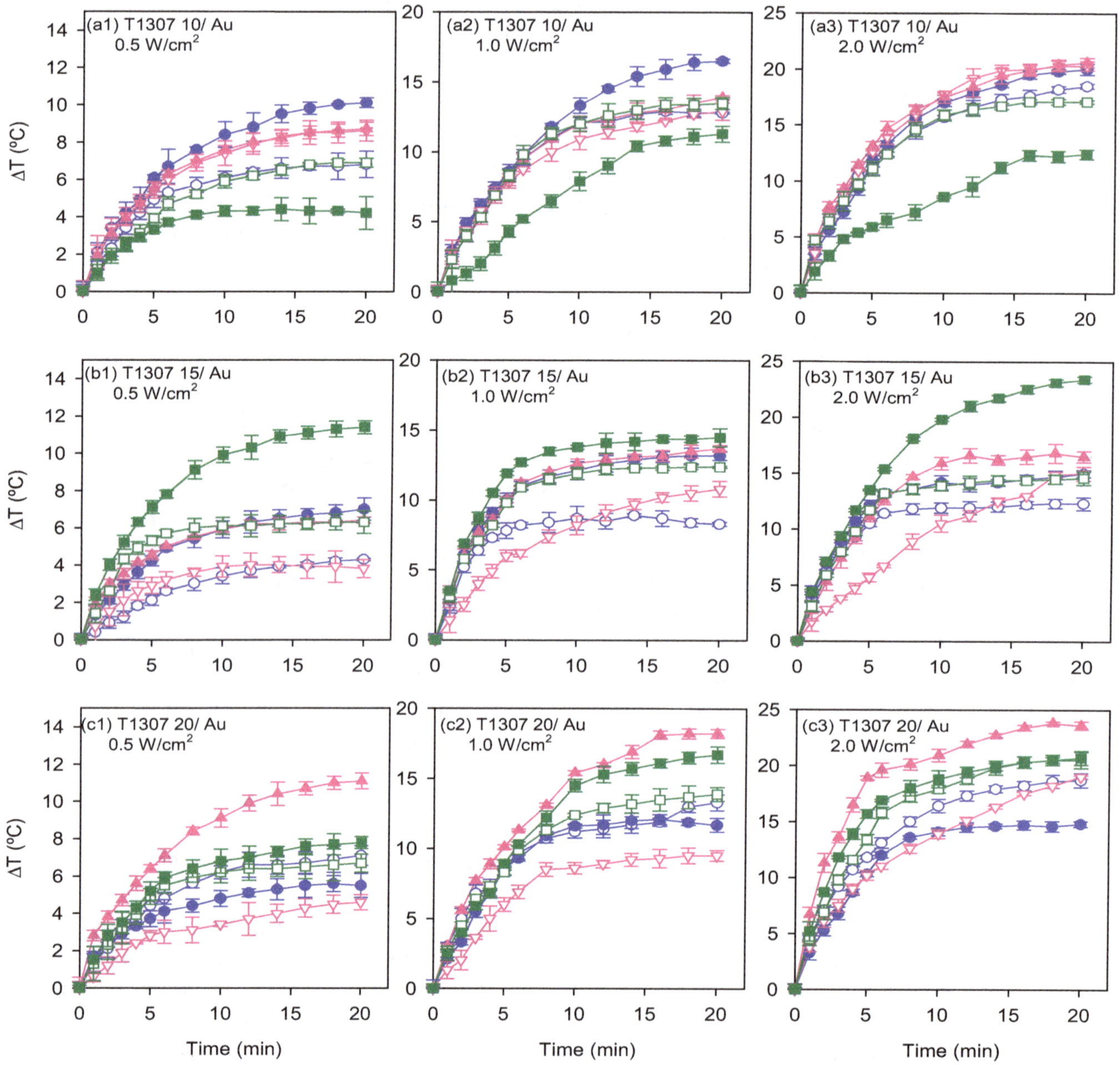

Figure 4. NIR-induced temperature increase (from a basal value of 37 °C) as a function of time for T1307/Au dispersions prepared with (**a**) 10 mM, (**b**) 15 mM, and (**c**) 20 mM T1307, and a final Au concentration of 0.05 (open symbols) or 0.5 (full symbols) mM in water (blue symbols) and in 0.154 M (pink symbols) and 1 M (green symbols) of NaCl aqueous media. The dispersions were exposed to NIR light irradiation using a 980 nm laser at 0.5, 1, and 2 W/cm^2 for 20 min.

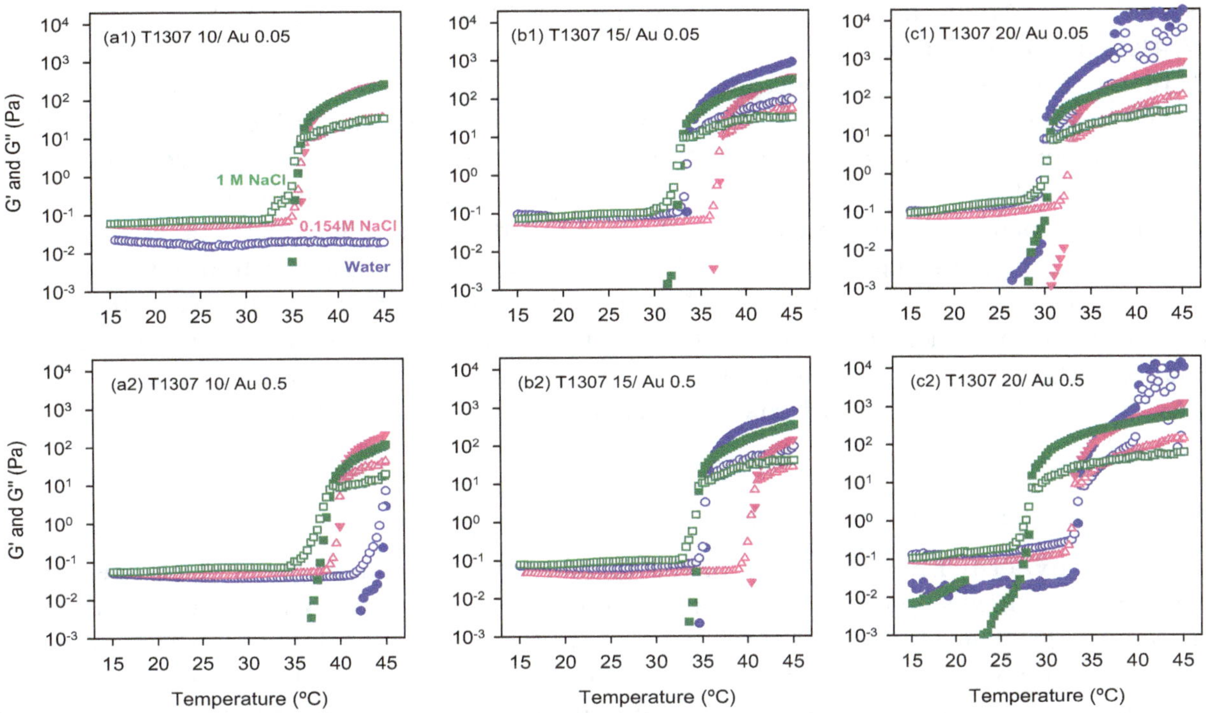

Figure 5. Effect of the temperature on the storage (G′, full symbols) and loss (G″, open symbols) moduli of (**a**) 10 mM, (**b**) 15 mM, and (**c**) 20 mM T1307 dispersions prepared with 0.05 (1) or 0.5 (2) mM gold salt in water (blue symbols) and in 0.154 M (pink symbols) and 1 M (green symbols) NaCl aqueous solutions.

3.4. Rheological Behavior

Once confirmed that the spontaneously formed AuNPs in the T1307 dispersions are sensitive to NIR, the next step was to investigate whether the dispersions can still undergo sol-to-gel transitions in the presence of the AuNPs and behave as gel depots at body temperature. Rheological characterization of T1307 (10, 15 and 20 mM) dispersions in water and in 0.125 M and 1 M NaCl media with and without gold was carried out in the 15–45 °C range (Figure 5).

Ten millimole T1307 dispersions prepared in water did not form gels, and the presence of AuNPs did not modify that behavior. This finding is in good agreement with previous reports and means that this hydrophilic copolymer in a good solvent, such as water, requires a higher concentration or further increase in temperature to trigger the micelle self-association [25]. Differently, in 0.154 M and 1 M NaCl media, the sol-to-gel transition of T1307 (10 mM)/Au (0.05 mM) was observed at 36.8 °C and 36.4 °C, respectively, while the transition of T1307 (10 mM)/Au (0.5 mM) occurred at 40.3 and 39.3 °C, respectively (Figure 5a). The shift in the gelling temperature observed in the presence of the highest Au concentration tested (0.5 mM) suggests that some copolymer unimers involved in the stabilization of the AuNPs may be not available to contribute to the micellization and subsequent in situ gelling.

The sol-to-gel transitions of T1307 (15 mM)/Au (0.05 mM) dispersions in water and 0.154 M NaCl and 1 M NaCl media were recorded at 33.9, 37.5, and 33.2 °C, respectively (Figure 5b). These results suggest that the salting-out effect caused by NaCl at a low concentration may cause the PEO corona to be in a less extended conformation, making the contact among micelles more difficult. It should be noted that 0.154 M NaCl caused a minor decrease in the CMC of T1307 compared to that recorded in water [31]. Differently, the CMC was one order of magnitude lower in 1 M NaCl, and thus more unimers are participating in micelle formation and also in the gelling process, which explains the decrease in the gelling temperature. As observed for the less concentrated T1307 dispersions, increasing the Au concentration led to an increase in the gelling temperature. The sol-to-gel transition of T1307 (15 mM)/Au (0.5 mM) dispersions in water and 0.154 M NaCl and 1 M NaCl media occurred at 35.7, 41.1, and 35.0 °C, respectively.

A further increase in T1307 concentration up to 20 mM did not modify the pattern of behavior of the dispersions, but a decrease in the gelling temperature was recorded. T1307 (20 mM)/Au (0.05 mM) dispersions in water and 0.154 M NaCl and 1 M NaCl media underwent the sol-to-gel transition at 30.3, 32.8, and 30.7 °C, respectively, while the gelling temperatures of T1307 (20 mM)/Au (0.5 mM) dispersions in the same media were 33.9, 33.2, and 28.5 °C (Figure 5c). Therefore, in terms of temperature-induced in situ gelling, T1307 (15 mM)/Au (0.05 or 0.5 mM) systems either formulated in water or in 1 M NaCl may be valid as well as any combination of T1307 (20 mM) with Au (0.05 or 0.5 mM). Relevantly, it has been previously shown that similarly highly concentrated T1307 gels (without AuNPs) exhibit a good balance between syringeability, depot consistency, and erosion rate under in vivo conditions [28], which make them suitable for the pursued purpose.

3.5. Performance under Irradiation Cycles at 37 °C

Once the hyperthermia capability of the formulations after a single shot of NIR light was demonstrated, the next step was to elucidate whether the formulations could be useful as depots of gold nanoparticles that provide localized elevations of temperature each time the zone is irradiated. The reproducibility of the photothermal effects has been barely reported in literature [37] and for some materials, irreversible changes and inactivation after the first shot of radiation have been observed [38]. Therefore, for a biomedical application, the reproducibility of the NIR-induced heating should be verified. Consequently, T1307/Au dispersions were subjected to irradiation cycles. The irradiation was maintained until a temperature plateau was achieved. The highest increase in temperature, applying 2 W/cm^2, was recorded for T1307 (15 mM)/Au (0.5 mM) prepared in 1 M NaCl medium (Figure 6a). In the case of T1307 (20 mM)/Au (0.5 mM) dispersions, the highest increase in temperature was 20 °C when prepared in the isotonic 0.154 M NaCl medium (Figure 4b). The maximum temperature was achieved after 10 min of irradiation. When the laser was switched off, the temperature progressively decreased until near the basal level. Successive laser switch on and off allowed a reproducible response to be recorded. The photothermal effect of all systems tested was maintained after being exposed to three irradiation cycles, which means that the formed AuNPs did not degrade after the first irradiation shot and that they can provide superimposable heating responses (when the laser was on or off).

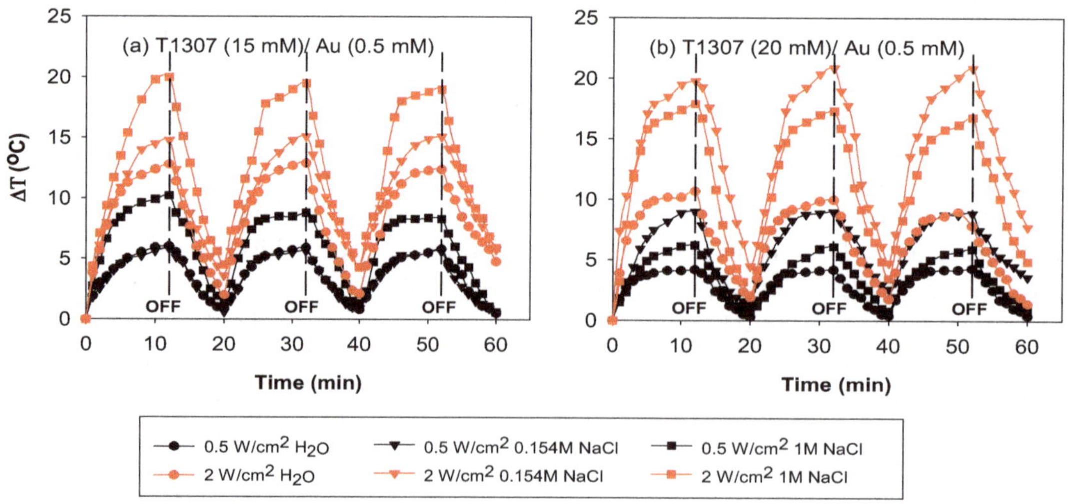

Figure 6. Temperature increase as a function of time under NIR irradiation during three cycles of 12 min irradiation and 8 min of non-irradiation with a 980 nm laser at 0.5 and 2 W/cm^2 on (**a**) 15 mM T1307 and (**b**) 20 mM T1307 dispersions.

4. Conclusions

Tetronic 1307 systems have been demonstrated to be able to transform gold salt into AuNPs directly in the final formulation under mild conditions, providing injectable systems with built-in temperature and light responsiveness. Adequate gold salt concentrations are in the 0.05 to 0.5 mM range; higher gold salt proportions may hinder the reduction, probably due to an extremely acid pH and insufficient copolymer. The information gathered points out that (i) the poloxamine concentration plays a key role on AuNPs' size and shape under isotonic conditions; the typical LSPR of gold nanoplates was recorded for T1307 concentrations equal to or above 10 mM. Interestingly, different morphologies of AuNPs (e.g., triangles, nanoprisms, and spheres) coexist in the same dispersion and seem to be encapsulated in the copolymer aggregates. (ii) The AuNPs cause minor shifts in the temperature-induced gelling transition of T1307 towards slightly higher temperatures, which may be related to the consumption of some copolymer unimers in the stabilization of the AuNPs and, therefore, less unimers are available for the micellization and subsequent in situ gelling. (iii) The spontaneously formed AuNPs exhibit remarkable photothermal responsiveness using a NIR laser of relatively low power, causing increments in temperature which surpass the required threshold for thermal ablation when needed. The gelling of the copolymer dispersion seems to facilitate the efficiency of the responsiveness, probably because of the larger size of the copolymer–AuNP aggregates. Similarly, an increase in NaCl concentration also enhances the photothermal effect. Remarkably, isotonic dispersions of T1307 (15–20 mM) containing AuNPs can undergo the sol-to-gel transition under physiological conditions and may retain the AuNPs for exploitation of the photothermal effects under successive NIR light irradiation cycles. The reproducible photoresponsiveness of the obtained T1307/AuNPs systems may be exploited for ablation of tumor cells or bacteria, but also for other applications such as the photo-controlled release of therapeutic substances.

Author Contributions: Conceptualization, C.A.-L., A.C., S.B. and P.T.; methodology, S.C.-M. and C.A.-L.; validation, S.C.-M., P.T. and S.B.; resources, C.A.-L., P.T.; writing—original draft preparation, S.C.-M.; writing—review and editing, C.A.-L., A.C., S.B. and P.T.; supervision, C.A.-L. and A.C.

Acknowledgments: The authors thank Raquel Antón Segurado from RIAIDT USC for help with SEM and EDX analysis, and BASF for kind donation of Tetronic samples.

References

1. Melancon, M.P.; Zhou, M.; Li, C. Cancer theranostics with near-infrared light-activatable multimodal nanoparticles. *Acc. Chem. Res.* **2011**, *44*, 947–956. [CrossRef] [PubMed]
2. Mieszawska, A.J.; Mulder, W.J.M.; Fayad, Z.A.; Cormode, D.P. Multifunctional gold nanoparticles for diagnosis and therapy of disease. *Mol. Pharm.* **2013**, *10*, 831–847. [CrossRef]
3. Barbosa, S.; Topete, A.; Alatorre-Meda, M.; Villar-Alvarez, E.M.; Alvarez-Lorenzo, C.; Concheiro, A.; Taboada, P.; Mosquera, V. Targeted combinatorial therapy using gold nanostars as theranostic platforms. *J. Phys. Chem. C* **2014**, *118*, 26313–26323. [CrossRef]
4. Liu, T.M.; Yu, J.; Chang, A.; Chiou, A.; Chiang, H.K.; Chuang, Y.C.; Wu, C.H.; Hsu, C.H.; Chen, P.A.; Huang, C.C. One-step shell polymerization of inorganic nanoparticles and their applications in SERS/nonlinear optical imaging, drug delivery, and catalysis. *Sci. Rep.* **2014**, *4*, 5593. [CrossRef] [PubMed]
5. Polo, E.; Poupard, M.F.N.; Guerrini, L.; Taboada, P.; Pelaz, B.; Alvarez-Puebla, R.A.; del Pino, P. Colloidal bioplasmonics. *Nano Today* **2018**, *20*, 58–73. [CrossRef]
6. Adnan, N.N.M.; Cheng, Y.Y.; Ong, N.M.N.; Kamaruddin, T.T.; Rozlan, E.; Schmidt, T.W.; Duong, H.T.T.; Boyer, C. Effect of gold nanoparticle shapes for phototherapy and drug delivery. *Polym. Chem.* **2016**, *7*, 2888–2903. [CrossRef]

7. Choi, C.H.J.; Alabi, C.A.; Webster, P.; Davis, M.E. Mechanism of active targeting in solid tumors with transferrin-containing gold nanoparticles. *Proc. Natl. Acad. Sci. USA* **2010**, *107*, 1235–1240. [CrossRef] [PubMed]
8. Alvarez-Lorenzo, C.; Garcia-Gonzalez, C.A.; Bucio, E.; Concheiro, A. Stimuli-responsive polymers for antimicrobial therapy: Drug targeting, contact-killing surfaces and competitive release. *Expert Opin. Drug Deliv.* **2016**, *13*, 1109–1119. [CrossRef]
9. Cabana, S.; Lecona-Vargas, C.S.; Melendez-Ortiz, H.I.; Contreras-Garcia, A.; Barbosa, S.; Taboada, P.; Magariños, B.; Bucio, E.; Concheiro, A.; Alvarez-Lorenzo, C. Silicone rubber films functionalized with poly(acrylic acid) nanobrushes for immobilization of gold nanoparticles and photothermal therapy. *J. Drug Deliv. Sci. Technol.* **2017**, *42*, 245–254. [CrossRef]
10. Espinosa, A.; Kolosnjaj-Tabi, J.; Abou-Hassan, A.; Sangnier, A.P.; Curcio, A.; Silva, A.K.A.; Di Corato, R.; Neveu, S.; Pellegrino, T.; Liz-Marzan, L.M.; et al. Magnetic (hyper)thermia or photothermia? Progressive comparison of iron oxide and gold nanoparticles heating in water, in cells, and in vivo. *Adv. Funct. Mater.* **2018**, *28*, 1803660. [CrossRef]
11. Zhao, M.X.; Cai, Z.C.; Zhu, B.J.; Zhang, Z.Q. The apoptosis effect on liver cancer cells of gold nanoparticles modified with lithocholic acid. *Nanoscale Res. Lett.* **2018**, *13*, 304. [CrossRef] [PubMed]
12. Simpson, C.A.; Salleng, H.J.; Cliffel, D.E.; Feldheim, D.L. In vivo toxicity, biodistribution, and clearance of glutathione-coated gold nanoparticles. *Nanomedicine* **2013**, *9*, 257–263. [CrossRef] [PubMed]
13. Fraga, S.; Brandão, A.; Soares, M.E.; Morais, T.; Duarte, J.A.; Pereira, L.; Soares, L.; Neves, C.; Pereira, E.; Bastos, M.L.; et al. Short- and long-term distribution and toxicity of gold nanoparticles in the rat after a single-dose intravenous administration. *Nanomedicine* **2014**, *10*, 1757–1766. [CrossRef] [PubMed]
14. Yook, S.; Cai1, Z.; Lu, Y.; Winnik, M.A.; Pignol, J.P.; Reilly, R.M. Intratumorally injected 177Lu-labeled gold nanoparticles: Gold nanoseed brachytherapy with application for neoadjuvant treatment of locally advanced breast cancer. *J. Nucl. Med.* **2016**, *57*, 936–942. [CrossRef] [PubMed]
15. Lai, P.; Lechtman, E.; Mashouf, S.; Pignol, J.P.; Reilly, R.M. Depot system for controlled release of gold nanoparticles with precise intratumoral placement by permanent brachytherapy seed implantation (PSI) techniques. *Int. J. Pharm.* **2016**, *515*, 729–739. [CrossRef] [PubMed]
16. Li, H.; Liu, X.; Huang, N.; Ren, K.; Jin, Q.; Ji, J. Mixed-charge Self-Assembled Monolayers as a facile method to design pH-induced aggregation of large gold nanoparticles for near-infrared photothermal cancer therapy. *ACS Appl. Mater. Interfaces* **2014**, *6*, 18930–18937. [CrossRef] [PubMed]
17. Sun, M.; Peng, D.; Hao, H.; Hu, J.; Wang, D.; Wang, K.; Liu, J.; Guo, X.; Wei, Y.; Gao, W. Thermally triggered in situ assembly of gold nanoparticles for cancer multimodal imaging and photothermal therapy. *ACS Appl. Mater. Interfaces* **2017**, *9*, 10453–10460. [CrossRef] [PubMed]
18. Sakai, T.; Alexandridis, P. Mechanism of gold metal ion reduction, nanoparticle growth and size control in aqueous amphiphilic block copolymer solutions at ambient conditions. *J. Phys. Chem. B* **2005**, *109*, 7766–7777. [CrossRef] [PubMed]
19. Khullar, P.; Singh, V.; Mahal, A.; Kumar, H.; Kaur, G.; Bakshi, M.S. Block copolymer micelles as nanoreactors for self-assembled morphologies of gold nanoparticles. *J. Phys. Chem. B* **2013**, *117*, 3028–3039. [CrossRef]
20. Alexandridis, P.; Tsianou, M. Block copolymer-directed metal nanoparticle morphogenesis and organization. *Eur. Polym. J.* **2011**, *47*, 569–583. [CrossRef]
21. Goy-Lopez, S.; Taboada, P.; Cambon, A.; Juarez, J.; Alvarez-Lorenzo, C.; Concheiro, A.; Mosquera, V. Modulation of size and shape of Au nanoparticles using amino-X-shaped poly(ethylene oxide)-poly(propylene oxide) block copolymers. *J. Phys. Chem. B* **2010**, *114*, 66–77. [CrossRef] [PubMed]
22. Rey-Rico, A.; Frisch, J.; Venkatesan, J.K.; Schmitt, G.; Rial-Hermida, I.; Taboada, P.; Concheiro, A.; Madry, H.; Alvarez-Lorenzo, C.; Cucchiarini, M. PEO–PPO–PEO carriers for rAAV-mediated transduction of human articular chondrocytes in vitro and in a human osteochondral defect model. *ACS Appl. Mater. Interfaces* **2016**, *8*, 20600–20613. [CrossRef] [PubMed]
23. Ribeiro, A.; Sosnik, A.; Chiappetta, D.A.; Veiga, F.; Concheiro, A.; Alvarez-Lorenzo, C. Single and mixed poloxamine micelles as nanocarriers for solubilization and sustained release of ethoxzolamide for topical glaucoma therapy. *J. R. Soc. Interfaces* **2012**, *9*, 2059–2069. [CrossRef]
24. Gonzalez-Lopez, J.; Alvarez-Lorenzo, C.; Taboada, P.; Sosnik, A.; Sández-Macho, I.; Concheiro, A. Self-associative behavior and drug-solubilizing ability of poloxamine (Tetronic) block copolymers. *Langmuir* **2008**, *24*, 10688–10697. [CrossRef] [PubMed]

25. Rey-Rico, A.; Silva, M.; Couceiro, J.; Concheiro, A.; Alvarez-Lorenzo, C. Osteogenic efficiency of in situ gelling poloxamine systems with and without bone morphogenetic protein-2. *Eur. Cells Mater.* **2011**, *21*, 317–340. [CrossRef]
26. Vyas, B.; Pillai, S.A.; Bahadur, A.; Bahadur, P. A comparative study on micellar and solubilizing behavior of three EO-PO based star block copolymers varying in hydrophobicity and their application for the in vitro release of anticancer drugs. *Polymers* **2018**, *10*, 76. [CrossRef]
27. Puig-Rigall, J.; Obregon-Gomez, I.; Monreal-Perez, P.; Radulescu, A.; Blanco-Prieto, M.J.; Dreiss, C.A.; Gonzalez-Gaitano, G. Phase behaviour, micellar structure and linear rheology of tetrablock copolymer Tetronic 908. *J. Colloid Interfaces Sci.* **2018**, *524*, 42–51. [CrossRef] [PubMed]
28. Rodriguez-Evora, M.; Reyes, R.; Alvarez-Lorenzo, C.; Concheiro, A.; Delgado, A.; Evora, C. Bone regeneration induced by an in situ gel-forming poloxamine, bone morphogenetic protein-2 system. *J. Biomed. Nanotechnol.* **2014**, *10*, 959–969. [CrossRef]
29. Sandez-Macho, I.; Casas, M.; Lage, E.V.; Rial-Hermida, M.I.; Concheiro, A.; Alvarez-Lorenzo, C. Interaction of poloxamine block copolymers with lipid membranes: Role of copolymer structure and membrane cholesterol content. *Colloids Surf. B Biointerfaces* **2015**, *133*, 270–277. [CrossRef]
30. Wang, W. Tolerability of hypertonic injectables. *Int. J. Pharm.* **2015**, *490*, 308–315. [CrossRef]
31. Bahadur, A.; Cabana-Montenegro, S.; Aswal, V.K.; Lage, E.V.; Sandez-Macho, I.; Concheiro, A.; Alvarez-Lorenzo, C.; Bahadur, P. NaCl-triggered self-assembly of hydrophilic poloxamine block copolymers. *Int. J. Pharm.* **2015**, *494*, 453–462. [CrossRef] [PubMed]
32. Pandit, N.; Trygstad, T.; Croy, S.; Bohorquez, M.; Koch, C. Effect of salts on the micellization, clouding, and solubilization behavior of Pluronic F127 solutions. *J. Colloid Interface Sci.* **2000**, *222*, 213–220. [CrossRef] [PubMed]
33. Sakai, T.; Enomoto, H.; Torigoe, K.; Sakai, H.; Abe, M. Surfactant- and reducer-free synthesis of gold nanoparticles in aqueous solutions. *Colloids Surf. A Physicochem. Eng. Asp.* **2009**, *347*, 18–26. [CrossRef]
34. Hirsch, L.R.; Stafford, R.J.; Bankson, J.A.; Sershen, S.R.; Rivera, B.; Price, R.E.; Hazle, J.D.; Halas, N.J.; West, J.L. Nanoshell-mediated near-infrared thermal therapy of tumors under magnetic resonance guidance. *Proc. Natl. Acad. Sci. USA* **2003**, *100*, 13549–13554. [CrossRef] [PubMed]
35. Jaque, D.; Martínez Maestro, L.; del Rosal, B.; Haro-Gonzalez, P.; Benayas, A.; Plaza, J.L.; Martín Rodríguez, E.; Solé, J.G. Nanoparticles for photothermal therapies. *Nanoscale* **2014**, *6*, 9494–9530. [CrossRef] [PubMed]
36. Meng, D.; Yang, S.; Guo, L.; Li, G.; Ge, J.; Huang, Y.; Bielawski, C.W.; Geng, J. The enhanced photothermal effect of graphene/conjugated polymer composites: Photoinduced energy transfer and applications in photocontrolled switches. *Chem. Commun.* **2014**, *50*, 14345–14348. [CrossRef] [PubMed]
37. Rahoui, N.; Jiang, B.; Hegazy, M.; Taloub, N.; Wang, Y.; Yu, M.; Huang, Y.D. Gold modified polydopamine coated mesoporous silica nano-structures for synergetic chemo-photothermal effect. *Colloid Surf. B Biointerfaces* **2018**, *171*, 176–185. [CrossRef]
38. Klekotko, M.; Olesiak-Banska, J.; Matczyszyn, K. Photothermal stability of biologically and chemically synthesized gold nanoprisms. *J. Nanopart. Res.* **2017**, *19*, 327. [CrossRef]

14

Gadolinium-Doped Gallic Acid-Zinc/Aluminium-Layered Double Hydroxide/Gold Theranostic Nanoparticles for a Bimodal Magnetic Resonance Imaging and Drug Delivery System

Muhammad Sani Usman [1,*], Mohd Zobir Hussein [1,*], Sharida Fakurazi [2,3], Mas Jaffri Masarudin [4] and Fathinul Fikri Ahmad Saad [5]

1 Materials Synthesis and Characterization Laboratory, Institute of Advanced Technology (ITMA), Serdang 43400, Selangor, Malaysia
2 Laboratory of Vaccines and Immunotherapeutics, Institute of Bioscience, Serdang 43400, Selangor, Malaysia; sharida.fakurazi@gmail.com
3 Department of Human Anatomy, Faculty of Medicine and Health Sciences, Serdang 43400, Selangor, Malaysia
4 Department of Cell & Molecular Biology, Faculty of Biotechnology and Biomolecular Sciences, Serdang 43400, Selangor, Malaysia; masjaffri@upm.edu.my
5 Centre for Diagnostic and Nuclear Imaging, Faculty of Medicine and Health Sciences, Universiti Putra Malaysia, Serdang 43400, Selangor, Malaysia; ahmadsaadff@gmail.com
* Correspondence: muhusma@gmail.com (M.S.U.); mzobir@upm.edu.my (M.Z.H.);

Abstract: We have developed gadolinium-based theranostic nanoparticles for co-delivery of drug and magnetic resonance imaging (MRI) contrast agent using Zn/Al-layered double hydroxide as the nanocarrier platform, a naturally occurring phenolic compound, gallic acid (GA) as therapeutic agent, and $Gd(NO_3)_3$ as diagnostic agent. Gold nanoparticles (AuNPs) were grown on the system to support the contrast for MRI imaging. The nanoparticles were characterized using techniques such as Hi-TEM, XRD, ICP-ES. Kinetic release study of the GA from the nanoparticles showed about 70% of GA was released over a period of 72 h. The in vitro cell viability test for the nanoparticles showed relatively low toxicity to human cell lines (3T3) and improved toxicity on cancerous cell lines (HepG2). A preliminary contrast property test of the nanoparticles, tested on a 3 Tesla MRI machine at various concentrations of GAGZAu and water (as a reference) indicates that the nanoparticles have a promising dual diagnostic and therapeutic features to further develop a better future for clinical remedy for cancer treatment.

Keywords: Zn/Al LDH; gallic acid; therapeutic; diagnostic; theranostic

---

1. Introduction

Nano-based materials or nanotechnology research has become a hot zone of material science research globally, due to the various advantages that come with nanomaterials [1], especially in numerous biomedical applications [2–6]. Chemotherapy remains the best choice of cancer treatment, due the availability of various anticancer agents. Nevertheless, the challenge of toxicities posed by these agents still exits [7]. Over a decade or so, various nanotechnology platforms have been explored in overcoming this challenge. Some of the areas of interest are the nanodrug delivery systems (NDDS). However, multimodal delivery systems (MDS) are recently gaining more attention [8], where drugs are simultaneously loaded along with other active agents on the same nanocarrier platform [7,9]. For instance, in theranostic research, the concept of MDS is employed where a nanocarrier is used as a delivery agent for therapeutic agents and diagnostic agents, such as magnetic resonance imaging (MRI) contrast agents [6], for a non-invasive concurrent delivery [10].

MRI is a non-invasive and non–ionizing important imaging tool used for cancer clinical diagnosis. Since the 1970s, MRI has been one of the most recognized powerful imaging techniques due to its high spatial resolution and tissue penetrating ability [8,11]. However, the use of MRI often requires contrast agents. Gadolinium-based (Gd) contrast agents are the commonly used contrast agents for MRI, which improve the T1 and T2 relaxation times of the images produced [8]. T1 and T2 relaxations are the main signals among others generated during MR imaging, which have distinctive grey-scale color contrasts reflecting the fluid and soft tissue composition of human subject. The signals represent spin–lattice relaxation and spin–spin relaxation for T1 and T2, respectively [12]. Zn/Al-layered double hydroxide (LDH) is one of the candidates capable of simultaneously intercalating and adsorbing theranostic agents due to their exchangeable interlayer anions. LDH is one of the group of two-dimensional layered structures materials [13] and has the general formula of $[M^{2+}_{1-x}\ M^{3+}_{x}\ (OH)_2]_x + [A^{n-}]\ x/n{\cdot}mH_2O]$ [14], where divalent and trivalent metal cations are represented by M^{2+} and M^{3+}, respectively, and interlayer exchangeable anions are represented by $[A^{n-}]$, and water as x/n [8,15–17]. Gallic acid is the therapeutic agent employed in this research; it is a naturally occurring polyhydroxyl phenolic compound, often found in different kinds of fruits. It is believed to have anticancer properties as well as other activities in a range of cells [18]. Although there are various research publications on drug intercalation using LDH in drug delivery as reviewed by Kura et al. [19], only a few works have so far been done on theranostic applications using LDH-based nanocarriers. Those articles have also been reviewed by Usman et al. [8], amongst which none has reported synthesis of theranostic nanocomposite using drug intercalation process.

Herein, we synthesized theranostic nanoparticles by Gd doping onto Zn/Al-LDH. Gallic acid was first intercalated into the interlayers of the LDH-Gd and AuNPs were then grown on the surface of the LDH nanoparticles. The LDH prepared via co-precipitation method was used as the nanocarrier, while Gd and AuNPs were used as the main contrast agent and booster for MRI, respectively.

2. Results and Discussion

The final GAGZAu nanoparticles were subjected to various characterizations as will be reported later, although the analyses were done at every step of the synthesis, starting with the LDH nanocarrier itself. Figure 1 is a representative of a typical multimodal theranostic setting, similar to a host–guest reaction in supramolecular chemistry, where a nano-carrier, a 2D host was first loaded with therapeutic agent (the first guest) by the intercalation process, gallic acid. Following the formation of pure phase, diagnostic agents (the second guests), Gd, and AuNPs were loaded. A third guest, a targeting agent, can be also loaded, resulting in the formation of a multimodal theranostic nanodelivery system [8]. However, the loading of a targeting agent will be done in our near future work. The mechanism of bonding between the LDH and the GA is via hydrogen bonding due the surplus OH groups in the anionic guest as well as ion exchange with the interlayer anions [20]. Whereas the contrast agents are bonded to the LDH through van der Waals forces of attraction.

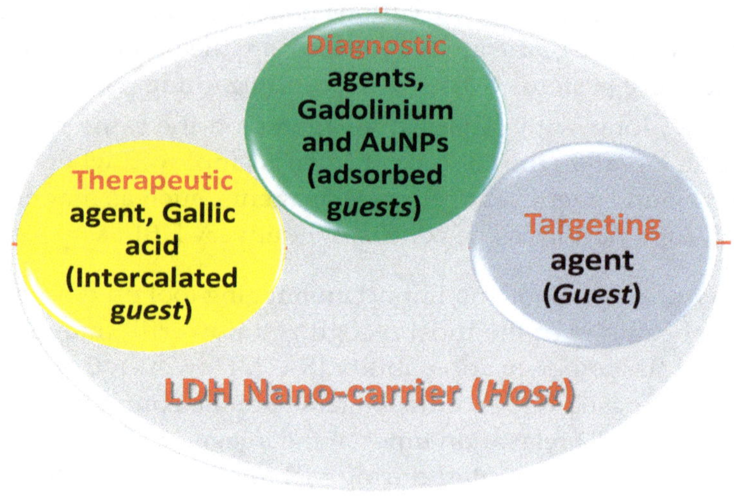

Figure 1. Schematic arrangement of GAGZAu nanocomposite in respect to theranostic delivery system in a typical host–guest relationship.

2.1. *X-ray Diffraction*

The diffractograms in Figure 2a indicate various patterns of the different stages of the nanocomposite synthesis, from the starting material to the final nanocomposite (A–E respectively). The diffractogram (A) represents the $Gd(NO_3)_3$, (B) represents LDH, (C) is for gallic acid, which are all in a pristine state. Further, the pattern of GAGZA (D) represents the first stage of the formation of theranostic nanocomposite, that is, the anticancer drug was intercalated into the LDH/Gd (A) interlayers at this stage. This as a result shows increase in basal spacing up to 9.9 Å, that is much higher than 7.7 Å of the LDH basal spacing; which strongly indicates the drug intercalation had taken place. In addition, the slight shift to a lower 2θ angle also implies the intercalation of the therapeutic agent GA into the interlayers of the LDH has taken place. The diffractogram of the theranostic GAGZAu (E) nanoparticles however, did not indicate most of the reflections of the LDH. This is presumably due to the surface coating of the AuNPs on the surface of the theranostic nanoparticles. Nonetheless, the pattern (Pattern 4-784) observed match with FCC (111, 200, and 220) of pure AuNPs [21].

2.2. *Drug Release Profile and Kinetics from GAGZA Nanocomposite*

The amount of drug loaded and in vitro drug release in the nanoparticles was calculated using a standard curve of the UV–Vis spectrometer at λ_{max} of the drug, 264 nm. As seen in Figure 2b, the maximum percentage of about 60% of the drug is released over a period of 5000 min (84 h) with 50% drug loading. The release was done using PBS buffer solution at pH 4.8 and 7.4. The release in the slightly alkaline pH is observed to be significantly lower (10%) than in the acidic pH (60%); which could be attributed to ion exchange occurring in the buffer media between the anions in the drug and the LDH nanocarrier [22]. Nonetheless, the sustained release profiles suggest safe release of the drug from the nanocarrier to the solution under acidity of pH 4.8 and less release at the higher pH 7.4. The huge difference in the release pattern of the pH is attributed to the mechanism or behavior of the nanocarrier in buffer solutions, as it is a common attribute of LDH interlayers to dissolve in acidic media together with the anionic guest on the external surface of the LDH [15], hence resulting in more release of the intercalated guest. This indicates the suitability of the nanohybrid as a good candidate for anticancer research, as rightly reported in literature where LDH nanoparticles was reported to have penetrated the cervical cancer cells via mediated endocytosis [23]. Furthermore, to understand the mechanism of the drug release, the data from the release study was fitted to three different kinetics models, namely

$$\text{Pseudo-first order: } \ln(q_e - q_t) = \ln q_t - kt \tag{1}$$

$$\text{Pseudo-second order: } \frac{t}{q_t} = \frac{1}{kq_e^2} + \frac{t}{q} \quad (2)$$

$$\text{Parabolic diffusion: } (1 - M_t/M_o)/t = kt^{-0.5} + b \quad (3)$$

The parameters used in the fitting equations are the drug content in the nanocarrier during release which are represented as M_t and M_o, the amount released at equilibrium and time t designated as q_e and q_t respectively; and the release constant k [15].

The three models as represented in Equations (1)–(3), gave different kinetic processes, the model that best describes the kinetic release of the gallic acid from the nanocomposite at both pH (7.4 and 4.8) is the pseudo-second order model, as expressed in Equation (2). The parameter $\frac{t}{q_t}$ is plotted against the time t, which gave correlation coefficients (R^2) of 0.994 at both pH 7.4 and 4.8 (Figure 2c,d). The rate constants (k) were determined to be 4.7×10^{-2} and 8.5×10^{-3} g/mg h, for pH 7.4 and 4.8, respectively. These results are consistent with other reported findings on drug release using LDH nanocarriers [15] and other nanocarriers [24]. Table 1 is a compilation of the fitted data of correlation coefficients (R^2), rate constants (k), and half-lives ($t_{1/2}$), as well as saturation points (%) of gallic acid released from GAGZA at pH 7.4 and 4.8.

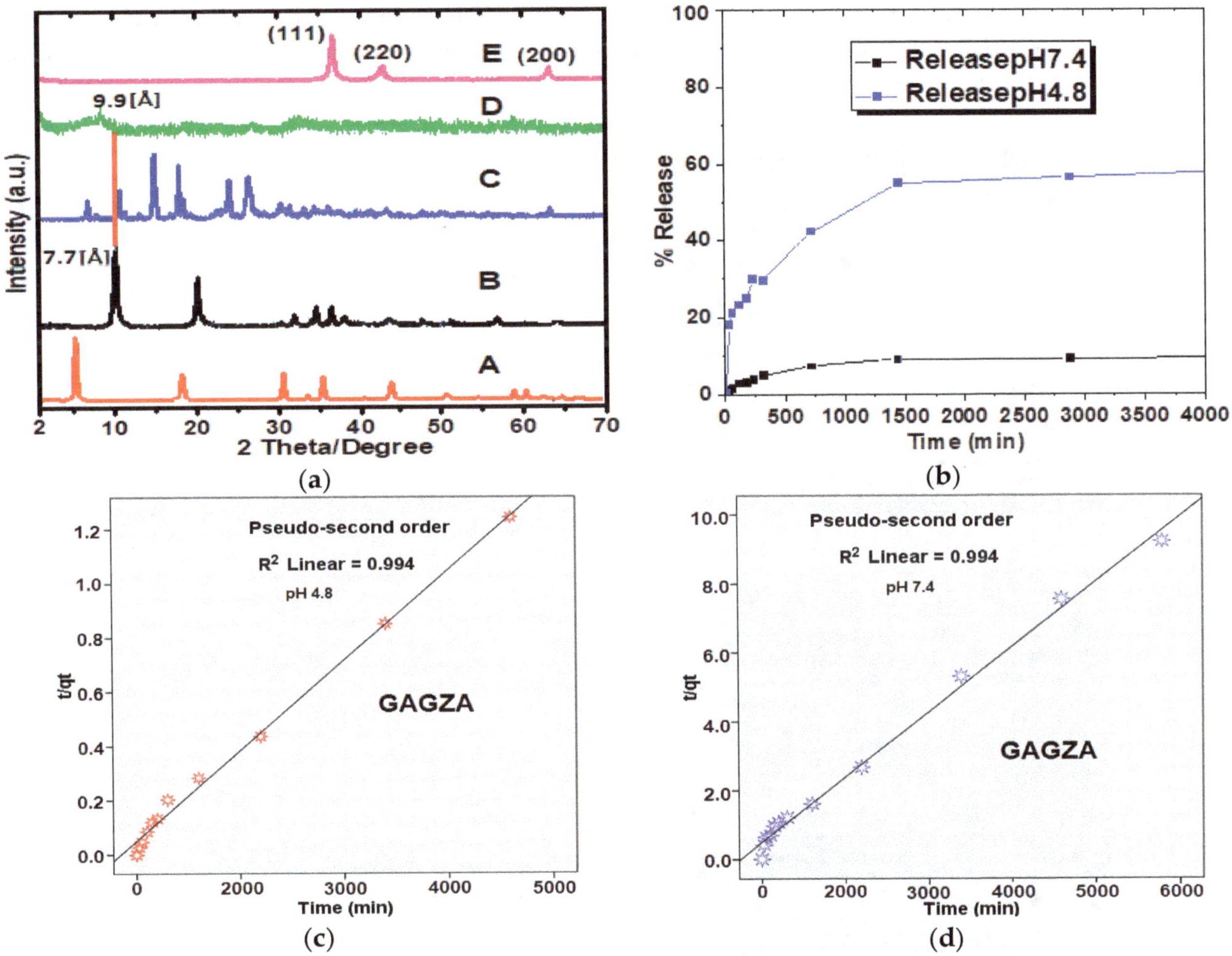

Figure 2. (**a**) X-ray diffractograms of (A) $Gd(NO_3)_3$, (B) Zn/Al-LDH, (C) pure gallic acid, (D) gallic acid-Zn/Al-LDH-Gd nanocomposite (GAGZA), (E) gallic acid-Zn/Al-LDH/Gd-Au nanocomposite (GAGZAu); (**b**) Release profiles of gallic acid intercalated into Zn/Al-LDH-Gd nanoparticles (GAGZA) in phosphate-buffered solutions at pH 4.8 and pH 7.4; (**c**) Data of gallic acid released from GAGZA obtained at pH 4.8 fitted to pseudo-seconder order; (**d**) Data of gallic acid released from GAGZA obtained at 7.4 fitted to pseudo-seconder order.

Table 1. Fitted data of correlation coefficients (R^2), rate constants (k), and half-lives ($t_{1/2}$) of gallic acid released from GAGZA at pH 7.4 and 4.8.

Medium pH	Release Saturation (%)	(R^2)	(R^2)	(R^2)	Rate Constant (k)	$t_{1/2}$ (min)
		Pseudo-First Order	Pseudo-Second Order	Parabolic Diffusion		
7.4	18	0.432	0.994	0	4.7×10^{-2}	520
4.8	62	0.094	0.994	0.7	8.5×10^{-3}	400

2.3. Surface Morphology and Elemental Content Analysis

The morphology of the nanoparticles was studied before and after the addition of AuNPs, that is for GAGZA and GAGZAu. Figure 3a depicts micrographs of GAGZAu and Figure 3c shows GAGZA micrographs. Though evenly distributed, the nanoparticles are observed to be agglomerated at dry state. The agglomeration may be due to surface energy, a phenomenon associated with small sized nanoparticles [25]. As observed in Figure 3a, the AuNPs coated on the GAGZA nanocomposite appears to have covered the LDH structure which has affected the thermal stability of the final GAGZAu nanocomposite as discussed in the TGA analysis chapter, as well as the MRI contrast due to increased surface area to volume ratio in the nanohybrid. The FESEM micrographs of the nanoparticles analyzed with EDX indicated the presence of the all the active elements in the nanoparticles (Zn, Al, O, C, Gd, and Au).

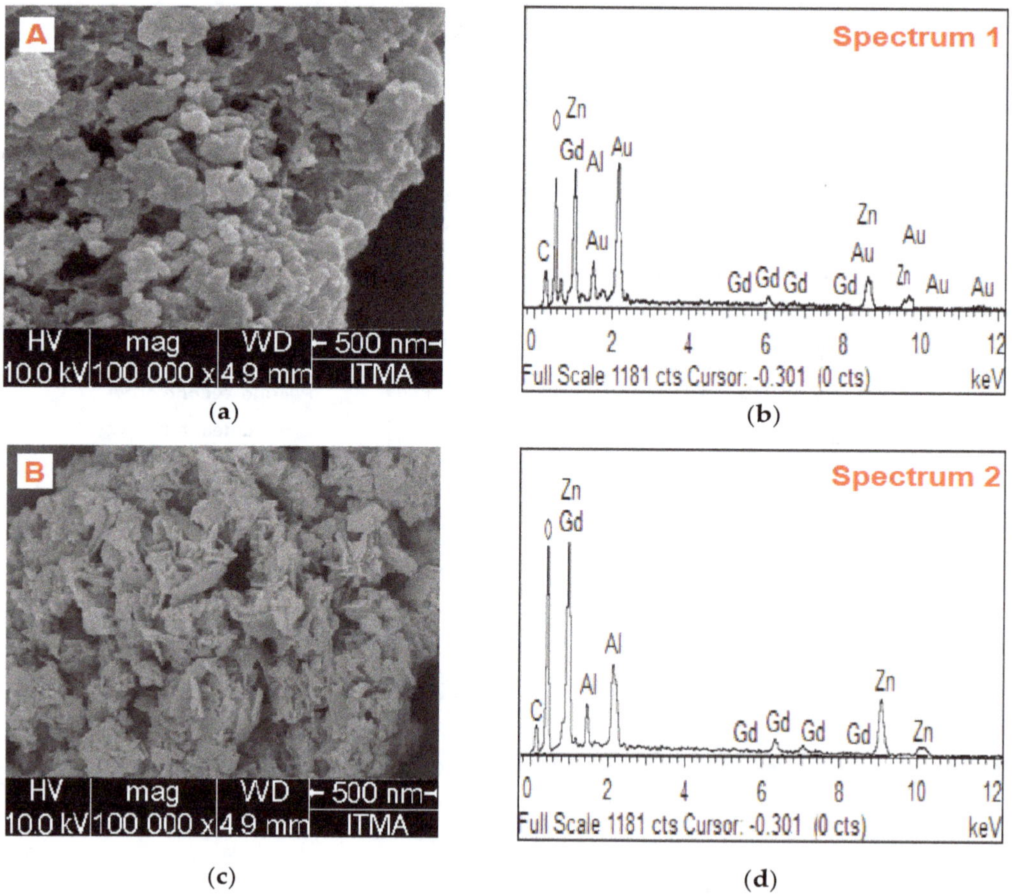

Figure 3. (**a**) Field emission scanning electron microscopy (FESEM) micrograph (A) and (**b**) Energy dispersive X-ray (EDX) spectrum (1) of gallic acid intercalated in LDH/Gd nanoparticles coated with AuNPs (GAGZAu); (**c**) micrograph (B); and (**d**) EDX spectrum (2) of gallic acid intercalated in LDH/Gd nanoparticles (GAGZA).

The EDX spectra were generated via random capture of the whole area of the FESEM micrographs attached to the spectra. As anticipated, the elements contained in spectrum 1 (Figure 3b) obtained from GAGZAu contain various reflections of Au which appeared to dominate the Gd reflections in spectrum 2 (Figure 3d), indicting the coating of the LDH surface with AuNPs. The few reflections of Gd are also suggesting the presence of the element in the micrograph. However, as expected also, the spectrum 2 obtained from GAGZA micrograph, before the addition of AuNPs (Figure 3d) showed dominant reflections from Gd with no sign of Au signals, which confirms the initial formation of LDH-Gd nanocomposites. Likewise, the Zn and Al reflections which appeared in both spectra confirm the structure of Zn/Al-Gd LDH. Further, aside from the C and O signals that appeared in the spectra, which are likely from the intercalated GA drug, no other reflections are observed. This shows the high percentage of purity of the nanocomposite at various stages of synthesis. The results appear to be in conformity with ICP-ES elemental composition analysis carried out on the samples, which showed presence of all the intended elements in the nanocomposite.

2.4. Size, Shape, and Distribution Analysis

TEM was used to analyze size and shape/distribution of the nanoparticles. The GAGZA micrograph (Figure 4b) indicates various sizes of the nanoparticles in different shapes, including rod-shaped nanoparticles which are conspicuously seen throughout the micrographs at different magnifications. All the nanoparticles are found to be within the nanorange (1–100 nm) [1].

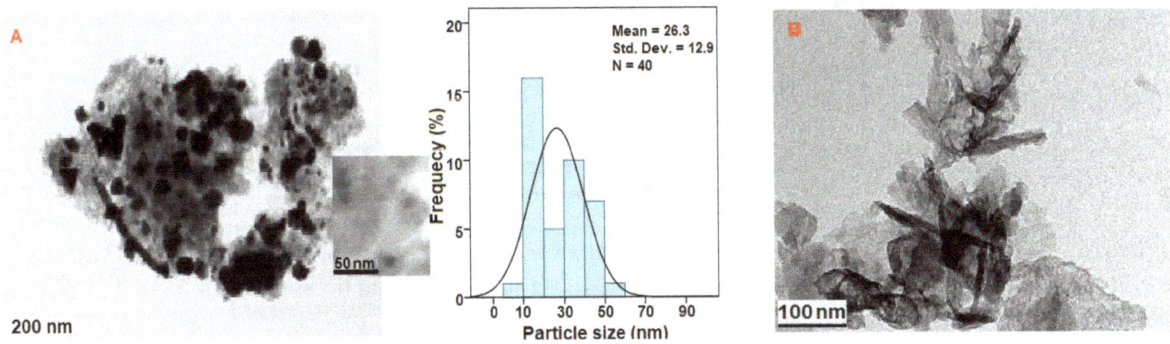

(a) (b)

Figure 4. (**a**) Transmission electron microscopy (TEM) micrograph (A) and particle size distribution of gallic acid-intercalated in Zn/Al-LDH/Gd nanoparticles coated with AuNPs (GAGZAu) and micrograph (B); (**b**) of gallic acid intercalated in Zn/Al-LDH/Gd nanoparticles (GAGZA).

The micrograph of the sample containing AuNPs (GAGZAu) (Figure 4a) evidently indicates the presence of the AuNPs in various sizes and shapes—such as hexagonal, triangular, and spherical shapes—thus confirming the growth of the AuNPs as indicated by other characterization results of the sample. The mean size of the AuNPs is approximately 26.3 nm as indicated in the histogram in Figure 4a, which are predominantly evenly distributed on the surface of the LDH nanocomposite across all shapes and sizes.

2.5. Chemical Interaction Studies (FT-IR Analysis)

The chemical interactions and changes between the nanocarriers and nanoparticles were studied using FT-IR spectroscopy. The changes in functional groups, chemical bonds and shifts in wavenumbers are the indication that some of the interactions have taken place. For easy comparison, the analysis was done on the pristine samples and the nanoparticles. Figure 5 depicts the FT-IR spectra of the Zn/Al-LDH, $Gd(NO_3)_3$, GA, GAGZA, and GAGZAu (A–E). The bands between 3307–3391 cm^{-1} which appear in all the FT-IR spectra are associated with OH stretching vibrations [26]; 1736 and 1702 cm^{-1} are characteristic absorptions of C=O; C=C aromatic ring stretching modes are represented by the bands 1541 and 1441, and 1541 and 1449 cm^{-1} in the GAGZA and GA spectra respectively; the band at 595 cm^{-1} represents bending vibration of OH carboxylic group. The bands at 1232, 1089, and 1025 cm^{-1} which appear in the GAGZA spectrum and at 1246 and 1026 cm^{-1} in the GA spectrum, are of C–O stretching vibrations [27]. The nitrate group stretching mode appears as a band at 1384 cm^{-1} of the Zn/Al spectrum; the band is noticeably absent in all other spectra; this is due to the loss of the nitrate anion in the bonding process, while H_2 bending vibration band can be seen at 1640 cm^{-1}. Furthermore, as expected the spectra of GAGZAu (E) appeared to be similar to spectra D of GAGZA, with the only difference is blue-shift in the band positions to higher wavenumbers. Generally, there are all shifts in the absorptions of the bands which are as a result of the bonding that took place between the guests and the LDH host at different stages of synthesis.

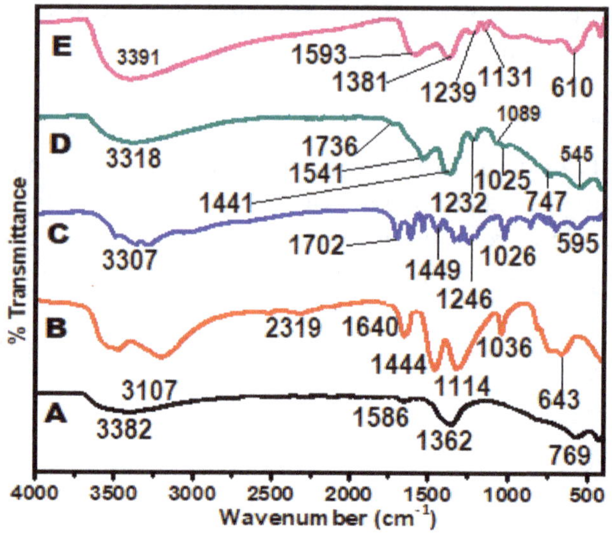

Figure 5. Fourier transform infrared spectroscopy (FT-IR) spectra (A) LDH, (B) $Gd(NO_3)_3$, (C) pure gallic acid, (D) gallic acid-Zn/Al-LDH/Gd nanoparticles (GAGZA), (E) Gallic acid-Zn/Al-LDH/Gd-Au nanoparticles (GAGZAu).

2.6. Thermal Stability Analysis (TGA/DTG)

The thermal stability of the nanoparticles and the pristine materials (GA and LDH) was tested with thermogravimetric and differential thermogravimetric analyses (TGA/DTG). To have more understanding of the thermal changes that occur, the TGA/DTG patterns of Zn/Al-LDH, GA, GAGZA, and GAGZAu were obtained as shown in Figure 6, and some key parameters have been highlighted in Table 2, which are: maximum peak temperature (Tmax), decomposition temperature range (Trange), and change in mass [(decomposed mass) Delta m] [28]. The peak at 88 °C which corresponds with weight loss of 5.9% in the Zn/Al-LDH thermogram (Figure 6a) is representative of physisorbed water loss on the surface and interlayer of the LDH.

The second peak at 243 °C with 16.3% mass loss and the third peak with 8.7% weight loss are reflective of nitrate decomposition and metal hydroxide layers dehydroxylation. The GA thermogram in Figure 6b shows three significant peaks, the first peak at 86 °C with 8.8% weight loss is attributed to absorbed water, while the peak at 264 °C which accounts to substantial weight loss of 41.0% is due to the dihydroxylation and decomposition of gallic acid structure, and lastly the one at 325 °C (22.5%) which represents residue decomposition.

Figure 6c depicts the thermogram of the GAGZA nanoparticles. The peak at 112 °C which represents 10.6% weight loss is related to removal of water. The peak next to it at 250 °C representing 17.4% loss of weight is due to dehydroxylation of the intercalated gallic acid as well as partial decomposition of nitrate. The peak at 600 °C indicating 8.2% weight loss could be attributed to the decomposition of $Gd(NO_3)_3$ together with the nitrate ions of LDH layers in the nanocomposite.

The sharp peak at 851 °C (8.3%) indicates the collapse of hydrotalcite-like layers and complete decomposition of the nanoparticles [29], which shows improved thermal stability that took place in comparison with the individual components. This is due to electrostatic attraction bonding that occurred between the negatively charged gallic acid functional groups and the positively charged LDH interlayer surfaces. Interestingly, the thermogram of the final nanocomposite which is the gold coated GAGZAu (Figure 6d), showed less thermal stability compared to the GAGZA thermogram. For instance, the first two peaks (99 and 198 °C) which represent loss of water and that of dihydroxylation respectively, appear to be at lower temperatures in comparison with GAGZA composite (112 and 250 °C). The peak at 602 °C and 1.59% weight loss of GAGZAu is associated with nitrate ions decomposition in nanocomposite. The peak associated with AuNPs surface decomposition is at 334 °C [30], amounting to about 2.2% weight loss. Generally however, the nanohybrid appear to be less thermally stable after coating with the AuNPs as depicted in Table 2. Nonetheless, the AuNPs could be more thermally stable when synthesized separately in their pure nanoparticles form using capping agents. As reported in literature, thermal stability of AuNPs depends on certain factors, such as the capping or stabilizing agents used in the synthesis and the type of bonding that occur between them determine the thermal stability, thus, weak bonds result in less stability and vice versa [31–34]. In our case, the reduction in thermal stability after AuNPs coating is presumably due to weak interaction between the AuNPs and the LDH nanocomposite surface, since no capping agent was used for the AuNPs synthesis.

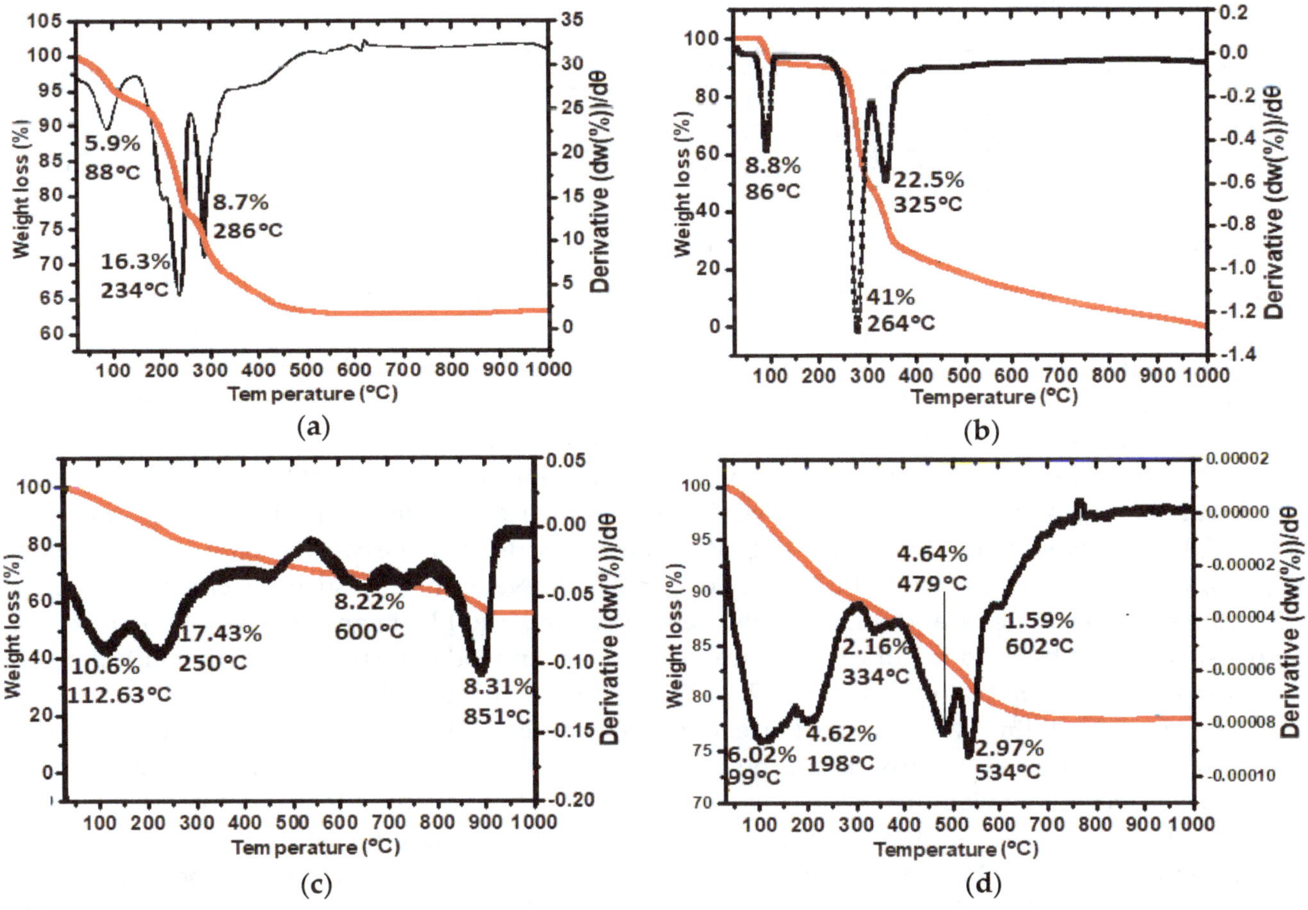

Figure 6. (**a**) Thermogravimetric and differential thermogravimetric analyses (TGA/DTG) thermograms of pure LDH; (**b**) pure gallic acid; (**c**) gallic acid-LDH/Gd nanoparticles (GAGZA); (**d**) gallic acid-LDH/Gd-Au nanoparticles (GAGZAu).

Table 2. Maximum peak temperature (Tmax) decomposition temperature range (Trange) and change in mass (Delta m).

Sample	Tmax (°C)	Trange (°C)	Delta m (%)
(A) LDH	234	88–286	30.9
(B) Gallic acid	264	86–325	72.3
(C) GAGZA	851	112–851	44.6
(D) GAGZAu	534	99–602	22.2

2.7. CHNS-ICP-ES Analyses

The composition of the GAGZAu nanocomposite was determined by combining CHNS and ICP-ES analyses, the individual data acquired were used to estimate the percentage content of each element. As indicated in Table 3, the constituents of the nanocomposite have, as obtained from the results, indicated successful intercalation of the guest drug (gallic acid) into LDH interlayer gallery. Additionally, the mole ratio of the Zn^{2+}/Al^{3+} in the GAGZAu nanocomposite and in the LDH was observed to be the same (0.1%). The ICP-ES data also shows presence of Gd and Au, indicating successful integration of Gd in the LDH-Gd block as well as coating of the surface with AuNPs. Moreover, the results are a validation of the EDX results reported earlier in this paper, which similarly confirms the presence of the aforesaid elements in the nanocarrier.

Table 3. Elemental analysis results for Zn/Al-layered double hydroxide (LDH) nanocarrier and GAGZAu nanocomposite.

Sample	C% •	H% •	N% •	Zn% ••	Al% ••	Gd% ••	Au% ••	Zn^{2+}/Al^{3+}% ••	Drug% •
Zn/Al-LDH	-	-	7.3	45	5.2	-	-	0.1	-
GAGZA-Au	8.714	2.186	0.4208	8.82	1.02	1.56	3.0	0.1	50

• Calculated from CHNS analysis; •• Calculated from ICP-ES analysis.

2.8. In Vitro Cytotoxicity Studies against HepG2 and 3T3 Cell Lines

The toxicities of the GAGZAu, the free drug and the nanocarrier were tested via cell viability study against liver cancer cell lines and normal human cell lines, HepG2 and 3T3, respectively. The cell lines were exposed to different concentrations of the aforementioned samples, starting with 0 (control) to 100 μ/mL. As observed in Figure 7, the free drug, the LDH and the GAGZAu nanohybrid tested against the 3T3 cell lines indicate nearly 100% cell viability in most of the concentrations. The 50 and 100 μ/mL dosage of the free drug however, shows slightly lower viability. This is expected as anticancer drugs are known to be cytotoxic and have certain undesirable side effects on normal cells [35,36]. Likewise, Gd-based contrast agent has been reported to have caused nephrogenic systemic fibrosis, which is associated with the toxicity of Gd [37,38]. Nevertheless, such toxicities are reduced when the anticancer agents and other agents are intercalated into LDH nanocarriers [39] or adsorbed on the surface, as observed in our case, the toxicities of GA and Gd have been virtually neutralized in the nanoparticles form, that is in the GAGZAu tested for the normal cell lines.

The HepG2 cell lines were similarly treated with different concentrations of the free drug, LDH and GAGZAu. Although the toxicity of the gallic acid against the HepG2 cell lines decreased in the nanoparticles form, the viability of the cells treated with GAGZAu still indicates cytotoxicity against HepG2 cell lines. Moreover, the LDH nanocarrier affects the therapeutic activity of the gallic acid; the nanoparticles could be more cytotoxic to other cancer cell lines. Nonetheless, the cells treated at 50 μ/mL of GAGZAu show the highest anticancer activity, which is due to higher release of the anticancer compounds contained inside the nanocomposite. Even though both 3T3 and HepG2 cells lines are non-phagocytic and have negatively charged cell surfaces, only the cancer cell lines will be susceptible to anticancer activity effects of the nanocomposite. The general mechanism of GA uptake by the cells is through electrostatic attraction which is prompted by cellular endocytosis between the positively charged GAGZAu surface and the negatively charged cell surface [20]. The individual specific mechanism through which the GAGZAu intake occurs in the 3T3 and HepG2 cannot be described via simple MTT assay alone, other more precise experiments such as flow cytometry have to be applied.

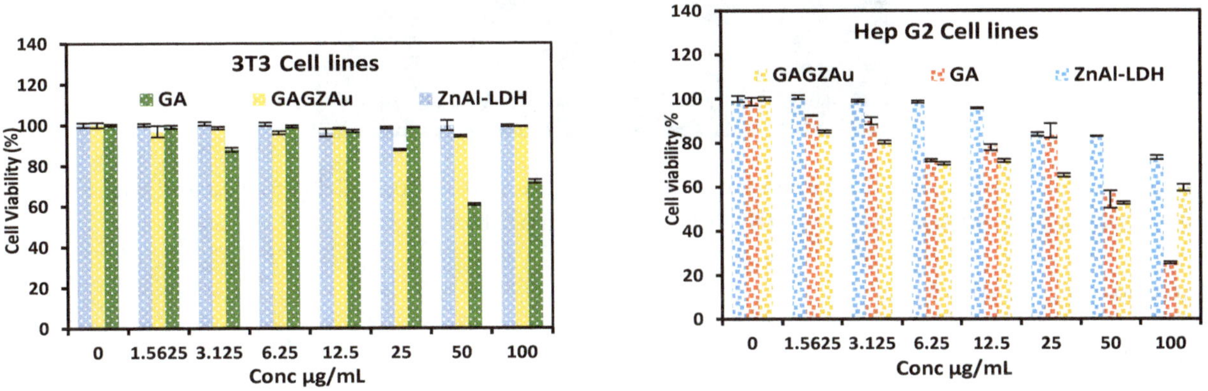

(a) (b)

Figure 7. Cytotoxicity study of GAGZAu, LDH, and free drug at various concentrations exposed to (**a**) cancer cell lines (HepG2) and; (**b**) normal cell lines (3T3).

2.9. Magnetic Resonance Imaging

The magnetic resonance image of the samples was captured as shown in Figure 8, where five tubes were arranged, each representing GAGZAu nanoparticle solutions at different concentrations in order of increasing Gd^{3+} concentration; 0.2, 0.5, and 2.0 w/v, $Gd(NO_3)_3$ and distilled water (as the reference). The average intensity of each tube was measured using Syngovia MRI software, and signal mean intensities were calculated. The signals intensities of each concentrate tube was documented to increase steadily and proportionally as the concentration of Gd^{3+} in the nanohybrid, that is 322.44, 297.70, and 262.00 for 2.0, 0.5, and 0.2 w/v concentration, respectively. In addition, the R1 signal intensity of GAGZAu at the lowest dosage (0.2 w/v) indicates higher R1 signal intensity (262.00) than $Gd(NO_3)_3$ (235.45) at 0.5 concentration and the water reference (228.66). This is indicative that R1 signal increase is as a result of the formation of Gd-based nanoparticles. The boost occurred as a result of the shortening of the longitudinal relaxation time (T1) [40,41] due higher surface area to volume ratio of AuNPs coated on the surface of the nanoparticles, which improves water solubility [41] and molecule movement, and proton exchange within the Gd^{3+}/LDH lattice [42,43]. The phenomenon is suspected to be connected with the change in structure of the nanohybrid after AuNPs surface coating, as observed in the GAGZAu TEM and FESEM micrographs. The free movement of water molecules through the nanohybrid results in shortening of the longitudinal relaxation time as well as reduces short circulation in the system, which in turn increases the R1 value of the recorded MR image. The longitudinal relaxation time as stated earlier in this work is responsible for the contrast effect of MR imaging [44]. Similar outcome was reported by previous works done using Gd/LDH-Au nanoparticles [8].

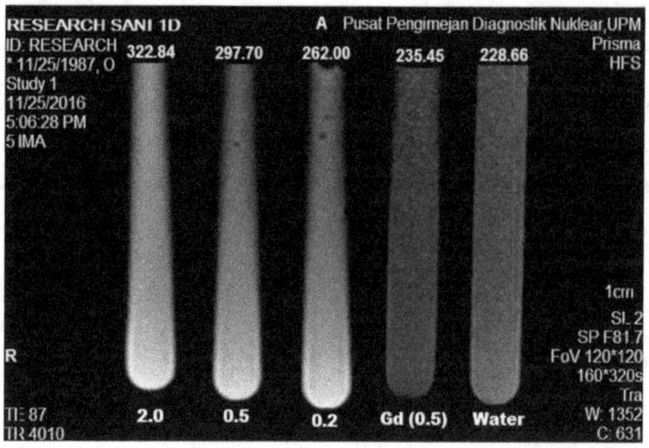

Figure 8. GAGZAu image at different Gd^{3+} concentrations (2.0, 0.5, 0.2), Gd (0.5) *w/v* and water taken from magnetic resonance imaging MRI Prisma 3-Tesla machine.

3. Materials and Methods

3.1. Materials

Gallic acid with molecular weight of 170.12 g/mol and 98% purity, sodium hydroxide molecular weight of 40.00 g/mol and 98% purity and phosphate-buffered saline were purchased from Sigma-Aldrich (St. Louis, MO, USA). Zinc nitrate hexahydrate molecular weight of 297.47 g/mol, 98% purity, and aluminium nitrate hexahydrate molecular weight of 375.13 g/mol, 98% purity, were purchased from Systerm ChemPur (Shah Alam, Selangor Darul Ehsan, Malaysia). Gadolinium (III) nitrate hexahydrate and molecular weight of 451.4 g/mol with 99.9% purity and tetrachloroauric(III) acid trihydrate, 393.83 g/mol and 49% Au purity were purchased from Acros Organics (Morris Plains, NJ, USA). Sodium borohydride molecular weight of 37.83 g/mol, and 99% purity was purchased from Fluka Analytical (St. Gallen, Switzerland). All chemicals were used as received without further purification. Deionized water was used throughout the experiment.

3.2. Synthesis of Gd-Zn/Al-Layered Double Hydroxide

Zn/Al-layered double hydroxide was synthesized using $Zn(NO_3)_2$ and $Al(NO_3)_3$ at a molar ratio of 4:1 of Zn^{2+} to Al^{3+}. $Gd(NO_3)_3$ (0.0008 M) was firstly dissolved in 250 mL deionized water before the addition of the Zn/Al nitrate salts. Dropwise addition of NaOH (2 M) was immediately followed until a pH of 7 was reached. The synthesis was conducted under nitrogen flow and vigorous stirring. The slurry obtained at the end of the process was aged for 18 h at 70 °C, centrifuged, washed with deionized water (three times), and oven dried at 60 °C.

3.3. Loading of Gallic Acid into Gd-Zn/Al-LDH Nanoparticles (GAGZA)

Briefly, gallic acid, 0.2 M solution was prepared by dissolving 3.6 g of the drug into 50 mL deionized water while stirring and heating at 45 °C. Under continuous nitrogen flow with vigorous stirring, the drug solution was simultaneously added dropwise with NaOH (2 M) into the 250 mL solution of Gd-Zn/Al-layered double hydroxide. The solution was kept until pH 7 was reached and the drug was completely loaded. The mixture was then aged for 18 h at approximately 70 °C. The resultant slurry obtained was filtered, washed/centrifuged using deionized water, and oven dried at 60 °C for 12 h.

3.4. Doping of Gold Nanoparticles (AuNPs) onto Zn/Al-Gd GA LDH (GAGZAu)

Appropriate amount of GAGZA was ultrasonically dispersed for 5 min, under gentle stirring; 2% $HAuCl_4$ (6 mL) solution was added. After 5 min stirring, 0.125 M NaOH (4 mL) was added; the dispersion was allowed to stir for 5 min before the temperature of the solution was raised to 60 °C and stirred for 24 h in dark conditions. The resulting precipitate was obtained after centrifuge/filtration, the mixture was re-dispersed in 30 mL deionized water; 1 M $NaBH_4$ (20 mL) was added and stirred for an hour. The final suspension obtained was washed six times using a centrifuge, filtered, and dried at 70 °C in an oven.

3.5. Characterization

An XRD-6000 (Shimadzu, Tokyo, Japan) X-ray diffraction (XRD) instrument was used for crystallographic analysis of the powdered samples. CuK_α radiation (λ = 1.5418 Å) at scan speed of 4°/min, using a range of 2–70 °C at 30 kV and 30 mA was used in obtaining the XRD patterns. A ultraviolet–visible (UV–Vis) spectrophotometer (PerkinElmer, Singapore) (Lambda35) was used for the controlled release and optical property studies. Fourier transform infrared (FT-IR) spectra of the materials were obtained using a Thermo Nicolet, Nicolet 6700 model (Thermo Scientific, Waltham, MA, USA). The spectra were obtained using the potassium bromide (KBr) discs at 10 ton pellet pressing and a resolution of 4 cm^{-1} over a range of 400–4000 cm^{-1}. A PerkinElmer spectrophotometer (PerkinElmer, Wellesley, MA, USA) (model Optima2000DV) inductively coupled plasma atomic emission spectrometry (ICP-ES) was employed in studying the composition of zinc, aluminum, gadolinium, and gold content of the nanoparticles. A CHNS-932 LECO (LECO, St. Joseph, Michigan, USA) instrument was used in determining carbon, hydrogen, nitrogen, and sulphur (CHNS) content in the sample. A Mettler-Toledo instrument (METTLER TOLEDO, Shah Alam, Selangor, Malaysia) was used for thermogravimetric and differential thermogravimetric (TGA/DTG) analyses. A sample heating rate of 10 °C/min and a range of 20–1000 °C were used in this work. The analysis was carried out at a continuous nitrogen flow at 50 mL/min flow rate. High resolution transmission electron microscope (Hi-TEM) (FEI Tecnai TF20 X-Twin, Hillsboro, OR, USA) and FEI Nova NanoSEM 230 field emission scanning electron microscope (FESEM) (FEI, Hillsboro, OR, USA) were employed for shape/sizes analyses and morphological analyses, respectively while energy dispersive X-ray spectroscopy (EDX) (FEI, Hillsboro, OR, USA) was used for elemental analysis of the FESEM micrographs.

3.6. Drug Release Study

As mentioned earlier, gallic acid release from GAGZA was studied using a PerkinElmer Lambda 35 UV-Vis spectrophotometer (PerkinElmer, Singapore). Firstly, standard solutions of gallic acid at different concentrations were prepared. Appropriate amount of GAGZA was dissolved in 5 mL of HCl (1 mol/L) and then diluted with 45 mL deionized water. The lambda max of the drug in the solution was found to be 264 nm, which was used in determining the standard curve for the standard solutions and drug loading capacity of GA. Kinetic release of the loaded GA from GAGZA was done at pH 7.4 and 4.8 in a phosphate-buffered solution (PBS). Briefly, 25 mg of the sample was dispersed in 30 mL of the PBS in tubes. The tubes were placed in an oil bath shaker at 37 °C and 3 mL of the solutions were withdrawn and replaced with 3 mL of pure PBS at time intervals of 0.5, 1.0, 2.0, 3.0, 4.0, 5.0, 6.0, 12.0, 24.0, 48.0, 72.0, 92.0, and 120.0 h. The release media extracted were analyzed at lambda max = 264 nm wavelength with a UV–Vis spectrophotometer (PerkinElmer, Singapore).

3.7. Cell Culture

The cell lines used for cancer study was HepG2 (human liver hepatocellular carcinoma cell line) and normal cell lines, 3T3 (standard fibroblast cell line) for toxicity study, which were obtained from ATCC. RPMI 1640 was used as a medium for cell lines growth, which contains 1% penicillin/streptomycin and 10% fetal bovine serum (FBS). Cells culture was done at approximately 80% confluence, as adherent monolayers. Temperature was set at 37 °C and in a 5% CO_2 humidified atmosphere. Cell harvest was done via trypsinization (in brief) with trypsin-EDTA solution. All reagents are research grade and were used as received.

3.8. MTT Cell Viability Assays

RPMI 1640 was also used as a medium for the cancer cell lines and normal cells, which were grown in a humidified incubator at 37 °C and 5% CO_2. The cells were grown and were harvested and counted. Prior to 24 h incubation, the cells were transferred to 96-well plates (1 × 104 cells/well) and then the GAGZAu nanoparticles, LDH, and free GA were added. The medium was kept for 24 h to allow the cells to attach to the surface before treatment. The cells containing the GAGZAu, Zn/Al-LDH, and free drug were administered and applied in different concentrations prior to treatment and 72 h incubation. For MTT, 5 mg of (3-[4,5-dimethylthiazol-2-yl]-2, 5-diphenyltetrazolium bromide was dissolved in PBS (2 mL). To each of the 96-well plates, 20 µL of the MTT solution was added and incubated at 37 °C for 3 h until formazan product was developed (purple-colored). Suction method was employed to remove the solution in each well containing media, unbound MTT, and dead cells; 100 µL of DMSO was added to each well. The optical densities of the cells were obtained with the use of a microplate reader at 570 nm. Prior to the measurements, the cells were shaken. All analyses were done in triplicate and the cell viabilities/increase was presented in percentage in reference to control cells.

3.9. MR Imaging Analysis

The GAGZAu nanocomposite was tested for MRI signal intensity using 3.0 T MRI clinical instrument (3.0 T Siemens Magnetom, Erlangen, Germany). Prior to the analysis, GAGZAu was prepared in various concentrations (2.0, 0.5, and 0.2 w/v) according Gd^{3+} concentration. $Gd(NO_3)_3$ (0.5 w/v) and water together with samples were then placed in a 1 mL tube. The MR image was acquired by attaching the tubes to an MRI phantom, and then the phantom was placed in the instrument. The T1-weighted images of the samples were captured at TR/TE: (83/9000) 224 × 220 s, field of view (FOV): 120 × 120. The MR image was analyzed and signal intensities of the individual samples were extracted with Syngovia (MRI and CT reporting software, syngo MR E11, Siemens, Erlangen, Germany, 2013).

4. Conclusions

Gd-based nanocomposite (GAGZAu) was developed in this work, which was painstakingly analyzed to understand and ascertain its theranostic properties. The results obtained from different stages of the nanoparticles synthesis until the final nanocomposite GAGZAu shows the potentiality of the nanohybrid to be used as a theranostic bimodal delivery agent. The in vitro drug release study shows higher drug release in pH 4.8 (pH of cancer cells), indicating the capability of the platform to convey the GA into cancer cells and prevent premature release in the blood stream. Moreover, the nanocomposite shows reasonable cytotoxicity to HepG2 cancer cell lines and negligible toxicity to 3T3 normal cell lines. The preliminary MR imaging analysis conducted on the developed theranostic nanohydrid also indicates improved MRI contrast of T1-weighted image obtained as compared to pure $Gd(NO_3)_3$ and water. Based on the promising outcome of this work, further works such as in vivo testing could be done on the GAGZAu nanocomposite, which would improve its theranostic prospects, such as reducing artefact formations like short circulation and tissue specificity that are associated with gadolinium-based contrast agents as well as toxicities of chemotherapeutic agents.

Acknowledgments: The authors acknowledge Universiti Putra Malaysia (UPM) and the Ministry of Higher Education of Malaysia (MOHE) for providing the funds to conduct this research under NanoMITe grant Vot No. 5526300. We also acknowledge the assistance provided by Nor Kamalia Binti Abdul Jalil of Centre for Diagnostic and Nuclear Imaging, Universiti Putra Malaysia, during the MR imaging test of this research.

Author Contributions: Muhammad Sani Usman and Mohd Zobir Hussein conceived and designed the experiments; Muhammad Sani Usman performed the experiments; Sharida Fakurazi and Mas Jaffri Masarudin analyzed the data; Fathinul Fikri Ahmad Saad and Mohd Zobir Hussein contributed reagents/materials/analysis tools; Muhammad Sani Usman wrote the paper. All authors read and edited the paper before submission.

References

1. Usman, M.S.; Ibrahim, N.A.; Shameli, K.; Zainuddin, N.; Yunus, W.M.Z.W. Copper nanoparticles mediated by chitosan: Synthesis and characterization via chemical methods. *Molecules* **2012**, *17*, 14928–14936. [CrossRef] [PubMed]
2. Kovanda, F.; Jindova, E.; Dousova, B.; Kolousek, D.; Plestil, J.; Sedlakova, Z. Layered double hydroxides intercalated with organic anions and their application in preparation of l dh/polymer nanocomposites. *Acta Geodyn. Geomater.* **2009**, *6*, 111–119.
3. Swierczewska, M.; Liu, G.; Lee, S.; Chen, X. High-sensitivity nanosensors for biomarker detection. *Chem. Soc. Rev.* **2012**, *41*, 2641–2655. [CrossRef] [PubMed]
4. Yoo, D.; Lee, J.-H.; Shin, T.-H.; Cheon, J. Theranostic magnetic nanoparticles. *Acc. Chem. Res.* **2011**, *44*, 863–874. [CrossRef] [PubMed]
5. Xu, W.; Kattel, K.; Park, J.Y.; Chang, Y.; Kim, T.J.; Lee, G.H. Paramagnetic nanoparticle T_1 and T_2 MRI contrast agents. *Phys. Chem. Chem. Phys.* **2012**, *14*, 12687–12700. [CrossRef] [PubMed]
6. Jeong Kim, T.; Seok Chae, K.; Chang, Y.; Ho Lee, G. Gadolinium oxide nanoparticles as potential multimodal imaging and therapeutic agents. *Curr. Top. Med. Chem.* **2013**, *13*, 422–433. [CrossRef]
7. Usman, M.S.; Hussein, M.Z.; Fakurazi, S.; Ahmad Saad, F.F. Gadolinium-based layered double hydroxide and graphene oxide nano-carriers for magnetic resonance imaging and drug delivery. *Chem. Cent. J.* **2017**, *11*, 47. [CrossRef]
8. Cherry, S.R. Multimodality imaging: Beyond PET/CT and SPECT/CT. *Semin. Nucl. Med.* **2009**, *39*, 348–353. [CrossRef] [PubMed]
9. Srinivasan, M.; Rajabi, M.; Mousa, S.A. Multifunctional nanomaterials and their applications in drug delivery and cancer therapy. *Nanomaterials* **2015**, *5*, 1690–1703. [CrossRef] [PubMed]
10. Elgqvist, J. Nanoparticles as Theranostic Vehicles in Experimental and Clinical Applications—Focus on Prostate and Breast Cancer. *Int. J. Mol. Sci.* **2017**, *18*, 1102. [CrossRef] [PubMed]
11. Kim, K.S.; Park, W.; Hu, J.; Bae, Y.H.; Na, K. A cancer-recognizable MRI contrast agents using pH-responsive polymeric micelle. *Biomaterials* **2014**, *35*, 337–343. [CrossRef] [PubMed]
12. Campbell, J.L.; Arora, J.; Cowell, S.F.; Garg, A.; Eu, P.; Bhargava, S.K.; Bansal, V. Quasi-cubic magnetite/silica core-shell nanoparticles as enhanced MRI contrast agents for cancer imaging. *PLoS ONE* **2011**, *6*, e21857. [CrossRef] [PubMed]
13. Gwak, G.-H.; Kim, M.-K.; Oh, J.-M. Composites of quasi-colloidal layered double hydroxide nanoparticles and agarose hydrogels for chromate removal. *Nanomaterials* **2016**, *6*, 25. [CrossRef] [PubMed]
14. Zhang, Y.; Liu, X.; Zhang, C.; He, M.; Lu, X. Interlayer Structures and Dynamics of Arsenate and Arsenite Intercalated Layered Double Hydroxides: A First Principles Study. *Minerals* **2017**, *7*, 53. [CrossRef]
15. Barahuie, F.; Hussein, M.Z.; Arulselvan, P.; Fakurazi, S.; Zainal, Z. Drug delivery system for an anticancer agent, chlorogenate-Zn/Al-layered double hydroxide nanohybrid synthesised using direct co-precipitation and ion exchange methods. *J. Solid State Chem.* **2014**, *217*, 31–41. [CrossRef]
16. Saifullah, B.; Hussein, M.Z.; Hussein-Al-Ali, S.H.; Arulselvan, P.; Fakurazi, S. Sustained release formulation of an anti-tuberculosis drug based on para-amino salicylic acid-zinc layered hydroxide nanocomposite. *Chem. Cent. J.* **2013**, *7*, 72. [CrossRef] [PubMed]
17. Bullo, S.; Hussein, M.Z. Inorganic nanolayers: Structure, preparation, and biomedical applications. *Int. J. Nanomed.* **2015**, *10*, 5609. [CrossRef] [PubMed]
18. Dorniani, D.; Hussein, M.Z.B.; Kura, A.U.; Fakurazi, S.; Shaari, A.H.; Ahmad, Z. Preparation of Fe_3O_4 magnetic nanoparticles coated with gallic acid for drug delivery. *Int. J. Nanomed.* **2012**, *7*, 5745–5756. [CrossRef] [PubMed]
19. Kura, A.U.; Hussein, M.Z.; Fakurazi, S.; Arulselvan, P. Layered double hydroxide nanocomposite for drug delivery systems; bio-distribution, toxicity and drug activity enhancement. *Chem. Cent. J.* **2014**, *8*. [CrossRef] [PubMed]
20. Choi, S.-J.; Choi, G.E.; Oh, J.-M.; Oh, Y.-J.; Park, M.-C.; Choy, J.-H. Anticancer drug encapsulated in inorganic lattice can overcome drug resistance. *J. Mater. Chem.* **2010**, *20*, 9463–9469. [CrossRef]
21. Long, N.N.; Kiem, C.D.; Doanh, S.C.; Nguyet, C.T.; Hang, P.T.; Thien, N.D.; Quynh, L.M. Synthesis and optical properties of colloidal gold nanoparticles. *J. Phys. Conf. Ser.* **2009**, *187*, 012026. [CrossRef]

22. Hussein, M.Z.B.; Zainal, Z.; Yahaya, A.H.; Wong Vui Foo, D. Controlled release of a plant growth regulator, α-naphthaleneacetate from the lamella of Zn-Al-layered double hydroxide nanocomposite. *J. Control. Release* **2002**, *82*, 417–427. [CrossRef]
23. Oh, J.-M.; Choi, S.-J.; Kim, S.-T.; Choy, J.-H. Cellular uptake mechanism of an inorganic nanovehicle and its drug conjugates: Enhanced efficacy due to clathrin-mediated endocytosis. *Bioconjug. Chem.* **2006**, *17*, 1411–1417. [CrossRef] [PubMed]
24. Dorniani, D.; Kura, A.U.; Hussein-Al-Ali, S.H.; Bin Hussein, M.Z.; Fakurazi, S.; Shaari, A.H.; Ahmad, Z. In vitro sustained release study of gallic acid coated with magnetite-PEG and magnetite-PVA for drug delivery system. *Sci. World J.* **2014**, 416354. [CrossRef]
25. Raffi, M.; Mehrwan, S.; Bhatti, T.M.; Akhter, J.I.; Hameed, A.; Yawar, W.; ul Hasan, M.M. Investigations into the antibacterial behavior of copper nanoparticles against *Escherichia coli*. *Ann. Microbiol.* **2010**, *60*, 75–80. [CrossRef]
26. Kong, X.; Jin, L.; Wei, M.; Duan, X. Antioxidant drugs intercalated into layered double hydroxide: Structure and in vitro release. *Appl. Clay Sci.* **2010**, *49*, 324–329. [CrossRef]
27. Zhang, Z.; Liu, W.; Zheng, Y.; Jin, L.; Yao, W.; Gao, X. SGP-2, an acidic polysaccharide from Sarcandra glabra, inhibits proliferation and migration of human osteosarcoma cells. *Food Funct.* **2014**, *5*, 167–175. [CrossRef] [PubMed]
28. Chieng, B.W.; Ibrahim, N.A.; Yunus, W.M.Z.W.; Hussein, M.Z. Poly (lactic acid)/poly (ethylene glycol) polymer nanocomposites: Effects of graphene nanoplatelets. *Polymers* **2013**, *6*, 93–104. [CrossRef]
29. Ghotbi, M.Y.; bin Hussein, M.Z. Gallate–Zn–Al-layered double hydroxide as an intercalated compound with new controlled release formulation of anticarcinogenic agent. *J. Phys. Chem. Solids* **2010**, *71*, 1565–1570. [CrossRef]
30. Mukherjee, P.; Bhattacharya, R.; Bone, N.; Lee, Y.K.; Patra, C.R.; Wang, S.; Lu, L.; Secreto, C.; Banerjee, P.C.; Yaszemski, M.J. Potential therapeutic application of gold nanoparticles in B-chronic lymphocytic leukemia (BCLL): Enhancing apoptosis. *J. Nanobiotechnol.* **2007**, *5*, 4. [CrossRef] [PubMed]
31. Zarabi, M.F.; Arshadi, N.; Farhangi, A.; Akbarzadeh, A. Preparation and Characterization of Gold Nanoparticles with Amino Acids, Examination of Their Stability. *Indian J. Clin. Biochem.* **2014**, *29*, 306–314. [CrossRef] [PubMed]
32. King, S.R.; Shimmon, S.; Gentle, A.R.; Westerhausen, M.T.; Dowd, A.; McDonagh, A.M. Remarkable thermal stability of gold nanoparticles functionalised with ruthenium phthalocyanine complexes. *Nanotechnology* **2016**, *27*, 215702. [CrossRef] [PubMed]
33. Patra, J.K.; Baek, K.H. Novel green synthesis of gold nanoparticles using Citrullus lanatus rind and investigation of proteasome inhibitory activity, antibacterial, and antioxidant potential. *Int. J. Nanomed.* **2015**, *10*, 7253. [CrossRef]
34. Zawada, K.; Waldemar, T.; Elżbieta, M. A smart synthesis of gold/polystyrene core–shell nanohybrids using TEMPO coated nanoparticles. *RSC Adv.* **2014**, *4*, 23876–23885. [CrossRef]
35. Sugano, K.; Kansy, M.; Artursson, P.; Avdeef, A.; Bendels, S.; Di, L.; Ecker, G.F.; Faller, B.; Fischer, H.; Gerebtzoff, G. Coexistence of passive and carrier-mediated processes in drug transport. *Nat. Rev. Drug Discov.* **2010**, *9*, 597–614. [CrossRef] [PubMed]
36. Xu, Z.P.; Lu, G. Layered double hydroxide nanomaterials as potential cellular drug delivery agents. *Pure Appl. Chem.* **2006**, *78*, 1771–1779. [CrossRef]
37. Tian, X.; Shao, Y.; He, H.; Liu, H.; Shen, Y.; Huang, W.; Li, L. Nanoamplifiers synthesized from gadolinium and gold nanocomposites for magnetic resonance imaging. *Nanoscale* **2013**, *5*, 3322–3329. [CrossRef] [PubMed]
38. Thomsen, H.S. Nephrogenic systemic fibrosis: A serious late adverse reaction to gadodiamide. Nephrogenic systemic fibrosis: A serious late adverse reaction to gadodiamide. *Eur. Radiol.* **2006**, *5*, 2619–2621. [CrossRef] [PubMed]
39. Sparreboom, A.; Baker, S.D.; Verweij, J. Paclitaxel repackaged in an albumin-stabilized nanoparticle: Handy or just a dandy? *J. Clin. Oncol.* **2005**, *23*, 7765–7767. [CrossRef] [PubMed]
40. Atabaev, T.S.; Lee, J.H.; Shin, Y.C.; Han, D.-W.; Choo, K.S.; Jeon, U.B.; Hwang, J.Y.; Yeom, J.A.; Kim, H.-K.; Hwang, Y.-H. Eu, Gd-Codoped Yttria Nanoprobes for Optical and T1-Weighted Magnetic Resonance Imaging. *Nanomaterials* **2017**, *7*, 35. [CrossRef] [PubMed]
41. Le, W.; Cui, S.; Chen, X.; Zhu, H.; Chen, B.; Cui, Z. Facile synthesis of gd-functionalized gold nanoclusters as potential MRI/CT contrast agents. *Nanomaterials* **2016**, *6*, 65. [CrossRef] [PubMed]

42. Zhang, L.; Liu, T.; Xiao, Y.; Yu, D.; Zhang, N. Hyaluronic acid-chitosan nanoparticles to deliver Gd-DTPA for MR cancer imaging. *Nanomaterials* **2015**, *5*, 1379–1396. [CrossRef] [PubMed]
43. Caravan, P. Strategies for increasing the sensitivity of gadolinium based MRI contrast agents. *Chem. Soc. Rev.* **2006**, *35*, 512–523. [CrossRef] [PubMed]
44. Shen, A.J.; Li, D.L.; Cai, X.J.; Dong, C.Y.; Dong, H.Q.; Wen, H.Y.; Dai, G.H.; Wang, P.J.; Li, Y.Y. Multifunctional nanocomposite based on graphene oxide for in vitro hepatocarcinoma diagnosis and treatment. *J. Biomed. Mater. Res. A* **2012**, *100*, 2499–2506. [CrossRef] [PubMed]

Permissions

All chapters in this book were first published by MDPI; hereby published with permission under the Creative Commons Attribution License or equivalent. Every chapter published in this book has been scrutinized by our experts. Their significance has been extensively debated. The topics covered herein carry significant findings which will fuel the growth of the discipline. They may even be implemented as practical applications or may be referred to as a beginning point for another development.

The contributors of this book come from diverse backgrounds, making this book a truly international effort. This book will bring forth new frontiers with its revolutionizing research information and detailed analysis of the nascent developments around the world.

We would like to thank all the contributing authors for lending their expertise to make the book truly unique. They have played a crucial role in the development of this book. Without their invaluable contributions this book wouldn't have been possible. They have made vital efforts to compile up to date information on the varied aspects of this subject to make this book a valuable addition to the collection of many professionals and students.

This book was conceptualized with the vision of imparting up-to-date information and advanced data in this field. To ensure the same, a matchless editorial board was set up. Every individual on the board went through rigorous rounds of assessment to prove their worth. After which they invested a large part of their time researching and compiling the most relevant data for our readers.

The editorial board has been involved in producing this book since its inception. They have spent rigorous hours researching and exploring the diverse topics which have resulted in the successful publishing of this book. They have passed on their knowledge of decades through this book. To expedite this challenging task, the publisher supported the team at every step. A small team of assistant editors was also appointed to further simplify the editing procedure and attain best results for the readers.

Apart from the editorial board, the designing team has also invested a significant amount of their time in understanding the subject and creating the most relevant covers. They scrutinized every image to scout for the most suitable representation of the subject and create an appropriate cover for the book.

The publishing team has been an ardent support to the editorial, designing and production team. Their endless efforts to recruit the best for this project, has resulted in the accomplishment of this book. They are a veteran in the field of academics and their pool of knowledge is as vast as their experience in printing. Their expertise and guidance has proved useful at every step. Their uncompromising quality standards have made this book an exceptional effort. Their encouragement from time to time has been an inspiration for everyone.

The publisher and the editorial board hope that this book will prove to be a valuable piece of knowledge for researchers, students, practitioners and scholars across the globe.

List of Contributors

Dimitrios Skourtis, Dimitra Stavroulaki, Varvara Athanasiou and Hermis Iatrou
Industrial Chemistry Laboratory, Department of Chemistry, National and Kapodistrian University of Athens, Panepistimiopolis, Zografou, GR-15771 Athens, Greece

Panagiota G. Fragouli
Dyeing, Finishing, Dyestuffs and Advanced Polymers Laboratory, University of West Attica, DIDPE, 250 Thevon Street, GR-12241 Athens, Greece

Francesca Marzoli, Paola Minosi and Stefano Pieretti
Istituto Superiore di Sanità, National Center for Drug Research and Evaluation, 00161 Rome, Italy

Carlotta Marianecci and Maria Carafa
Department of Drug Chemistry and Technology, Sapienza University of Rome, 00185 Rome, Italy

Federica Rinaldi
Center for Life Nano Science@Sapienza, Istituto Italiano di Tecnologia (ITT), 00161 Rome, Italy

Daniele Passeri
Department of Basic and Applied Sciences for Engineering, Sapienza University of Rome, 00161 Rome, Italy

Marco Rossi
Department of Basic and Applied Sciences for Engineering, Sapienza University of Rome, 00161 Rome, Italy
Research Center for Nanotechnology Applied to Engineering, Sapienza University of Rome (CNIS), 00185 Rome, Italy

Dominik Weber, Frank Momburg and Reinhard Schwartz-Albiez
Deutsches Krebsforschungszentrum (DKFZ), Clinical Cooperation Unit Applied Tumor Immunology, D-69120 Heidelberg, Germany

Bernhard Torger
Institute of Plant and Wood Chemistry, Technische Universität Dresden, D-01737 Tharandt, Germany

Karsten Richter and Michelle Nessling
Deutsches Krebsforschungszentrum (DKFZ), Central Unit Electron Microscopy, D-69120 Heidelberg, Germany

Beatrice Woltmann
Institute of Physiological Chemistry, Faculty of Medicine Carl Gustav Carus, Technische Universität Dresden, 01307 Dresden, Germany

Martin Müller
Department Polyelectrolytes and Dispersions, Leibniz-Institut für Polymerforschung Dresden e.V., Hohe Straße 6, D-01069 Dresden, Germany
Department of Chemistry and Food Chemistry, Technische Universität Dresden, D-01062 Dresden, Germany

Martina Asprea, Vieri Piazzini, Maria Camilla Bergonzi and Anna Rita Bilia
Department of Chemistry, University of Florence, Via U. Schiff 6, 50019 Sesto Fiorentino, Florence, Italy

Francesca Tatini and Francesca Rossi
Institute of Applied Physics "N. Carrara" (IFAC-CNR), Via Madonna del Piano 10, 50019 Sesto Fiorentino, Italy

Natalia Zashikhina, Mariia Antipchik, Irina Tarasenko and Evgenia Korzhikova-Vlakh
Institute of Macromolecular Compounds, Russian Academy of Sciences, Saint-Petersburg 199004, Russia

Vladimir Sharoyko, Yurii Anufrikov and Tatiana Tennikova
Institute of Chemistry, Saint-Petersburg State University, Saint-Petersburg 198584, Russia

Antonina Lavrentieva
Institute of Technical Chemistry, Leibniz University, Hannover 30167, Germany

Antonio Lopalco, Annalisa Cutrignelli, Angela Lopedota, Massimo Franco and Valentino Laquintana
Department of Pharmacy–Drug Sciences, University of Bari "Aldo Moro", 4 E. Orabona st, 70125 Bari, Italy

Nunzio Denora
Department of Pharmacy–Drug Sciences, University of Bari "Aldo Moro", 4 E. Orabona st, 70125 Bari, Italy
Institute for Physical and Chemical Processes (IPCF)-CNR, SS Bari, 4 E. Orabona st, 70125 Bari, Italy

Valentina Coccè, Loredana Cavicchini and Augusto Pessina
CRC StaMeTec, Department of Biomedical, Surgical and Dental Sciences, University of Milan, 20133 Milan, Italy

Silvia Franzè and Francesco Cilurzo
Department of Pharmaceutical Science, University of Milan, 20133 Milan, Italy

Anna Teresa Brini
CRC StaMeTec, Department of Biomedical, Surgical and Dental Sciences, University of Milan, 20133 Milan, Italy
IRCCS Orthopedic Institute Galeazzi, 20161 Milan, Italy

Aldo Bruno Giannì
IRCCS Orthopedic Institute Galeazzi, 20161 Milan, Italy
Maxillo-Facial and Dental Unit, Fondazione Ca' Granda IRCCS Ospedale Maggiore Policlinico, 20122 Milan, Italy

Luisa Pascucci
Department of Veterinary Medicine, University of Perugia, 06123 Perugia, Italy

Emilio Ciusani
Laboratory of Clinical Pathology and Medical Genetics, Fondazione IRCCS Istituto Neurologico "C. Besta", 20133 Milan, Italy

Giulio Alessandri
Cellular Neurobiology Laboratory, Department of Cerebrovascular Diseases, IRCCS Neurological Institute C. Besta, 20133 Milan, Italy

Giampietro Farronato
IRCCS Orthopedic Institute Galeazzi, 20161 Milan, Italy
Unit of Orthodontics and Paediatric Dentistry, Fondazione Ca' Granda IRCCS Ospedale Maggiore Policlinico, 20122 Milan, Italy

Valeria Sordi
Diabetes Research Institute, IRCCS San Raffaele Scientific Institute, 20132 Milan, Italy

Rita Paroni and Michele Dei Cas
Department of Health Sciences of the University of Milan, 20142 Milan, Italy

Roberta Guagliardo, Pieterjan Merckx, Agata Zamborlin, Lynn De Backer, Stefaan C. De Smedt and Koen Raemdonck
Ghent Research Group on Nanomedicines, Laboratory of General Biochemistry and Physical Pharmacy, Department of Pharmaceutics, Ghent University, Ottergemsesteenweg 460, 9000 Ghent, Belgium

Mercedes Echaide and Jesus Pérez-Gil
Departamento de Bioquímica y Biología Molecular, Facultad de Biologia, and Research Institute Hospital 12 de Octubre, Universidad Complutense, José Antonio Novais 12, 28040 Madrid, Spain

Valeria De Matteis and Chiara Cristina Toma
Dipartimento di Matematica e Fisica "E. De Giorgi", Università del Salento, Via Monteroni, 73100 Lecce, Italy

Mariafrancesca Cascione
Dipartimento di Scienze Biomediche e Oncologia Umana, Università degli Studi di Bari "Aldo Moro", p.zza G. Cesare, 70124 c/o Policlinico Bari, Italy

Stefano Leporatti
CNR Nanotec-Istituto di Nanotecnologia, c/o Campus Ecotekne, Via Monteroni, 73100 Lecce, Italy

Nathalie Goergen, Matthias Wojcik, Shashank Reddy Pinnapireddy, Jana Brüßler, Udo Bakowsky and Jarmila Jedelská
Department of Pharmaceutics and Biopharmaceutics, University of Marburg, 35037 Marburg, Germany

Simon Drescher
Institute of Pharmacy, Biophysical Pharmacy, Martin Luther University Halle-Wittenberg, 06120 Halle (Saale), Germany
Institute of Pharmacy, University of Greifswald, 17489 Greifswald, Germany

Magdalena Osial, Paulina Rybicka, Marek Pękała, Grzegorz Cichowicz, Michał K. Cyrański and Paweł Krysiński
Faculty of Chemistry, University of Warsaw, Pasteura 1 Street, 02-093 Warsaw, Poland

Sonia Cabana-Montenegro, Angel Concheiro and Carmen Alvarez-Lorenzo
Departamento de Farmacología, Farmacia y Tecnología Farmacéutica, R+D Pharma Group (GI-1645), Facultad de Farmacia and Health Research Institute of Santiago de Compostela (IDIS), Universidade de Santiago de Compostela, 15782 Santiago de Compostela, Spain

Silvia Barbosa and Pablo Taboada
Área de Física de la Materia Condensada, Facultad de Física, Universidade de Santiago de Compostela, 15782 Santiago de Compostela, Spain

Muhammad Sani Usman and Mohd Zobir Hussein
Materials Synthesis and Characterization Laboratory, Institute of Advanced Technology (ITMA), Serdang 43400, Selangor, Malaysia

Sharida Fakurazi
Laboratory of Vaccines and Immunotherapeutics, Institute of Bioscience, Serdang 43400, Selangor, Malaysia
Department of Human Anatomy, Faculty of Medicine and Health Sciences, Serdang 43400, Selangor, Malaysia

Mas Jaffri Masarudin
Department of Cell & Molecular Biology, Faculty of Biotechnology and Biomolecular Sciences, Serdang 43400, Selangor, Malaysia

Fathinul Fikri Ahmad Saad
Centre for Diagnostic and Nuclear Imaging, Faculty of Medicine and Health Sciences, Universiti Putra Malaysia, Serdang 43400, Selangor, Malaysia

Index

A

Amino Acids, 43, 85, 87, 89, 93, 95-96, 108, 228

Analgesia, 26, 32

Analgesic Drug, 26

Andrographis Paniculata, 71, 73, 84

Andrographolide, 71, 73, 79, 84

Angiogenesis, 3, 9-10, 19, 24, 54-55, 68, 70, 128, 179, 182-183

Antibiotics, 169, 176

Antibodies, 3, 44, 47-48, 58, 130, 147

B

Biocompatibility, 8, 13, 38-40, 49, 55, 67, 71, 81, 87, 131, 170, 173, 178-180, 186, 197, 203

Biodegradability, 8, 38-39, 71, 85, 87, 170

Biodistribution, 1-2, 20, 38, 43, 68, 73, 159, 167, 212

Biogenesis, 117, 126

Biological Membranes, 26, 34, 72, 130

Biomedical Applications, 2, 50, 146, 181, 185, 196-197, 214, 227

Blood-brain Barrier, 44, 49, 84, 107, 114-115

Bloodstream, 2, 20, 47, 200

C

Cancer Cells, 39, 43, 50, 115, 117-118, 122, 124-125, 127, 129, 135, 147, 153-159, 166, 207, 212, 216, 226

Capsaicin, 26, 29, 31-32, 34, 36-37

Cardiomyocyte, 2, 6, 8-9, 11-13, 18-19, 21, 25

Cardiovascular Diseases, 1, 9, 20-23

Cardiovascular System, 1

Cell Membrane, 20, 65, 71-72, 82-83, 87, 114, 153

Cell Proliferation, 9, 12, 54, 58, 65-66, 104, 118, 121-122, 125

Cellular Uptake, 5, 12, 45, 51, 54-55, 57, 61, 68, 81, 83, 132, 135-136, 139-140, 142, 145, 161, 228

Cellulose Sulfate, 54-56, 58, 60-61, 64-65

Cholesterol, 5-8, 27-29, 71, 73, 75, 77, 82, 107, 109, 130-132, 137, 139, 143, 145, 175, 213

Clinical Use, 2, 5, 72

Coronary Artery Disease, 1, 9, 21

Cytotoxicity, 6, 12, 36, 55, 58, 67-68, 81, 85, 101, 103, 114, 129, 153-154, 156-157, 159, 165-166, 182, 184, 222-223, 226

D

Dextran Sulfate, 54-56, 58, 60-61, 134

Diabetes, 1, 12, 85-87, 104-106, 117

Dopamine, 107-109, 114-115

Drug Delivery, 1-3, 5, 12, 16, 19-23, 25, 27, 34, 36-40, 50-52, 54-55, 67-69, 71-72, 79, 83-84, 86, 99, 105, 107, 114-118, 126-129, 135, 144, 146, 158, 169-170, 179, 181, 183, 185-186, 196-197, 211, 214-215, 227-228

E

Echocardiography, 10-11, 18, 20

Endocytosis, 3-4, 6, 23, 27, 43-44, 61, 67, 69, 113-114, 130-131, 216, 222, 228

Endothelial Cells, 3, 5, 7, 9, 54-56, 58, 60-67, 69-70, 107-108, 111, 158

Erythrocyte, 85, 87, 91, 102, 105-106

Eukaryotic Cells, 38, 49

F

Fibroblasts, 16, 25, 71, 73, 81, 154-155, 165

G

Gingival Papilla, 118, 121, 125

H

Heart Failure, 1-2, 5, 9, 12, 22, 25

Heparin, 19, 25, 54-56, 58, 60-61, 67-70, 90-91, 99-101

Hydrophilic Drugs, 2, 8, 27, 114

Hyperalgesia, 26, 29-30, 32-34, 36

Hypertrophy, 2, 12, 16, 19

I

Ibuprofen, 26-36

Immune System, 2, 47-49

Immunogenicity, 38, 47, 49, 131

Inflammatory Pain, 26, 34

Inflammatory Response, 11, 155

Interdental Papilla, 117-118, 127

L

Lecithin, 5, 8, 27, 71

Liposomes, 1, 4-7, 23-24, 27, 34, 37-38, 71-73, 77-79, 82-83, 107-108, 112, 114-116, 118, 126, 128, 130, 132-134, 141-143, 145, 181-182

Lyoprotectants, 71, 74

M

Macromolecules, 3, 84, 130, 144, 183

Macrophages, 11, 18, 25, 47, 71, 73, 81, 83, 131, 135, 144, 153-155, 165

Mitosis, 54, 64, 67

Mortality, 1, 85, 159, 169

Myocardial Infarction, 1, 7, 21-25

Myocardium, 2, 5-9, 11, 13, 16, 18-20, 22-25

N

Nanocochleates, 71-73, 77-79, 84

Nanomaterials, 1-2, 9, 20, 69, 105, 146, 151, 156-158, 160-161, 165, 185, 214, 227-229

Nanomedicine, 1-3, 8-9, 22-23, 37-38, 47-51, 83, 144-146, 156, 161-162, 166-167, 212

Nanoparticles, 1-5, 8-12, 16, 19, 21-25, 36, 38-39, 44-46, 48-56, 58-69, 74, 81, 84-85, 88, 93-94, 98, 103-105, 114-115, 130-132, 142-147, 150-151, 155, 157, 159-168, 182-183, 185-193, 195-205, 207, 210-229

Necrosis, 9, 22, 154-155, 165

Neuropathy, 26, 30, 33, 86, 102, 104

Niosomes, 26-28, 30-31, 34-37, 112

Nociception, 26, 34, 36

P

Paclitaxel, 117-118, 121, 124, 127-129, 183, 228

Parkinson's Disease, 107, 114-115

Peptides, 3, 6, 39, 42-43, 45, 47-49, 89-90, 96, 100, 103-104, 106, 116, 166

Phagocytosis, 11, 72, 82, 84

Phosphatidylcholine, 6-7, 21, 34, 71, 73, 77-78, 131

Phosphatidylserine, 71-73, 77-78, 123, 138, 140

Photothermal Therapy, 25, 200-201, 212

Plasma Membrane, 3, 63, 81, 118, 159

Polyethylene Glycol, 3, 5, 23, 108, 161, 183

Polysaccharides, 54-55, 58, 67, 70, 73, 151

R

Ribonucleoprotein, 38, 40, 46, 51

S

Secretome, 117, 119-126

Small Unilamellar Vesicle, 72

Smooth Muscle, 3, 13, 19, 86, 104, 153-154

Squamous Cell Carcinoma, 117-118, 120, 122, 126-128

T

Therapeutics, 1-3, 9, 19-20, 22, 35, 50, 69, 107, 130-131, 143, 156, 166, 169, 185

Tissue Regeneration, 2, 54-55

Transferrin, 107-108, 112-113, 115-116, 212

Tumor Cells, 48, 55, 122, 156-157, 200, 211

V

Ventricular Dilation, 2, 9

Viruses, 38, 51, 150

Z

Zymosan, 26, 29-30, 32, 34-36

www.ingramcontent.com/pod-product-compliance
Lightning Source LLC
LaVergne TN
LVHW082156200926
848484LV00008B/2171